Informatik aktuell

Reihe herausgegeben von

Gesellschaft für Informatik e.V. (GI), Bonn, Deutschland

Ziel der Reihe ist die möglichst schnelle und weite Verbreitung neuer Forschungs- und Entwicklungsergebnisse, zusammenfassender Übersichtsberichte über den Stand eines Gebietes und von Materialien und Texten zur Weiterbildung. In erster Linie werden Tagungsberichte von Fachtagungen der Gesellschaft für Informatik veröffentlicht, die regelmäßig, oft in Zusammenarbeit mit anderen wissenschaftlichen Gesellschaften, von den Fachausschüssen der Gesellschaft für Informatik veranstaltet werden. Die Auswahl der Vorträge erfolgt im allgemeinen durch international zusammengesetzte Programmkomitees.

Thomas M. Deserno · Heinz Handels ·
Andreas Maier · Klaus Maier-Hein ·
Christoph Palm · Thomas Tolxdorff
(Hrsg.)

Bildverarbeitung für die Medizin 2023

Proceedings, German Workshop on
Medical Image Computing,
Braunschweig, July 2-4, 2023

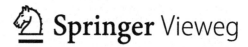

Hrsg.
Thomas M. Deserno ⓘ
Peter L. Reichertz Institut für Medizinische
Informatik der TU Braunschweig und der
Medizinischen Hochschule Hannover
Braunschweig, Deutschland

Andreas Maier ⓘ
Lehrstuhl für Mustererkennung
Friedrich-Alexander-Universität
Erlangen, Deutschland

Christoph Palm ⓘ
Fakultät für Informatik und Mathematik
Ostbayerische Technische Hochschule
Regensburg
Regensburg, Deutschland

Heinz Handels ⓘ
Institut für Medizinische Informatik
Universität zu Lübeck
Lübeck, Deutschland

Klaus Maier-Hein ⓘ
Medical Image Computing, E230
Deutsches Krebsforschungszentrum
(DKFZ)
Heidelberg, Deutschland

Thomas Tolxdorff ⓘ
Institut für Medizinische Informatik
Charité – Universitätsmedizin Berlin
Berlin, Deutschland

ISSN 1431-472X
Informatik aktuell
ISBN 978-3-658-41656-0   ISBN 978-3-658-41657-7   (eBook)
https://doi.org/10.1007/978-3-658-41657-7

Die Deutsche Nationalbibliothek verzeichnet diese Publikation in der Deutschen Nationalbibliografie;
detaillierte bibliografische Daten sind im Internet über http://dnb.d-nb.de abrufbar.

Planung/Lektorat: Petra Steinmueller
Springer Vieweg ist ein Imprint der eingetragenen Gesellschaft Springer Fachmedien Wiesbaden GmbH
und ist ein Teil von Springer Nature.
Die Anschrift der Gesellschaft ist: Abraham-Lincoln-Str. 46, 65189 Wiesbaden, Germany

Bildverarbeitung für die Medizin 2023

Veranstalter

PLRI   Peter L. Reichertz Institut für Medizinische Informatik der TU Braunschweig und der Medizinischen Hochschule Hannover

Unterstützende Fachgesellschaften

BVMI	Berufsverband Medizinischer Informatiker
CURAC	Computer- und Roboterassistierte Chirurgie
DAGM	Deutsche Arbeitsgemeinschaft für Mustererkennung
DGBMT	Fachgruppe Medizinische Informatik der Deutschen Gesellschaft für Biomedizinische Technik im Verband Deutscher Elektrotechniker
GI	Gesellschaft für Informatik – Fachbereich Informatik in den Lebenswissenschaften
GMDS	Gesellschaft für Medizinische Informatik, Biometrie und Epidemiologie
IEEE	Joint Chapter Engineering in Medicine and Biology, German Section

Tagungsvorsitz

Univ.-Prof. Dr. rer. nat. Dipl.-Ing. Thomas M. Deserno
Peter L. Reichertz Institut für Medizinische Informatik der TU Braunschweig und der Medizinischen Hochschule Hannover

Tagungssekretariat

Selin Celik und Christian Hilbert
Peter L. Reichertz Institut für Medizinische Informatik

Anschrift:	Mühlenpfordtstr. 23, 38106 Braunschweig
Telefon:	+49 531 391 2130
Fax:	+49 531 391 9502
Email:	orga-2023@bvm-workshop.org
Web:	https://bvm-workshop.org

Lokale BVM-Organisation

Prof. Dr. Thomas M. Deserno, Paulo Haas, Viktor Sobotta

Verteilte BVM-Organisation

Begutachtung	Heinz Handels und Jan-Hinrich Wrage – Institut für Medizinische Informatik, Universität zu Lübeck
Mailingliste	Klaus Maier-Hein – Medical Image Computing, Deutsches Krebsforschungszentrum (DKFZ) Heidelberg
Special Issue	Andreas Maier – Lehrstuhl für Mustererkennung, Friedrich-Alexander Universität Erlangen-Nürnberg
Tagungsband	Thomas M. Deserno, Nico Baumann, Paula Lüpke, Michael Völcker, Vivien Wegel – Peter L. Reichertz Institut für Medizinische Informatik, TU Braunschweig
Web & News	Christoph Palm, Leonard Klausmann, Alexander Leis und Sümeyye R. Yildiran – Regensburg Medical Image Computing (ReMIC), Ostbayerische Technische Hochschule Regensburg

BVM-Komitee

Prof. Dr. Thomas M. Deserno, Peter L. Reichertz Institut für Medizinische Informatik der TU Braunschweig und der Medizinischen Hochschule Hannover

Prof. Dr. Heinz Handels, Institut für Medizinische Informatik, Universität zu Lübeck

Prof. Dr. Andreas Maier, Lehrstuhl für Mustererkennung, Friedrich-Alexander-Universität Erlangen-Nürnberg

Prof. Dr. Klaus Maier-Hein, Medical Image Computing, Deutsches Krebsforschungszentrum Heidelberg

Prof. Dr. Christoph Palm, Regensburg Medical Image Computing (ReMIC), Ostbayerische Technische Hochschule Regensburg

Prof. Dr. Thomas Tolxdorff, Institut für Medizinische Informatik, Charité–Universitätsmedizin Berlin

Programmkomitee

Jürgen Braun, Charité-Universitätsmedizin Berlin
Thomas M. Deserno, PLRI Braunschweig
Jan Ehrhardt, Universität zu Lübeck
Sandy Engelhardt, Universitätsklinik Heidelberg
Friedrich Feuerhake, Medizinische Hochschule Hannover
Ralf Floca, DKFZ Heidelberg
Nils Forkert, University of Calgary, Calgary, Kanada
Michael Götz, Universitätsklinik Ulm

Sponsoren und Unterstützer des Workshops BVM 2023

Wir bedanken uns bei den Unterstützern und freuen uns sehr über die langjährige kontinuierliche Unterstützung mancher Firmen sowie auch über das neue Engagement anderer. Die BVM wäre ohne diese finanzielle Unterstützung in ihrer erfolgreichen Konzeption nicht durchführbar.

- **GuiG mbH & Co. KG**
  Rochusweg 8
  41516 Grevenbroich
  `https://entscheiderfabrik.com`

- **ID Information und Dokumentation im Gesundheitswesen GmbH & Co. KGaA**
  Platz vor dem Neuen Tor 2
  10115 Berlin
  `https://www.id-berlin.de`

- **Magrathea Informatik GmbH**
  Goseriede 1-5
  30159 Hannover
  `https://www.magrathea.eu`

- **Nexus Chili GmbH**
  Friedrich-Ebert-Str. 2
  69221 Dossenheim
  `https://nexus-chili.com`

- **Siemens Healthcare GmbH**
  Lindenplatz 2
  20099 Hamburg
  `https://www.siemens-healthineers.com`

- **Springer Vieweg**
  Abraham-Lincoln-Str. 46
  65189 Wiesbaden
  `https:///www.springer.com`

- **sysGen GmbH**
  Am Hallacker 48
  28327 Bremen
  `https://www.sysgen.de`

Preisträger der BVM 2022 in Heidelberg

BVM Award CHILI

Hristina Uzunova
(Institut für Medizinische Informatik, Universität zu Lübeck)
Generative Deep Learning Models for the Automatic Analysis and Synthesis of Medical Image Data Featuring Pathological Structures

Beste wissenschaftliche Arbeiten

1. **Richin Sukesh**
   (Pattern Recognition Lab, FAU Erlangen-Nürnberg)
   Sukesh R, Fieselmann A, Jaganathan S, Shetty K, Kärgel R, Kordon F, Kappler S, Maier A
   Training Deep Learning Models for 2D Spine X-rays using Synthetic Images and Annotations Created from 3D CT Volumes
2. **Maja Schlereth**
   (Department Artificial Intelligence in Biomedical Engineering, FAU Erlangen-Nürnberg)
   Schlereth M, Stromer D, Mantri Y, Tsujimoto J, Breininger K, Maier A, Anderson C, Garimella PS, Jokerst JV
   Initial Investigations Towards Non-invasive Monitoring of Chronic Wound Healing using Deep Learning and Ultrasound Imaging
3. **Mingxuan Gu**
   (Pattern Recognition Lab, FAU Erlangen-Nürnberg)
   Gu M, Vesal S, Kosti R, Maier A
   Few-shot Unsupervised Domain Adaptation for Multi-modal Cardiac Image Segmentation

Bester Vortrag

Michael Baumgartner
(Division of Medical Image Computing, German Cancer Research Center)
Baumgartner M, Jäger PF, Isensee F, Maier-Hein KH
nnDetection: A Self-configuring Method for Medical Object Detection

Bestes Poster

Sven Köhler
(Department of Internal Medicine III, Heidelberg University Hospital)
Köhler S, Sharan L, Kuhm J, Ghanaat A, Gordejeva J, Simon NK, Grell NM, André F, Engelhardt S
Comparison of Evaluation Metrics for Landmark Detection in CMR Images

Vorwort

Die Tagung Bildverarbeitung für die Medizin (BVM) wird seit weit mehr als 20 Jahren an wechselnden Orten Deutschlands veranstaltet. Inhaltlich fokussiert sich die BVM dabei auf die computergestützte Analyse medizinischer Bilddaten, die Anwendungsgebiete sind vielfältig, z.B. im Bereich der Bildgebung, der Diagnostik, der Operationsplanung, der computerunterstützten Intervention und der Visualisierung.

In dieser Zeit hat es bemerkenswerte methodische Weiterentwicklungen und Umbrüche gegeben, wie zum Beispiel im Bereich des maschinellen Lernens, an denen die BVM-Community intensiv mitgearbeitet hat. In der Folge dominieren inzwischen Arbeiten im Zusammenhang mit Deep Learning die BVM. Auch diese Entwicklungen haben dazu beigetragen, dass die Medizinische Bildverarbeitung an der Schnittstelle zwischen Informatik und Medizin als eine Schlüsseltechnologie zur Digitalisierung des Gesundheitswesens etabliert ist.

Zentraler Aspekt der BVM ist neben der Darstellung aktueller Forschungsergebnisse schwerpunktmäßig aus der vielfältigen deutschlandübergreifenden BVM-Community insbesondere die Förderung des wissenschaftlichen Nachwuchses. Die Tagung dient vor allem Doktorand*innen und Postdoktorand*innen aber auch Studierenden mit hervorragenden Bachelor- und Masterarbeiten als Plattform, um ihre Arbeiten zu präsentieren, dabei in den fachlichen Diskurs mit der Community zu treten und Netzwerke mit Fachkolleg*innen zu knüpfen. Trotz der vielen Tagungen und Kongresse, die auch für die Medizinische Bildverarbeitung relevant sind, hat die BVM deshalb nichts von ihrer Bedeutung und Anziehungskraft eingebüßt.

Inhaltlich kann auch bei der BVM 2023 wieder ein attraktives und hochklassiges Programm geboten werden. Es wurden aus 72 Einreichungen über ein anonymisiertes Reviewing-Verfahren mit jeweils drei Reviews 31 Vorträge, 31 Posterbeiträge und drei Softwaredemonstrationen angenommen. Die besten Arbeiten werden auch in diesem Jahr mit Preisen ausgezeichnet.

Die Webseite des Workshops findet sich unter:

https://www.bvm-workshop.org

Das Programm wird durch Tutorials und zwei eingeladene Vorträge ergänzt, für die wir uns herzlich bedanken. Als Referenten für die Vorträge begrüßen wir herzlich

- Prof. Dr. Bernhard Kainz, Intelligent Data Exploration and Analysis Lab, Friedrich-Alexander-Universität Erlangen-Nürnberg
- Dr. med. Hinrich B. Winther, Machine Learning Arbeitsgruppe am Institut für Diagnostische und Interventionelle Radiologie, Medizinische Hochschule Hannover.

An dieser Stelle möchten wir allen, die bei den umfangreichen Vorbereitungen zum Gelingen des Workshops beigetragen haben, unseren herzlichen Dank für ihr Engagement aussprechen: den Referent*innen der Gastvorträge, den Autor*innen der Beiträge, den Referent*innen der Tutorien, den Industrierepräsentant*innen, dem Programmkomitee, den Fachgesellschaften, den Mitgliedern des BVM-Organisationsteams und allen Mitarbeitenden des Peter L. Reichertz Instituts für Medizinische Informatik der TU Braunschweig und der Medizinischen Hochschule Hannover.

Wir wünschen allen Teilnehmer*innen des Workshops BVM 2023 spannende neue Kontakte und inspirierende Eindrücke aus der Welt der medizinischen Bildverarbeitung.

März 2023

Thomas M. Deserno (Braunschweig)
Heinz Handels (Lübeck)
Andreas Maier (Erlangen)
Klaus Maier-Hein (Heidelberg)
Christoph Palm (Regensburg)
Thomas Tolxdorff (Berlin)

Inhaltsverzeichnis

Die fortlaufende Nummer am linken Seitenrand entspricht den Beitragsnummern, wie sie im endgültigen Programm des Workshops zu finden sind. Dabei steht V für Vortrag, P für Poster und S für Softwaredemonstration.

Session 2: Segmentation

Session 3: Image Generation & Enhancement

Software Demonstrationen

Postersession 1

Session 4: Object Detection & Datasets

Session 5: Digital Pathology

Postersession 2

Session 6: Beyond Supervised Learning

Keynote: Beyond Supervised Learning
Exploring Novel Machine Learning Approaches for Robust Medical Image Analysis

Bernhard Kainz

Friedrich-Alexander-Universität Erlangen-Nürnberg, Germany
bernhard.kainz@fau.de

Machine learning has been widely regarded as a solution for diagnostic automation in medical image analysis, but there are still unsolved problems in robust modelling of normal appearance and identification of features pointing into the long tail of population data. In this talk, I will explore the fitness of machine learning for applications at the front line of care and high throughput population health screening, specifically in prenatal health screening with ultrasound and MRI, cardiac imaging, and bedside diagnosis of deep vein thrombosis. I will discuss the requirements for such applications and how quality control can be achieved through robust estimation of algorithmic uncertainties and automatic robust modelling of expected anatomical structures. I will also explore the potential for improving models through active learning and the accuracy of non-expert labelling workforces. However, I will argue that supervised machine learning might not be fit for purpose, as it cannot handle the unknown and requires a lot of annotated examples from well-defined pathological appearance. This categorization paradigm cannot be deployed earlier in the diagnostic pathway or for health screening, where a growing number of potentially hundred-thousands of medically catalogued illnesses may be relevant for diagnosis. Therefore, I introduce the idea of normative representation learning as a new machine learning paradigm for medical imaging. This paradigm can provide patient-specific computational tools for robust confirmation of normality, image quality control, health screening, and prevention of disease before onset. I will present novel deep learning approaches that can learn without manual labels from healthy patient data only. Our initial success with single class learning and self-supervised learning will be discussed, along with an outlook into the future with causal machine learning methods and the potential of advanced generative models [1].

References

1. Web: https://bernhard-kainz.com/.

Keynote: Fully Automated Bone Removal in CBCT of the Lower Body Stem

Hinrich B. Winther, Sabine Maschke, Lena Becker, Cornelia Dewald, Marcel Eicke, Bernhard C. Meyer

winther.hinrich@mh-hannover.de

Introduction: The use of well-established bone removal (BRM) techniques is crucial for CT angiography (CTA) of the head, body, and lower limbs. The lower body stem, which includes the abdomen and pelvis, does not have a BRM for cone beam CT (CBCT). This frequently necessitates the interventionist doing a manual BRM, particularly in the pelvic area, as in the case of a prostate embolization, necessitating his exit from the interventional room.The aim of this study is to create and clinically test a BRM method for CBCT of the lower body stem that is high-quality, totally automated, and uses a convolutional neural network.

Materials and methods: Medical students with training manually segmented the ground truth images, and a radiologist with at least five years of expertise evaluated their accuracy. A convolutional neural network (3D U-Net, Içek, et al.) was trained using the image data and ground truth of 534 training examples. Five percent of the training data were used for the online evaluation. The top-performing model was selected based on overlap measures generated during the online validation. The test set consists of 30 cases for which the BRM was produced using the final model. Three interventional radiologists with at least ten years of experience visually assessed the test cases for comprehensiveness and overall quality.

Results: The bone mask was rated as complete in 100 % (n=30) with no overhanging, truncating the vascular tree, or soft tissue in 100 % (n=30) of the test cases, with either no or very minor residuals in the maximum intensity projection (MIP) or VRT. Each BRM test case was of good diagnostic quality and did not need any manual intervention. One CBCT takes about 20 seconds to process.

Discussion: The AI-based bone removal approach relieves the interventionist of performing a manual bone removal, allowing him to maximize the time spent in the intervention, potentially reducing total intervention time for the patient. BRM can also be used for CBCT image guidance, such as prostatic artery embolization.

Extending Tempcyclegan for Virtual Augmentation of Gastrointestinal Endoscopy Training Simulators

Moritz Wallrodt[1], Maximilian Schulz-Alsen[1], Hanno Ehlken[3], Thomas Rösch[3],
Rüdiger Schmitz[1,2,3,4,5], René Werner[1,2,5]

[1]Department of Computational Neuroscience, University Medical Center Hamburg-Eppendorf
[2]Center for Biomedical Artificial Intelligence, University Medical Center Hamburg-Eppendorf
[3]Department for Interdisciplinary Endoscopy, University Medical Center Hamburg-Eppendorf
[4]I. Department of Medicine, University Medical Center Hamburg-Eppendorf
[5]Equal contribution
r.werner@uke.de

Abstract. Simulator training is a core part of gastrointestinal (GI) endoscopy training. Based on rubber or silicon dummies, training lacks a realistic visual appearance. Aiming at a hyperrealistic training environment, we propose a CycleGAN-based framework to translate the training videos into realistically appearing GI endoscopy videos. We build on the concept of tempCycleGAN and (i) extend it to a generic framework to simultaneously work on n subsequent video frames in order to increase temporal consistency of generated videos and (ii) formulate a conditional variant of it to selectively incorporate pathologies into the generated videos. Extension (i) will be shown to increase temporal consistency and realism of the generated GI endoscopy videos. Feasibility and potential of (ii) is illustrated with superficial and deep duodenal ulcer as conditional classes.

1 Introduction

Simulator training is an essential part of endoscopic training. Central diagnostic examination procedures like gastroscopy and colonoscopy are practiced using rubber and silicon training models, i.e., physical phantoms that mimic the shape of the structures of interest. Despite confirmed success [1], this training approach is limited to simple mechanical procedures and lacks realistic visual appearance; the step to performing an actual gastroscopy on a patient remains high.

To narrow the gap between training phantoms and real patients, approaches to deep unpaired image-to-image translation originating from the field of computer vision appear promising. In the context of minimally invasive heart valve interventions, Engelhardt et al. introduced the term *hyperrealism* and defined a hyperrealistic environment as an environment in which "parts of the physical phantom that look unnatural are replaced by realistic appearances" [2]. Based on CycleGAN [3], they introduced the concept of *tempCycleGAN* to temporally consistently translate between phantom and real patient video image domain, and extended the CycleGAN framework to stereoscopic phantom images [4] as well as combined image translation and suture detection [5].

The contributions of our work are as follows:

- we transfer the concept of hyperrealism to the field of gastrointestinal (GI) endoscopy training models,

T. M. Deserno et al. (Hrsg.), *Bildverarbeitung für die Medizin 2023*,
Informatik aktuell, https://doi.org/10.1007/978-3-658-41657-7_3

- we extend the original tempCycleGAN to an n-frame framework that accounts for a larger history to increase the temporal consistency of the generated videos, and
- we propose to extend the tempCycleGAN framework to selectively incorporate pathological structures into the generated videos.

2   Materials and methods

2.1   Proposed extensions of the tempCycleGAN

2.1.1 n-frame tempCycleGAN. The setup of the n-frame tempCycleGAN (nf-tC-GAN) is sketched in Fig. 1. X denotes the GI training model (dummy) image domain, and Y the real patient image domain. Each nf-tC-GAN training step is based on a list of n time points $\tau := \{t_1, \ldots, t_n\}$. In a standard setup, t_1 is the time point of interest and $t_2, \ldots, t_n$ its temporal predecessors. For each t_i in τ, an ordered frame set $\underline{X}(t_i) := \{X_{t_i}, \ldots, X_{t_{i+(n-1)}}\}$ is defined, consisting of a video frame X_{t_i} and its $n - 1$ temporal predecessors. Each frame set is input to the generator G_Y, which generates a corresponding set $\underline{Y}(t_i)$ of n temporally consecutive video frames with the appearance of domain Y. Following the idea of CycleGAN, based on $\underline{Y}(t_i)$, G_X then generates a frame set $\underline{X}'(t_i)$ with the appearance of domain X, and discriminators D_Y and D_X try to differentiate between the generated frame sets and actual sets of the corresponding domain. In total, G_X, D_Y, and G_Y are run n-times (i.e., an individual run for each frame set $\underline{X}(t_i)$; shared weights for all runs). Optimization is based on the CycleGAN loss functions but extended to frame sets: adversarial losses $\mathcal{L}_{\text{adv}}(G_X, D_X, \underline{X}, \underline{Y})$ and

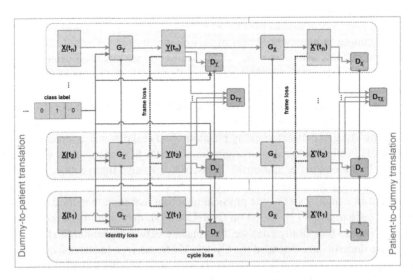

Fig. 1. Training setup for the proposed n-frame conditional tempCycleGAN; for details see the main text. Blue: shared weights. Identity and cycle losses are also computed for the frame sets $\underline{X}(t_i), i > 1$, but omitted for clarity.

$\mathcal{L}_{\text{adv}}(G_{\underline{Y}}, D_{\underline{Y}}, \underline{X}, \underline{Y})$, an L1-based identity loss $\mathcal{L}_{\text{identity}}(G_{\underline{X}}, G_{\underline{Y}})$, and an L1-based cycle loss $\mathcal{L}_{\text{cyc}}(G_{\underline{Y}}, G_{\underline{X}})$.

Following [2], temporal discriminators $D_{T\underline{Y}}$ and $D_{T\underline{X}}$ are introduced. $D_{T\underline{Y}}$ takes as input a temporal sequence of n consecutive frames defined as $\{\underline{Y}(t_1)[1], \ldots, \underline{Y}(t_n)[1]\}$ with $\underline{Y}(t_i)[1]$ as the first element of $\underline{Y}(t_i)$. The generated sequences are to be differentiated from corresponding real sequences; training is based on $\mathcal{L}_{\text{adv}}(G_{\underline{Y}}, D_{T\underline{Y}}, \underline{X}, \underline{Y})$. $D_{T\underline{X}}$ is similarly defined. In addition, a frame loss $\mathcal{L}_{\text{frame}}(G_{\underline{Y}}, G_{\underline{X}})$ is introduced to increase the consistency of the outputs for the different frame sets by minimizing $\sum_{j=2}^{n} \|\underline{Y}(t_j)[1] - \underline{Y}(t_1)[j]\|_1$ and $\sum_{j=2}^{n} \|\underline{X}'(t_j)[1] - \underline{X}'(t_1)[j]\|_1$. The total loss results as $\mathcal{L}_{\text{total}} = \mathcal{L}_{\text{adv}}(G_{\underline{Y}}, D_{\underline{Y}}) + \mathcal{L}_{\text{adv}}(G_{\underline{X}}, D_{\underline{X}}) + \lambda_1 \mathcal{L}_{\text{identity}}(G_{\underline{X}}, G_{\underline{Y}}) + \lambda_2 \mathcal{L}_{\text{cyc}}(G_{\underline{Y}}, G_{\underline{X}}) + \lambda_3 \mathcal{L}_{\text{adv}}(G_{\underline{Y}}, D_{T\underline{Y}}) + \lambda_3 \mathcal{L}_{\text{adv}}(G_{\underline{X}}, D_{T\underline{X}}) + \lambda_4 \mathcal{L}_{\text{frame}}(G_{\underline{Y}}, G_{\underline{X}})$ with λ_{1-4} as weighting factors.

During inference, for a given time point $\hat{t} =: t_1$ and the corresponding video frame X_{t_1}, the desired output is $\underline{Y}(t_1)[1]$.

For $n = 2$, the described setup is identical to the original tempCycleGAN. The CycleGAN can also be understood as a particular case of the nf-tC-GAN with $n = 1$ and without temporal discriminators/loss and frame loss. Generators and discriminators were largely similar to [3] ($G_{\underline{X}}$: encoder-decoder structure with residual blocks; discriminators: 70×70 patchGAN approach). For the translation $X \rightarrow Y$, a U-net structure was used (experiments showed better results for this configuration). In each case, the networks have a $n \times 3$ ($n \times$ RGB) channel input.

2.1.2 Conditional n-frame tempCycleGAN.

The integration of specific virtual pathologies into the generated videos is realized using a conditional U-net for $G_{\underline{Y}}$. The c intended pathology classes are represented by one hot encoding. The vector of size $c + 1$ (c pathology classes + no pathology) is integrated into the network through adaptive instance normalization (AdaIN) layers [6] that are added at each U-net level to adaptively compute class-specific representations. Additionally, the discriminator G_Y is extended by an auxiliary classifier, i.e., in addition to the differentiation of generated and real frame sets, the discriminator is forced to learn the correct class [7], implemented as a cross entropy loss $\lambda_5 \mathcal{L}_{\text{class}}(D_{\underline{Y}})$.

2.2 Data set and training

The experiments are based on 19 videos with a total of 96,132 frames of the dummy and 61 patient videos with a total of 202,780 videos frames (all cropped to a size of 1245×954 px to remove patient name information etc.; acquired with Olympus GIF-H190 or FujiFilm EG-760R; frame rate 25 Hz). 6 videos contained pathologies (4 videos with in total 1098 frames contained superficial and 2 videos with 988 frames deep ulcer). Before processing the data, the frames were square-cropped and resized to a size of 256×256 px. Horizontal and vertical flipping were applied for data augmentation. Optimization was performed with the Adam method with standard settings and batch size of 3. Training (hardware: Geforce RTX 3090) comprises 100 epochs and results for epochs 70-100 were inspected to find the visually most attractive results [2]. Weighting parameters were $\lambda_1 = 5$, $\lambda_2 = 10$, $\lambda_3 = 1$ and $\lambda_4 = 1$, and $\lambda_5 = 1$ (selection based on experiments).

Tab. 1. Temporal consistency rating results (0: very bad; 4: compelling; format: median (IQR) across all ratings; best results highlighted in bold). Video 1: Z line; video 2: inversion; video 3: pylorus and stomach; video 4: duodenum; video 5: esophagus. No temporal consistency rating was performed for the dummy video (assumed to be perfectly consistent).

$|\tau|$	Video 1	Video 2	Video 3	Video 4	Video 5	All
1 ($\equiv$ CycleGAN)	2.3 (1.8)	3.0 (0.7)	2.0 (0.9)	2.0 (0.9)	2.3 (1.4)	2.5 (1.5)
2 ($\equiv$ tempCycleGAN)	2.7 (0.7)	2.8 (0.5)	1.3 (1.1)	2.0 (0.6)	**2.4 (1.0)**	2.2 (1.4)
3 (proposed approach)	**3.0 (0.5)**	**3.5 (0.5)**	**3.0 (0.4)**	**3.0 (0.5)**	1.8 (1.2)	**3.0 (1.0)**

Tab. 2. Realism rating results (see Tab. 1 for explanations).

$|\tau|$	Video 1	Video 2	Video 3	Video 4	Video 5	All
n/a (dummy video)	1.0 (0.8)	1.0 (0.6)	1.0 (0.8)	1.0 (0.5)	1.2 (0.9)	1.0 (0.9)
1 ($\equiv$ CycleGAN)	2.5 (0.7)	2.4 (1.3)	2.0 (0.5)	2.3 (0.5)	**3.0 (0.5)**	2.5 (1.0)
2 ($\equiv$ tempCycleGAN)	2.8 (0.5)	3.0 (0.5)	1.0 (1.2)	2.5 (1.0)	2.3 (0.5)	2.5 (1.4)
3 (proposed approach)	**3.0 (0.8)**	**3.3 (0.5)**	**3.0 (0.6)**	**3.0 (0.4)**	2.0 (1.0)	**3.0 (1.0)**

2.3 Experiments and evaluation

The evaluation of the impact of the number of frames processed by the nf-tC-GAN was evaluated in a rater study. 11 raters (2 experts with > 2 years experience in GI endoscopy; 9 volunteers) were asked to rate temporal consistency and realism of mini-videos. 5 mini-videos (length of approximately 15 s) were acquired with the simulator and comprised the relevant anatomical parts in GI endoscopy: the Z line (video 1), stomach/inversion (endoscope rotated by 180 degree, instrument visible; video 2), pylorus and stomach (video 3), duodenum (video 4), and esophagus (video 5). The five videos were then translated using the nf-tC-GAN with $|\tau| = 1$ ($\equiv$ CycleGAN), $|\tau| = 2$ ($\equiv$ original tempCycleGAN), and $|\tau| = 3$. For $|\tau| > 3$, no considerable difference to $|\tau| = 3$ was observed during the experiments and corresponding videos not included in the rater study. Training was based on the videos without pathologies. Temporal consistency and realism were assessed using a 5-point scale (from 0 = very bad to 4 = compelling) [2, 8].

Feasibility of the selective incorporation of pathologies using the conditional nf-tC-GAN variant was studied using three classes: no pathology, deep ulcer, superficial ulcer. Due to the limited number of videos with pathologies, we also limited the training data for the no pathology class to 7 videos with in total 4123 frames.

3 Results

The results for the rater study are summarized in Tables 1 and 2. The 3-frame tempCycleGAN (3f-tC-GAN) ratings were higher than the CycleGAN and the tempCycleGAN implementations for both temporal consistency and realism for 4/5 videos. Only the ratings for the esophagus video (video 5) differ. Ratings of the experts and non-experts are consistent, but expert ratings were lower particularly for CycleGAN and the tempCycleGAN (median across all videos, expert realism ratings: 2.0 (IQR 0.5) for CycleGAN,

1.9 (1.7) for tempCycleGAN, 3.0 (1.1) for 3f-tC-GAN; non-experts: 2.5 (1.0) for CycleGAN, 2.5 (1.0) for tempCycleGAN, 3.0 (1.0) for 3f-tC-GAN; expert temporal consistency rating: 2.0 (0.5) for CycleGAN, 1.9 (1.2) for tempCycleGAN, 3.0(0.0) for 3f-tC-GAN; non-experts: 2.5 (1.1) for CycleGAN, 2.5 (1.0) for tempCycleGAN, 3.0 (1.0) for 3f-tC-GAN). Temporal consistency and realism ratings were highly corre-lated.

Exemplary video frames for the conditional 3f-tC-GAN approach are shown in Fig. 2, demonstrating the feasibility of selective integration of pathologies (here: deep and superficial ulcer) in the generated videos. Especially taking into account the limited training data, the individual frames look realistic; however, while being temporally consistent, the translation partially fails to imprint the pathologies as spatially static objects (i.e., they move with endoscope).

Training time is approximately 20 h and inference time approximately 60 ms (Cy-cleGAN: 59 ms; 3f-tC-GAN: 63 ms) for the described hardware.

4   Discussion

We presented an approach to transfer the concept and idea of hyperrealism to gastroin-testinal endoscopy. Building on CycleGAN and tempCycleGAN [2], we presented a framework to handle a (in theory) arbitrary number of consecutive video frames. In our experiments, temporal consistency was considerably improved for $|\tau| = 3$ frames compared to direct application of CycleGAN ($|\tau| = 2$) and the original tempCycleGAN approach ($|\tau| = 1$). However, we would like to emphasize that there may be differences between the original tempCycleGAN and our implementation.

The lower ratings for the generated esophagus video did not come as a surprise, as the acquisition of high-quality endoscopic views is technically much harder in the motile

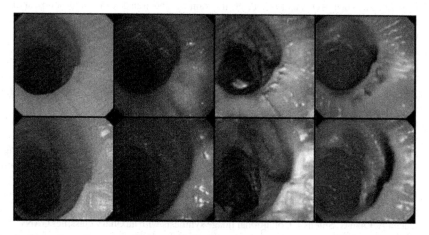

Fig. 2. Exemplary frames to illustrate the influence of the class condition on the dummy-to-patient domain frame translation. From left to right: original dummy frame; translation with class = healthy, class = deep ulcer, and class = superficial ulcer.

and narrow esophagus as compared to, e.g., the stomach. Therefore, in a typical video of a real examination, the portion of low-quality frames from the esophagus is much higher than from other anatomical sites. Only very few frames from an examination show a more or less "still", high-quality, wide view of the inflated esophagus. In the training dummy, on the contrary, the esophagus is found still and wide-open all the time. However, after the rating, we re-sorted the corresponding training data and removed low-quality frames, which led to visually more appealing outputs. Thus, as future work, automated quality-based selection of short video segments would help to extend the dataset.

This aspect already illustrates the importance of appropriate training sets for the proposed approach. Similarly, we assume that the undesired movement of the pathologies observed for the conditional nf-tC-GAN is mainly due to the very limited training data set available for the corresponding experiments. An obvious solution would be to include further videos in the training. If they are not available, the generation of synthetic videos could also help.

Furthermore, the present inference time of 60 ms does not meet real-time requirements yet. However, the usage of more powerful and dedicated hardware like tensor processing units should allow for the required additional speed-up.

Acknowledgement. The work was supported by the University of Hamburg (student research group GAIA, GAstroIntenstinal Augmented reality, to R.S.). The authors also thank A. Rohling of the Olympus Academy for providing access to the training simulators.

References

1. Haycock A, Koch AD, Familiari P, et al. Training and transfer of colonoscopy skills: a multinational, randomized, blinded, controlled trial of simulator versus bedside training. Gastrointest Endosc. 2010:298–307.
2. Engelhardt S, De Simone R, Full PM, et al. Improving surgical training phantoms by hyperrealism: deep unpaired image-to-image translation from real surgeries. Proc MICCAI. 2018:747–55.
3. Zhu JY, Park T, Isola P, et al. Unpaired image-to-image translation using cycle-consistent adversarial networks. Proc ICCV. 2017:2242–51.
4. Engelhardt S, Sharan L, Karck M, et al. Cross-domain generative adversarial networks for stereoscopic hyperrealism in surgical training. Proc MICCAI. 2019:155–63.
5. Sharan L, Romano G, Koehler S, et al. Mutually improved endoscopic image synthesis and landmark detection in unpaired image-to-image translation. IEEE J Biomed Health Inform. 2022:127–38.
6. Huang X, Belongie S. Arbitrary style transfer in real-time with adaptive instance normalization. Proc ICCV. 2017:1501–10.
7. Odena A, Olah C, Shlens J. Conditional image synthesis with auxiliary classifier GANs. Proc ICML. 2017:2642–51.
8. Yi Z, Zhang H, Tan P, et al. DualGAN: unsupervised dual learning for image-to-image translation. Proc ICCV. 2017:2868–76.

Abstract: Fiducial Marker Recovery and Detection From Severely Truncated Data in Navigation-assisted Spine Surgery

Fuxin Fan[1], Björn Kreher[2], Holger Keil[3], Andreas Maier[1], Yixing Huang[4]

[1]Fakultät für Pattern Recognition, FAU Erlangen-Nürnberg
[2]Siemens Healthcare GmbH, Forchheim
[3]Department of Trauma and Orthopedic Surgery, FAU Erlangen-Nürnberg
[4]Department of Radiation Oncology, Universitätsklinikum Erlangen, FAU Erlangen-Nürnberg
yixing.yh.huang@fau.de

Fiducial markers are commonly used in navigation-assisted minimally invasive spine surgery and they help transfer image coordinates into real-world coordinates. In practice, these markers might be located outside the field-of-view (FOV) of C-arm cone beam computed tomography (CBCT) systems. As a consequence, reconstructed markers in CBCT volumes suffer from artifacts and have distorted shapes, which sets an obstacle for navigation. In this work, we propose two fiducial marker detection methods: direct detection from distorted markers (direct method) and detection after marker recovery (recovery method) [1]. For direct detection from distorted markers in reconstructed volumes, an efficient automatic marker detection method using two neural networks and a conventional circle detection algorithm is proposed. For marker recovery, a task-specific data preparation strategy is proposed to recover markers from severely truncated data. Afterwards, a conventional marker detection algorithm is applied for position detection. The networks in both methods are trained only on simulated data and the two methods are evaluated on simulated data and real cadaver data. The direct method achieves 100% detection rates within 1 mm detection error on simulated data with normal truncation and simulated data with heavier noise, but only detect 94.6% markers in extremely severe truncation case. The recovery method detects all the markers successfully in three test data sets and around 95% markers are detected within 0.5 mm error. For real cadaver data, both methods achieve 100% marker detection rates with mean registration error below 0.2 mm. Our experiments demonstrate that the direct method is capable of detecting distorted markers accurately and the recovery method with the task-specific data preparation strategy has high robustness and generalizability on various data sets. The task-specific data preparation is able to reconstruct structures of interest outside the FOV from severely truncated data better than conventional data preparation.

References

1. Fan F, Kreher B, Keil H, Maier A, Huang Y. Fiducial marker recovery and detection from severely truncated data in navigation-assisted spine surgery. Med Phys. 2022.

T. M. Deserno et al. (Hrsg.), *Bildverarbeitung für die Medizin 2023*,
Informatik aktuell, https://doi.org/10.1007/978-3-658-41657-7_4

Abstract: C-arm Positioning for Standard Projections During Spinal Implant Placement

Lisa Kausch[1,2], Sarina Thomas[1], Holger Kunze[3], Tobias Norajitra[1], André Klein[1,2], Leonardo Ayala[2,4], Jan El Barbari[5], Maxim Privalov[5], Sven Vetter[5], Andreas Mahnken[6], Lena Maier-Hein[4], Klaus Maier-Hein[1]

[1]Medical Image Computing (MIC), German Cancer Research Center, Heidelberg
[2]Medical Faculty, Heidelberg University
[3]Advanced Therapy Systems Division, Siemens Healthineers, Erlangen
[4]Intelligent Medical Systems (IMSY), German Cancer Research Center, Heidelberg
[5]MINTOS Reseach Group, Trauma Surgery Clinic Ludwigshafen
[6]Division of Diagnostic and Interventional Radiology, University Hospital Marburg
l.kausch@dkfz-heidelberg.de

Fluoroscopy-guided trauma and orthopedic surgeries involve the repeated acquisition of correct anatomy-specific standard projections for guidance, monitoring, and evaluating the surgical result. C-arm positioning is usually performed by hand, involving repeated or even continuous fluoroscopy at a cost of radiation exposure and time. We propose to automate this procedure and estimate the pose update for C-arm repositioning directly from a first X-ray without the need for a patient-specific computed tomography scan (CT) or additional technical equipment. Our method is trained on digitally reconstructed radiographs (DRRs) which uniquely provide ground truth labels for an arbitrary number of training examples. The simulated images are complemented with automatically generated segmentations, landmarks, and with simulated k-wires and screws. To successfully achieve a transfer from simulated to real X-rays, and also to increase the interpretability of results, the pipeline was designed to closely reflect the actual clinical decision-making process followed by spinal neurosurgeons. It explicitly incorporates steps such as region-of-interest (ROI) localization, detection of relevant and view-independent landmarks, and subsequent pose regression. The method was validated on a large human cadaver study simulating a real clinical scenario, including k-wires and screws. The proposed procedure obtained superior C-arm positioning accuracy of $d\theta = 8.8° \pm 4.2°$ average improvement ($p_{t-test} \ll 0.01$), robustness, and generalization capabilities compared to the state-of-the-art direct pose regression framework [1].

References

1. Kausch L, Thomas S, Kunze H, Norajitra T, Klein A, Ayala L et al. C-arm positioning for standard projections during spinal implant placement. Med Image Anal. 2022;81:102557.

© Der/die Autor(en), exklusiv lizenziert an
Springer Fachmedien Wiesbaden GmbH, ein Teil von Springer Nature 2023
T. M. Deserno et al. (Hrsg.), *Bildverarbeitung für die Medizin 2023*,
Informatik aktuell, https://doi.org/10.1007/978-3-658-41657-7_5

Abstract: Shape-based Segmentation of Retinal Layers and Fluids in OCT Image Data

Timo Kepp[1,2], Julia Andresen[2], Claus von der Burchard[3], Johann Roider[3], Gereon Hüttmann[4], Heinz Handels[1,2]

[1]German Research Center for Artificial Intelligence, Lübeck, Germany
[2]Institute of Medical Informatics, University of Lübeck, Lübeck, Germany
[3]Department of Ophthalmology, University of Kiel, Kiel, Germany
[4]Institute of Biomedical Optics, University of Lübeck, Lübeck, Germany
timo.kepp@dfki.de

Optical coherence tomography (OCT) offers non-invasive imaging of the retina and has been well established in the field of ophthalmology for several decades. Based on its high-resolution cross-sectional images, OCT supports diagnosis of various eye diseases. For clinical examination and treatment planning, automated segmentation of individual retinal layers and pathologies is helpful. Retinal layers follow a strict topology that is not addressed by most state-of-the-art methods. While graph-based methods can be used to correct for topology errors, their application is costly and complex, especially in the presence of pathologies. In this work, we propose a segmentation method that uses shape information of retinal layers for improved topology preservation while providing a simple applicability. For this purpose, we use a multi-task framework based on the U-Net architecture that integrates regression of the shape information of the retinal layers in addition to pixel-wise classification. On the one hand, shape-based regression of retinal layers provides spatial regularization and enables the generation of plausible segmentations. On the other hand, the simultaneous classification results in sharper delineations of pathological structures. Furthermore, a task consistency enables semi-supervised training, allowing the use of unlabeled image data for training. A comprehensive evaluation of our segmentation method is performed using OCT image data from patients with diabetic macular edema. Both an ablation study and comparison with other methods have shown the advantages of our proposed segmentation framework. Learning multiple tasks via separate paths leads to higher generalization and prevents overfitting of network parameters. Simultaneously, feature representations preferred by both tasks are learned. Results also show improved preservation of retinal topology while maintaining sharp pathology delineation [1].

References

1. Kepp T, Andresen J, von der Burchard C, Roider J, Hüttmann G, Handels H. Shape-based segmentation of retinal layers and fluids in OCT image data. Proc SPIE Medical Imaging. 2023. Accepted.

Extending nnU-Net Is All You Need

Fabian Isensee[1,2,], Constantin Ulrich[1,4], Tassilo Wald[1,2], Klaus H. Maier-Hein[1,3]

[1]Division of Medical Image Computing, German Cancer Research Center (DKFZ)
[2]Helmholtz Imaging, German Cancer Research Center (DKFZ)
[3]Pattern Analysis and Learning Group, Department of Radiation Oncology, Heidelberg University Hospital, Heidelberg, Germany
[4]National Center for Tumor Diseases (NCT), NCT Heidelberg, a partnership between DKFZ and university medical center Heidelberg
f.isensee@dkfz-heidelberg.de

Abstract. Semantic segmentation is one of the most popular research areas in medical image computing. Perhaps surprisingly, despite its conceptualization dating back to 2018, nnU-Net continues to provide competitive out-of-the-box solutions for a broad variety of segmentation problems and is regularly used as a development framework for challenge-winning algorithms. Here, we use nnU-Net to participate in the AMOS-2022 challenge, which was a MICCAI22 challenge and comes with a unique set of tasks: not only is the dataset one of the largest ever created and boasts 15 target structures, but the second task of the competition also requires submitted solutions to handle both MRI and CT scans. Through careful modification of nnU-net's hyperparameters, the addition of residual connections in the encoder and the design of a custom postprocessing strategy, we were able to substantially improve upon the nnU-Net baseline. Advances in GPU memory capacity and processing speed allowed larger models and batch sizes than the default nnU-Net. Our final ensemble achieves Dice scores of 90.13 for Task 1 (CT) and 89.06 for Task 2 (CT+MRI) in a 5-fold cross-validation on the provided training cases. We submitted almost the same solution for both tasks, but adjusted the intensity normalization for task 2 to account for the additional MRI images. For the final testing stage, participants were asked to provide a docker container with their final solution to be applied to an unpublished test set. On both tasks, our nnU-Net extension achieved the first place by a wide margin.

1 Introduction

Automated delineation of all anatomical structures and pathologies in medical images is a long-standing goal in medical image computing. Due to the need of expert annotators and the time-intensive nature of 3D annotations, datasets have so far required careful balancing between the number of target structures and the number of training cases. Consequently, existing methods are either trained on many images and can robustly segment few structures or are trained on few images can segment many structures with reduced robustness. Thus, whenever a holistic perspective on a patients anatomy is required, multiple expert models must be pooled together from multiple sources. Not only does this increase the inference time, but it also creates new issues such as potentially conflicting predictions. Finally and perhaps most importantly, with each expert model being trained independently, label synergies cannot be exploited, thus

© Der/die Autor(en), exklusiv lizenziert an
Springer Fachmedien Wiesbaden GmbH, ein Teil von Springer Nature 2023
T. M. Deserno et al. (Hrsg.), *Bildverarbeitung für die Medizin 2023*,
Informatik aktuell, https://doi.org/10.1007/978-3-658-41657-7_7

potentially decreasing the label efficiency of the models as well as their robustness. In this context, the Abdominal Multi Organ Segmentation 2022 (AMOS2022) challenge [1], is set out to catalyzes the development of holistic segmentation methods. It comes with an unprecedented number of training images and annotated target structures: 15 organs of interest were labeled in 500 CT and 100 MRI scans, distributed into 200+40 (CT + MRI) training, 100+20 validation and 200+40 test images. The challenge poses two tasks: Task 1 is a classic multi-organ segmentation problem on just the CT images whereas Task 2 includes the MRI images and expects submitted methods to handle both modalities.

Within the context of medical image segmentation, nnU-Net [2] has stood the test of time. It consistently delivers state-of-the-art results on new segmentation datasets as they are released, despite its fully automated out-of-the-box nature. Moreover, nnU-Net was successfully used as a basis for task-specific method optimization, enabling not just us [3, 4] but also many other teams [5] to win highly contested challenges. Thus, it seems only natural to use nnU-Net for our participation in the AMOS2022 challenge as well.

2 Method

nnU-Net is a framework that automatically configures and trains U-Net [6] based segmentation pipelines. Through rigorous analysis of the target dataset, nnU-Net makes automated adaptations to the patch size, batch size, preprocessing, network topology and more. For a full description of nnU-Net, we refer to [2]. In this section we propose several modifications to nnU-net's automatically generated pipeline to maximize segmentation performance on the AMOS2022 challenge. Throughout method development we apply all modifications to both tasks with the sole difference being the intensity normalization scheme. For Task 1 we utilize nnU-Net's 'CT' scheme (data-driven clipping and normalization) and for Task 2 we use simple z-scoring of all images (nnU-Net's 'nonCT' setting).

2.1 Optimization of nnU-Net's segmentation pipeline to AMOS2022

Starting from the default '3d_fullres' configuration provided by nnU-Net we explore multiple improvements. We experimented with replacing the default encoder of the U-Net with a residual encoder (based on [7]). We furthermore optimized the preprocessing, specifically the batch size, patch size and target spacing. Advances in GPU memory capacity and processing speed allowed for larger models and batch sizes than the standard nnU-Net. Method development is performed by running 5-fold cross-validation on the provided training cases. All models are trained from scratch using the nnU-Net framework. Our experimentation resulted in three well-performing candidates for Task 1 and two candidates for Task 2 (Tab. 1). Fig. 1 shows the segmentation architectures used by our final configurations. They share the same topology but their feature map sizes differ due to nnU-Net's automatic configuration of convolutional strides and kernel sizes as a function of the patch size.

Tab. 1. Final configurations used in our submission. Table highlights changes to the nnU-Net defaults.

Task	Name	Patch Size	Spacing [mm]	Data Aug.	batch size	norm.	Arch.
-	'3d_fullres'	[64,160,160]	[2,0.69,0.69]	default	2	CT/z-score	-
1	Configuration 1	[128,192,192]	[1.5,1,1]	DA5	5	CT	A2
	Configuration 2	[80,224,192]	[2,0.69,0.69]	default	6	CT	A1
	Configuration 3	[128,192,192]	[1.5,1,1]	default	5	CT	A2
2	Configuration 4	[80,224,192]	[2,0.69,0.69]	default	6	z-score	A1
	Configuration 5	[128,192,192]	[1.5,1,1]	default	5	z-score	A2

2.2   Inference strategy

Prediction is carried out with the nnU-Net defaults (sliding window). For validation and test set prediction we use ensembling, using both the 5 models from our cross-validation as well as multiple different configurations (3 configurations for Task 1: 3 x 5 = 15 models in the ensemble). Ensembling is implemented as simple averaging of softmax outputs.

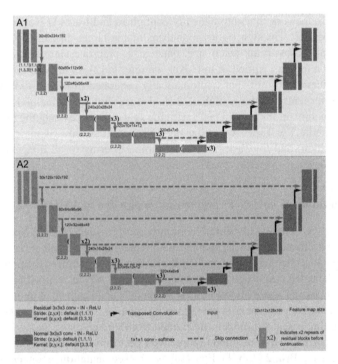

Fig. 1. The two architectures used by our final configurations. Due to nnU-Net's automatic configuration of kernel sizes and strides as a function of the patch size, their feature map sizes differ. Both architectures make use of residual connections in the encoder.

2.3 Postprocessing

The postprocessing offered by nnU-net was designed to cover a wide variety of use-cases. We believe that additional performance can be gained on AMOS2022 by specifically analyzing and targeting failure cases of our method. To identify those we generated a confusion matrix on our cross-validation results (Fig. 2) and performed rigorous visual inspection of our predicted segmentation maps.

Left-right confusion. Sometimes parts of the left kidney were classified as right kidney and vice-versa (same for adrenal glands). Here, removing disconnected small components is suboptimal because then parts of the kidneys would be labeled as background. Thus, we pooled the final kidney predictions into a joint class and use a connected component analysis to determine connected kidney regions. For each connected region we calculate its position within the image and assign its label (left/right) accordingly.

Connected component filtering. Just like the default nnU-Net we explore filtering of connected components. Specifically we determine whether removing all but the largest connected component can improve the Dice score.

Organ size constraints. Driven by the human anatomy, organs are expected to have a certain volume. This property can be exploited to filter small false positive predictions, for example in images in which the target organ is not present but false positive areas are. We use a parameter called 'rate' in combination with the minimum organ size observed in the training set. The rate is intended to be a safety margin: a rate of 0.75 indicates that components smaller than 75% of the minimum organ size are removed.

Component filtering with size constraints. We combine the two previous techniques and remove instances below a volume threshold unless its the only connected region.

Composition of post-processing steps In order to find the optimal post-processing scheme we create compositions of the previously mentioned post-processing schemes, namely:

1. PP1: Left right confusion (only kidneys & adrenal glands) followed by organ size constraints
2. PP2: Left right confusion (only kidneys & adrenal glands) followed by component filtering with size constraints

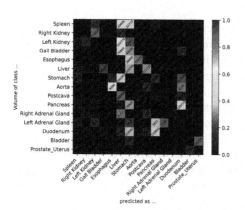

Fig. 2. Confusion of organs. The color encodes the relative percentage per row while the number represents the absolute volume over the entire cross validation dataset. We used this as an indicator which error cases exist and could be solved through postprocessing.

Tab. 2. Ablation results.

Method Metric	Task 1		Task 2	
	5-fold CV Dice	Val mean Score (Dice score)	5-fold CV Dice	Val mean Score (Dice score)
nnU-Net default	88.64	86.52 (90.31)	-	-
+ configuration improvements	89.08	-	-	-
+ residual encoder	89.45	-	88.43	-
+ increased batch size (bs 5) (corresponds to configs 3 & 5)	89.57	87.71 (91.43)	88.68	87.72 (90.97)

Tab. 3. 5-fold cross-validation results of all our configurations and their ensembles.

Task 1		Task 2	
Config.	Dice	Config.	Dice
Config. 1	89.60	Config. 4	88.56
Config. 2	89.59	Config. 5	88.69
Config. 3	89.57		
Ensemble	89.92	Ensemble	88.94
+ postprocessing	90.13	+ postprocessing	89.06

3. PP3: Left right confusion (only kidneys & adrenal glands) followed by connected component filtering.
4. PP4: Only left right confusion (only kidneys & adrenal glands).

We use the predictions of our ensemble on the 5-fold cross-validation (training images) to optimize the postprocessing scheme. Each organ is optimized independently and the best performing postprocessing strategy is retained. Note that we test multiple possible values for the 'rate' parameter where applicable.

3   Results

The proposed modifications to the default nnU-Net pipeline substantially improved the results both on the training set cross-validation as well as the official validation set. We perform ablation studies to highlight the contributions of each component (Tab. 2). Overall, we were able to increase the Dice for configuration 3 in table 1 by about 1% w.r.t. the nnU-Net baseline by modifying nnU-Net's automated configuration (specifically, target spacing, patch size) and using residual connections in the encoder of the U-Net. Increasing the batch size yielded further improvements.

For the sake of brevity we do not show detailed results of the remaining configurations. We summarize the cross-validation performance of all our configurations and their ensembles in table 3. As expected, ensembling provided a substantial gain in segmentation performance, as did our postprocessing.

4 Discussion

In this paper we performed task-specific optimizations of the default nnU-Net pipeline to maximize segmentation performance on the AMOS2022 challenge. Changing crucial hyperparameters such as the patch size, batch size and target spacing for resampling yielded substantial gains relative to the default configuration, as did the addition of residual connections in the encoder of the U-Net. Our final submission consists of three configurations for Task 1 and two for Task 2. Since each configurations was trained as a 5-fold cross-validation, our ensembles consist of 15 and 10 models, respectively. Naturally, the source code for training our models as well as the inference dockers will be made publicly available after the competition.

Acknowledgement. Part of this work was funded by Helmholtz Imaging, a platform of the Helmholtz Incubator on Information and Data Science.

References

1. Ji Y, Bai H, Yang J, Ge C, Zhu Y, Zhang R et al. AMOS: A large-scale abdominal multi-organ benchmark for versatile medical image segmentation. arXiv:2206.08023. 2022.
2. Isensee F, Jaeger PF, Kohl SAA, et al. nnU-Net: a self-configuring method for deep learning-based biomedical image segmentation. Nat Methods. 2021;18(2):203–11.
3. Isensee F, Jäger PF, Full PM, Vollmuth P, Maier-Hein KH. nnU-Net for brain tumor segmentation. International MICCAI Brainlesion Workshop. Springer. 2020:118–32.
4. Full PM, Isensee F, Jäger PF, Maier-Hein K. Studying robustness of semantic segmentation under domain shift in cardiac MRI. International Workshop on Statistical Atlases and Computational Models of the Heart. Springer. 2020:238–49.
5. Ma J. Cutting-edge 3D Medical Image Segmentation Methods in 2020: Are Happy Families All Alike? arXiv:2101.00232. 2021.
6. Ronneberger O, Fischer P, Brox T. U-Net: convolutional networks for biomedical image segmentation. Med Image Comput Comput Assist Interv 2015. (Lecture Notes in Computer Science). Springer International Publishing, 2015.
7. Heller N, Sathianathen N, Kalapara A, Walczak E, Moore K, Kaluzniak H et al. The KiTS19 challenge data: 300 kidney tumor cases with clinical context, CT semantic segmentations, and surgical outcomes. arXiv:1904.00445. 2020.

Abstract: Liver Tumor Segmentation in Late-phase MRI using Multi-model Training and an Anisotropic U-Net

Annika Gerken[1], Grzegorz Chlebus[1], Hans Meine[1,2], Felix Thielke[1], Farina Kock[1], Tobias Paulus[3], Nasreddin Abolmaali[3], Andrea Schenk[1,4]

[1]Fraunhofer-Institut für Digitale Medizin MEVIS, Bremen
[2]Universität Bremen, Medical Image Computing Group, Bremen
[3]Katholisches Klinikum Bochum, Universitätsklinikum der Ruhr Universität Bochum, Institut für Diagnostische und Interventionelle Radiologie und Nuklearmedizin, Bochum
[4]Medizinische Hochschule Hannover, Institut für Diagnostische und Interventionelle Radiologie, Hannover
andrea.schenk@mevis.fraunhofer.de

Automatic liver tumor segmentation can support the planning of liver interventions, such as selective internal radiation therapy (SIRT). Most studies on deep learning-based liver tumor segmentation have focused on contrast-enhanced CT, however dynamic contrast-enhanced MRI (DCE-MRI) can yield a higher sensitivity. In this work, we demonstrate the deep learning-based segmentation of liver tumors in the late hepatocellular phase of DCE-MRI. In particular, we employ an anisotropic 3D u-net architecture (aU-Net) and a multi-model training strategy: the training is started 16 times using different random weight initializations. After 5k, 10k, 20k and 40k iterations, the number of neural networks is reduced to the best performing half, based on validation data. This approach significantly improves the segmentation performance compared to a standard single-model training (mean Dice score 0.74 vs. 0.70), and is close to the inter-rater-agreement of three clinical experts (mean Dice score 0.78). Moreover, the aU-Net architecture alone improves the segmentation performance compared to our previous study using three 2D U-Nets working on orthogonal view directions (mean Dice score 0.65). In a qualitative rating, 66% of automatic segmentations from multi-model training are rated as good or very good, compared to 43% for the single-model training. However, the detection performance (F1-score 0.59) is still inferior to the inter-observer-agreement of the clinical experts (0.76). In summary, this study demonstrates that correctly detected liver tumors can be automatically segmented with high accuracy in late-phase DCE-MRI data, but the detection can still be improved, in particular of smaller lesions [1, 2].

References

1. Hänsch A, Chlebus G, Meine H, Thielke F, Kock F, Paulus T et al. Improving automatic liver tumor segmentation in late-phase MRI using multi-model training and 3D convolutional neural networks. Sci Rep. 2022;12(1):12262.
2. Chlebus G, Schenk A. Automatic liver and tumor segmentation in late-phase MRI using fully convolutional neural networks. Proc CURAC. 2018:195–200.

Automatic Vertebrae Segmentation in MR Volumes

A Comparison of Different Deep Learning-based Approaches

Orgest Xhelili[1], Miruna Gafencu[1], Francesca De Benetti[1], Nassir Navab[1],
Thomas Wendler[1,2]

[1]Chair for Computer Aided Medical Procedures and Augmented Reality, Technical University of
Munich, Garching, Germany
[2]SurgicEye GmbH & ScintHealth GmbH, Munich, Germany
francesca.de-benetti@tum.de

Abstract. Vertebrae segmentation is important in several clinical settings involving spine pathologies. In recent years, deep learning-based techniques have become popular in segmenting the spine in computed tomography (CT) volumes. However, few options have been tested for magnetic resonance (MR) imaging segmentation. In this paper, we provide a comparison of three deep learning methods tackling the automatic vertebrae segmentation in MR volumes. We selected three methods that were already established in the segmentation of CT images: 3D U-Net as our baseline, an iterative binary segmentation approach, and a multi-stage segmentation approach. Our experiments achieved a mean Dice score of 88.1% and demonstrate that CT segmentation methods are easily transferable to MR segmentation.

1 Introduction

Segmentation of vertebrae is a crucial step in assessment, diagnosis, and surgery planning of spine pathologies, and in the study of its biomechanics. As manual segmentation is time-consuming, error-prone, and requires expert knowledge, substantial research has been dedicated to fully automatic spine segmentation. In recent years, many deep learning approaches have been applied to the automatic segmentation and labeling of vertebrae in CT volumes. Among others, the large scale vertebrae segmentation challenge (VerSe) [1] provides benchmark datasets for tackling the problem of labeling and segmentation of vertebrae in CT volumes.

Despite the availability of a similar dataset for MR vertebrae segmentation called MRSpineSeg [2], fewer approaches have been brought forward for this task. In their work, Pang et al. use this dataset to train a combination of a 3D Graph Convolutional Network for 3D coarse segmentation and a 2D Residual U-Net for 2D segmentation refinement [2]. Lessmann et al. apply a modified 3D U-Net with two additional branches on MR volumes, which was initially developed for the segmentation of vertebrae in CT images [3]. In this paper, we implement three established methods for vertebrae segmentation in CT volumes and apply them to the same problem in MR volumes. Among the methods that were benchmarked against the VerSe dataset, we selected an iterative segmentation [3], and and a multi-stage approach [4]. We compared these two algorithms against a multi-class 3D U-Net, which we used as a baseline model.

© Der/die Autor(en), exklusiv lizenziert an
Springer Fachmedien Wiesbaden GmbH, ein Teil von Springer Nature 2023
T. M. Deserno et al. (Hrsg.), *Bildverarbeitung für die Medizin 2023*,
Informatik aktuell, https://doi.org/10.1007/978-3-658-41657-7_9

2 Materials and methods

2.1 Dataset

We used the MRSpineSeg dataset [2], which includes 172 T2-weighted MR images, with annotations of 19 structures (10 vertebrae, 9 intervertebral discs). The voxel size ranges from $0.3 \times 0.3 \times 4.4$ mm to $0.59 \times 0.59 \times 5.5$ mm. The annotated segmentation masks contain sacral (S), lumbar (L5-L1) and thoracic (T12-T9) vertebrae. As we did not tackle the problem of intervertebral discs segmentation, their labels were not considered. Moreover, the label for the T9 vertebra was removed because it is present in less than 10% of the volumes. The dataset was split randomly at a patient level, with 70% of it for training and the remaining part for validation (15%) and testing (15%).

2.2 Network 1: 3D U-net (baseline)

All the volumes went through a preprocessing stage, which included resampling to 1 mm isotropic spacing, cropping, padding, and normalization (in $[-1, 1]$). The images were cropped in the x axis to remove parts that do not contain the spine, and padded in the z axis to obtain a constant number of 72 slices. During training, we performed on-the-fly data augmentation, namely, Gaussian blur ($\sigma=1$), and Gaussian noise ($\mu=0$, $\sigma=0.05$) to the volumes.

Our baseline architecture is a standard 3D U-Net [5], with a 10-channel output and softmax as final activation. The network was trained on patches of size $128 \times 128 \times 72$ centered around specific vertebrae, for 10.000 iterations with a minibatch size of 2. For the baseline U-Net, we use an ADAM optimizer and a learning rate of 0.001. We trained the model with different losses: Dice loss, weighted Dice loss, and a combination of false positives and false negatives (Section 2.5).

2.3 Network 2: iterative model

This strategy is based on a network proposed by Lessmann et al. [3]. It performs iterative spine segmentation utilizing the anatomical knowledge that vertebrae are located one after the other. Compared to the original version, ours does not include the two branches used for anatomical identification and completeness classification, as it is reported that they do not improve the performance [3].

For this approach, we used a slightly modified 3D U-Net from Section 2.2. The network receives a 2-channel input composed of the nth MRI patch and the $(n-1)^{th}$ segmentation mask as memory component (Fig. 1). This means that for each iteration the network returns a binary segmentation map, which is then used to update the memory component for the next iteration. The preprocessing and training procedure is the same as in Section 2.2, including the use of the three loss functions: Dice loss, weighted Dice loss, and a combination of false positives and false negatives (Section 2.5).

2.4 Network 3: Payer et al.

This network requires the ground truth centroid of each vertebra, i.e. the center of mass of the vertebral body, which is not included in the MRSpineSeg dataset. Therefore, we compute it for each vertebra (except the sacrum) by calculating the center of mass of the whole vertebra and empirically shifting it towards the vertebral body. This shift accounts for the unwanted contribution of the vertebral arch to the position of the center of mass.

This third strategy is designed to handle both labeling and segmentation of the vertebrae in a three-step approach [4]:

- In the first stage, the network localizes the spine by predicting the line that passes through the vertebral centroids. It uses a modified 3D U-Net with average pooling in the contraction blocks and L2 as the loss function.
- The second stage is responsible for localizing the centroids of the vertebrae in the volume. In this step, a SpatialConfiguration-Net [6] model is trained to predict a Gaussian heatmap volume for each vertebra. In this case, a modified L2 loss function is used.
- The final stage performs the vertebrae segmentation and uses the same 3D U-Net as in the first stage. Because the second stage uniquely identifies the vertebrae, the segmentation network is designed to perform only binary segmentation of each vertebra from the background and is applied on vertebra-centered patches. For comparability reasons, this stage is not only trained with the originally proposed Binary Cross Entropy loss but also with two of the above-mentioned losses: Dice loss and weighted Dice loss (Section 2.5).

For training the networks from the three stages, we use an ADAM optimizer, a learning rate of 0.001, and a minibatch size of 1. Each stage network is trained for 10.000, 50.000, and 50.000 iterations respectively.

2.5 Loss functions

We define the binary dice score (DS) as

$$DS = 2\frac{\sum_{i \in N} w_i y_i \hat{y}_i + \epsilon}{\sum_{i \in N} w_i (y_i + \hat{y}_i) + \epsilon} \tag{1}$$

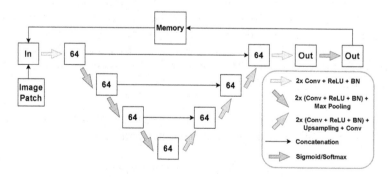

Fig. 1. 3D U-Net architecture for the iterative model. The number of channels per convolutional layer is denoted inside each block.

where y_i and $\hat{y}_i$ are respectively the ground truth and the prediction for a specific voxel and ϵ is an arbitrarily small number used to ensure numerical stability. This definition includes a voxel-specific weight w_i whose value depends on the loss function.

2.5.1 Dice loss. The dice loss (DL) is based on DS with $w_i = 1$, which is computed for all L output classes of the model

$$DL = 1 - \frac{1}{L} \sum_{l \in L} DS_l \tag{2}$$

2.5.2 Weighted dice loss. The weighted dice loss (wDL), is defined similarly as DL, but it uses a weighted DS instead of the conventional binary DS. The weighting gives more importance to pixels near the surface, as proposed by Lessmann et al. [3]

$$w_i = 8^{\left(-\delta_i^2 \frac{1}{36}\right)} + 1 \tag{3}$$

where δ_i denotes the distance of voxel i to the closest point in the surface.

2.5.3 Weighted FP and FN. The weighted FP and FN loss (wFPN) was introduced by Lessman et al. [3], and it uses information from false positives and false negatives

$$\text{wFPN} = \lambda \cdot FP + FN = \lambda \sum_{i \in N} w_i (1 - y_i)\hat{y}_i + \sum_{i \in N} w_i y_i (1 - \hat{y}_i) \tag{4}$$

where λ is a factor that converges to 1 during the training process.

2.6 Evaluation metrics

2.6.1 Vertebrae identification. We evaluated the capability of the networks to correctly identify the vertebrae. For each vertebra in the ground truth, we found the predicted vertebra with the biggest overlap. If the labels of the two vertebrae were the same, the vertebra is considered correctly identified. We call this metric true label percentage (TLP). In addition to this, we computed the identification (ID) rate, as defined in the VerSe challenge [1], for the model of Payer et al. In this case, a vertebra is considered correctly identified if the distance between ground truth and predicted centroid is smaller than 20 mm. Compared to TLP, the ID rate also considers the distance between the predicted and ground truth centroids.

2.6.2 Vertebrae segmentation. We use multi-class DS (mDS) and average symmetric surface distance (ASSD) to evaluate the segmentation performance

$$mDS = \frac{1}{L} \sum_{l \in L} DS_l \qquad \text{where } w_i = 1 \tag{5}$$

$$ASSD = \frac{\sum_{y_i} d(y_i, \hat{y}) + \sum_{\hat{y}_i} d(\hat{y}_i, y)}{|y| + |\hat{y}|} \qquad \text{where } d(x, Y) = \min_{y \in Y} ||x - y||_2 \tag{6}$$

Tab. 1. Evaluation metrics of the different segmentation methods (mean ± std). (* sacrum excluded).

	mDS (%) ↑	ASSD (mm) ↓	TLP (%) ↑	ID rate (%) ↑
Multi Class U-Net with DL	78.5 ± 16.5	5.0 ± 7.5	**94.5**	-
Multi Class U-Net with wDL	**81.2 ± 16.3**	**1.9 ± 2.3**	93.3	-
Multi Class U-Net with wFPN	77.3 ± 23.8	2.7 ± 8.1	90.3	-
Iterative model with DL	83.1 ± 16.6	1.3 ± 1.5	92.1	-
Iterative model with wDL	**88.1 ± 3.4**	**0.9 ± 0.43**	**100**	-
Iterative model with wFPN	87.1 ± 4.7	1.0 ± 0.7	**100**	-
Payer's et al. with DL*	84.4 ± 19.5	1.6 ± 3.4	93.8	**97.2**
Payer's et al. with wDL*	**84.4 ± 19.4**	**1.5 ± 3.4**	94.5	**97.2**
Payer's et al. with BCE*	84.1 ± 19.4	**1.5 ± 3.4**	94.5	**97.2**

3 Results

Tab. 1 shows the evaluation metrics for the different models. The best performing is the iterative model with wDL, with a mDS of 88.1 ± 3.4. For all three models, the wDL is the best-performing loss function in terms of mDS and ASSD metrics. However, the conventional DL leads to the best TLP results (94.5%) among the experiments that use the baseline model. On the other hand, the iterative model does not display differences between training with wDL and wFPN when analyzing the TLP (100%). Regarding the 3D U-Net and the iterative model, the choice of the loss function had a relevant impact on the DS, with an improvement of 3.9% in the baseline (wDL vs wFPN) and 5.0% in the iterative model (wDL vs DL). On the other hand, in Payer's model, the choice of the loss function only had a marginal impact on segmentation performance (mDS ∈ [84.1, 84.4] %, ASSD ∈ [1.5, 1.6] mm, TLP ∈ [93.8, 94.5] %). This can be explained by the large influence of this model's vertebrae localization stage (second stage) on the segmentation results. An example of one MR image, its ground truth, and the segmentation masks as predicted by all the considered models are shown in Fig. 2.

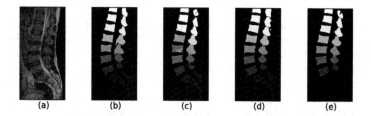

(a)   (b)   (c)   (d)   (e)

Fig. 2. Example of resulting segmentations for a middle slice on a test image: (a) Raw Image, (b) Ground Truth, (c) 3D U-Net model (baseline), (d) iterative model, (e) Payer et al. model.

4 Discussion

In all our experiments, the vertebrae identification was satisfactory (TLP > 90%). The iterative model is shown to be the best one (TLP = 100%), which can be explained by the fact that the labeling is performed using previous knowledge of the anatomy of the spine. However, choosing the wrong loss function can reduce the TLP.

Previous work on vertebrae segmentation on the same dataset [2] achieved a mean DS of $87.32 \pm 4.75\%$, whereas Lessmann et al. achieved $94.4\pm3.3\%$ on a different dataset. The iterative approach with wDL slightly improves the DS on the MRSpineSeg dataset (+0.78%). Indeed, the use of wDL improves the performance of all the models. For the model of Payer et al., a more thorough analysis showed that the labeling of T10 vertebra failed in most of the test images. Without T10 vertebra the performance of this model would be closer to the iterative model (mDS = 86.9%).

Finally, we computed the mDS for the iterative model without the sacrum (mDS = 88.3 %) to allow for a more accurate comparison with the networks trained on the VerSe dataset, which does not include annotations for the sacrum. Tab. 2 shows that methods developed for vertebrae segmentation in CT can be used for the same task in MR, without significant loss in performance. A similar performance gap reported in the VerSe results [1] can also be seen in our analysis here, pointing out that the choice of the model (as well as the choice of the loss function) has a great impact on the results.

| | CT* [1] | | MR* | |
	mDS (%)	ID rate (%)	mDS (%)	ID rate (%)
Iterative model	85.76	-	88.3	-
Payer et al.	89.80	94.25	84.4	97.2

Tab. 2. Comparison between segmentation approaches in CT and MR.

References

1. Sekuboyina A, Husseini ME, Bayat A, Löffler M, Liebl H, Li H et al. VerSe: a vertebrae labelling and segmentation benchmark for multi-detector CT images. Med Image Anal. 2021;73.
2. Pang S, Pang C, Zhao L, Chen Y, Su Z, Zhou Y et al. SpineParseNet: spine parsing for volumetric MR image by a two-stage segmentation framework with semantic image representation. IEEE T Med Imaging. 2020;40(1).
3. Lessmann N, Van Ginneken B, De Jong PA, Išgum I. Iterative fully convolutional neural networks for automatic vertebra segmentation and identification. Med Image Anal. 2019;53.
4. Payer C, Stern D, Bischof H, Urschler M. Coarse to fine vertebrae localization and segmentation with SpatialConfiguration-Net and U-Net. VISIGRAPP. 2020.
5. Çiçek Ö, Abdulkadir A, Lienkamp SS, Brox T, Ronneberger O. 3D U-Net: learning dense volumetric segmentation from sparse annotation. International conference on medical image computing and computer-assisted intervention (MICCAI). 2016.
6. Payer C, Štern D, Bischof H, Urschler M. Integrating spatial configuration into heatmap regression based CNNs for landmark localization. Med Image Anal. 2019;54.

Learnable Slice-to-volume Reconstruction for Motion Compensation in Fetal Magnetic Resonance Imaging

Constantin Jehn[1], Johanna P. Müller[1], Bernhard Kainz[1,2]

[1]IDEA Lab, Friedrich–Alexander University Erlangen–Nürnberg, DE
[2]Imperial College London, SW7 2AZ, London, UK
constantin.jehn@fau.de

Abstract. Reconstructing motion-free 3D magnetic resonance imaging (MRI) volumes of fetal organs comes with the challenge of motion artefacts due to fetal motion and maternal respiration. Current methods rely on iterative procedures of outlier removal, super-resolution (SR) and slice-to-volume registration (SVR). Long runtimes and missing volume preservation over multiple iterations are still challenges for widespread clinical implementation. We envision an end-to-end learnable reconstruction framework that enables faster inference times and that can be steered by downstream tasks like segmentation. Therefore, we propose a new hybrid architecture for fetal brain reconstruction, consisting of a fully differentiable pre-registration module and a CycleGAN model for 3D image-to-image translation that is pretrained on our custom-generated dataset of 209 pairs of low-resolution (LoRes) and high-resolution (HiRes) fetal brain volumes. Our results are evaluated quantitatively with respect to five different similarity metrics. We incorporate the learned perceptual image patch similarity (LPIPS) metric and apply it to quantify volumetric image similarity for the first time in literature. Furthermore, we evaluate the model outputs qualitatively and conduct an expert survey to compare our method's reconstruction quality to an established approach.

1 Introduction

Abnormalities in fetal development can indicate pathological long-term problems. They can impact the survival rates in the perinatal period and beyond, making accurate means of fetal organ reconstruction essential to counselling during pregnancy [1]. Due to its superior soft-tissue contrast and the absence of ionising radiation, MRI is the modality of choice for detailed structural imaging, for example, for the fetal brain. During the imaging process, multiple stacks in orthogonal slicing directions are acquired. These stacks are subject to inter-slice and inter-stack motion artefacts resulting from fetal and maternal motion. The problem formulation can be condensed to the successful generation of HiRes reconstructions from corrupted input data. The majority of established reconstruction methods uses a pre-registration step that brings all input stacks into approximate alignment by 3D-3D registration, followed by an iterative procedure as it was introduced in [2]: outlier-rejection aims to reject voxels that are likely motion artefacts; SR updates combine the information from the different input stacks into a common reconstruction volume. SVR steps iteratively register the single slices from the input stacks to the most recent reconstruction volume. [3] proposes a surrogate measure for intra-stack motion corruption to select the optimal stack during pre-registration and

T. M. Deserno et al. (Hrsg.), *Bildverarbeitung für die Medizin 2023*,
Informatik aktuell, https://doi.org/10.1007/978-3-658-41657-7_10

publishes a GPU implementation with significantly lower runtime. A pre-registration step based on CNNs and a new parametrization for the SVR is proposed in [4]. Most recently, Transformers have been proposed to regress the transformation parameters for the SVR [5]. In this work we present an end-to-end learnable hybrid reconstruction framework that combines a pre-registration module and a Cycle-GAN model for volume-to-volume translation.

2 Material and methods

2.1 Hybrid reconstruction framework

Registration-based reconstruction algorithms have advanced the image quality of fetal MRI imaging. Yet, long runtimes resulting from the high-dimensional optimisation problem and room for improvement in volume preservation over the iterations remain open challenges in the field. Motivated by these shortcomings and the urge to steer the process by downstream tasks such as segmentation, we strive for an end-to-end learnable reconstruction pipeline. It offers the possibility to incorporate neural network architectures as part of the reconstruction pipeline and profit from advances in learnable SR, image-to-image translation and generative models. We propose a hybrid framework for fetal brain reconstruction. Its structure is outlined in Fig. 1: the fully differentiable pre-registration module P^1 transforms the input stacks into a latent reconstruction space. Subsequently, a CycleGAN model[2], pretrained on our custom dataset, translates the LoRes volume into a high-quality reconstruction volume.

2.2 Pre-registration

The preregistration step combines the incoming stacks into a first approximate common volume. The outline of the algorithm is provided in Fig. 2. It reimplements the pre-registration steps from [3], allowing gradients to backpropagate to registration parameters. The first step gives a surrogate measure for the motion artefacts within one stack. The method is based on Singular Value Decomposition and the assumption that neighbouring slices of continuous volumes are highly correlated. The stack with the least artefacts is selected as template, and the remaining stacks are aligned using 3D-3D registration. Subsequently, the common volume undergoes an SR update.

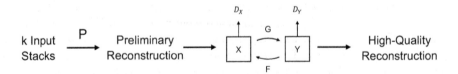

Fig. 1. The proposed hybrid architecture combines the preregistrator P with a pretrained CycleGAN model translating preliminary reconstructions into HiRes reconstructions.

---

[1]https://github.com/Constantin-Jehn/SVR_pytorch
[2]https://github.com/Constantin-Jehn/Cycle_GAN_3D

2.3 Image-to-image translation

The CycleGAN architecture is a variant of the GAN framework for unpaired image-to-image translation [6]. Unpaired models can be further improved by expert-approved HiRes reconstruction even without corresponding LoRes images. The model's structure is depicted in Fig. 1. The generators G and F translate between the set of LoRes volumes X and HiRes volumes Y, such that the results are not distinguishable from the target distribution. The discriminators D_X and D_Y aim to correctly classify true and synthetic samples. The key feature of the architecture is the additional cycle consistency loss, expressed in Eq. 1. It enforces $F(G(x)) \approx x$ and $G(F(y)) \approx y$, constraining the generators to mappings where input and output have a meaningful relationship. The complete objective function can be found in [6]

$$\mathcal{L}_{cyc} = \mathbb{E}_{x \sim p_{data}(x)}[\|F(G(x)) - x\|_1] + \mathbb{E}_{y \sim p_{data}(y)}[\|F(G(y)) - y\|_1] \qquad (1)$$

This additional constraint helps circumventing the introduction of random or artificial details during the image generation.

2.4 Data

We use a dataset containing 252 MRI studies from mothers in weeks 24-37 of their pregnancy acquired on a Philips Achieva 1.5 T and 3 T scanner. The volumes were acquired using single-shot fast spin echo T2-weighted sequences with half Fourier acquisition (ssFSE) and SENSE. The study was approved by the ethics committee at Imperial College London and the UK's NHS National Research Ethics Service.

2.5 Training details

Training the CycleGAN model requires two sets of volumes. However, our pre-registration module only generates approximate reconstructions. Therefore, we use an established slice-to-volume-reconstruction toolkit (SVRTK)[3] to generate surrugate HiRes reconstructions. All MRI stacks with manually generated brain segmentation masks are fed to SVRTK, and the HiRes reconstruction and its intermediate pre-registration result are extracted. The 209 MRI volumes with the respective segmentations are provided as input to our fully differentiable pre-registration module (FDPR). We include the 123 best

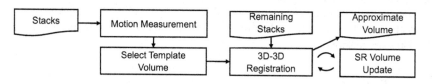

Fig. 2. The preregistration procedure selects the least motion-corrupted volume as a template. The remaining stacks are aligned by 3D-3D registration, followed by an SR update step.

---

[3]https://github.com/SVRTK/SVRTK

FDPR pre-registrations, together with 86 pre-registration results from SVRTK (SVPR) in the LoRes set X such that the complete dataset is covered. The generator networks are three-dimensional 9-block ResNet architectures, and the discriminators are fully convolutional networks. Using the Adam optimiser [7], the model is trained over 200 epochs with a linear learning rate (LR) decay after 100 epochs. Three starting LRs, 0.0002, 0.0004 and 0.001, are compared. With a train-test split of 169-40, the training takes approx. 24 hours on one NVIDIA A6000 (48GB) GPU.

3   Results

3.1   Quantitative results

Based on image similarity metrics, volumes generated by the CycleGAN model can be compared to target images from set Y, which allows quantifying the model's image-to-image translation performance. To facilitate comparisons, we assess the model with respect to four different global metrics: the peak signal-to-noise ratio (PSNR), the normalised mean square error (NMSE), the structural similarity index measure (SSIM) and normalized cross-correlation (NCC). Moreover, we incorporate the Learned Perceptual Image Patch Similarity (LPIPS) as a metric that has been shown to align better with human-perceived image similarity than standard metrics [8]. While LPIPS has been developed for 2D RGB-images, we aim to quantify similarity on volumetric one-channel data. To apply the 2D metric to our MRI volumes, all 2D slices in three orthogonal directions are extracted, and the channel values are assigned identically to all three RGB channels. We take the mean over all LPIPS values for the individual slices as the final measure. The mean results, with respect to the similarity metrics, on the subsets SVPR, FDPR and their union PR, are reported Table 1 for three different learning rates (0.0002, 0.0004 and 0.001). Each mean value is supplemented by the standard error of the mean (s.e.m.) $\frac{\sigma}{\sqrt{N}}$, with standard deviation σ and the number samples N, to quantify the variability of the mean values taking the size of the test data set into account. The rows SVPR, FDPR and PR report the mean similarity in their subset of X to its HiRes counterpart in Y. The three rows below state the mean similarity of the image-translation result of the generator G to the HiRes volumes for different LR on the subset name above in the table. Firstly, we can observe that the LR of 0.0004 performs best on three out of five metrics on the complete set. The PSNR measures a significant improvement on the complete set, mainly induced by the SVPR set. NMSE, SSIM and NCC indicate no significant improvement.The LPIPS metric improves over all the sets, which also aligns with the qualitative analysis revealing a similarity increase of the CycleGAN outputs to its targets. For the following evaluation steps, the results of the model trained with LR of 0.0004 are considered.

3.2   Qualitative results

Fig. 3 presents two example reconstructions taken from the test set. The upper row represents the preregistration inputs for the CycleGAN model, the second row depicts the CycleGAN result, and the last row visualises SVRTK's outputs for reference. For

Tab. 1. Image-to-image translation results with learning rates of 0.0002, 0.0004 and 0.001. For all rows, the result of three iterations of SVRTK is taken as a reference. The mean values, over the test set data, for different metrics are reported with standard error of the mean as a variability measure.

References	PSNR ↑	NMSE ↓	SSIM ↑	| NCC | ↑	LPIPS ↓
SVPR	23.11 ± 0.60	0.110 ± 0.010	**0.93** ± 0.010	**0.94** ± 0.009	0.10 ± 0.0064
G(lr=0.0002)	27.01 ± 0.40	0.069 ± 0.004	0.92 ± 0.010	0.91 ± 0.011	0.08 ± 0.0062
G(lr=0.0004)	**27.80** ± 0.27	**0.064** ± 0.002	0.92 ± 0.009	0.91 ± 0.011	**0.08** ± 0.0059
G(lr=0.001)	23.36 ± 0.23	0.140 ± 0.005	0.82 ± 0.011	0.85 ± 0.015	0.16 ± 0.0070
FDPR	21.80 ± 0.28	0.170 ± 0.009	0.82 ± 0.010	0.83 ± 0.010	0.19 ± 0.0060
G(lr=0.0002)	22.06 ± 0.28	0.181 ± 0.009	0.81 ± 0.011	0.83 ± 0.010	0.15 ± 0.0061
G(lr=0.0004)	22.10 ± 0.26	0.190 ± 0.009	0.82 ± 0.010	0.83 ± 0.010	0.14 ± 0.0059
G(lr=0.001)	21.99 ± 0.23	0.180 ± 0.006	0.79 ± 0.008	0.82 ± 0.099	0.19 ± 0.047
PR	22.39 ± 0.33	0.140 ± 0.008	0.87 ± 0.011	0.88 ± 0.069	0.15 ± 0.0085
G(lr=0.0002)	24.29 ± 0.46	0.132 ± 0.010	0.86 ± 0.011	0.87 ± 0.010	0.12 ± 0.0067
G(lr=0.0004)	24.66 ± 0.49	0.144 ± 0.012	0.87 ± 0.011	0.87 ± 0.010	0.11 ± 0.0065
G(lr=0.001)	22.61 ± 0.12	0.160 ± 0.005	0.81 ± 0.007	0.83 ± 0.009	0.17 ± 0.0046

FDPR and SVPR inputs, the CycleGAN model creates reconstructions with significantly improved image quality and increased visual similarity to the SVRTK result. The CycleGAN reconstructions with SVPR inputs are more similar to the target image, which can be explained by the input being an intermediate result of the target volume's reconstruction.

3.3 Expert survey

Any reconstruction is the result of either a complex optimisation problem or a deep neural network (NN), and therefore we have to acknowledge the absence of reliable ground truth data. To assess the reconstruction quality of our model compared to SVRKT, we conducted a survey among 16 domain experts. The survey is designed as two

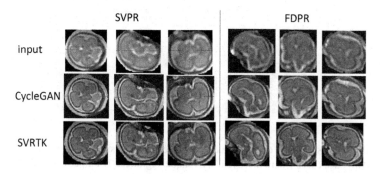

Fig. 3. The first row shows the LoRes input volumes, and the second row the CycleGAN volume-to-volume translation results. The third row gives SVRTK's reconstruction as a reference.

alternative-forced-choice (2AFC) test. The experts were shown three orthogonal views of a CycleGAN reconstruction and an SVRTK reconstruction of the same input. They had to answer which reconstruction they would prefer for interpretation. The indication of the methods was not given, and the answers were shuffled randomly over the survey. Fig. 4 shows that 19 out of 25 reconstruction comparisons were answered in favour of SVRTK, by the experts. There are only two edge cases where the CycleGAN significantly outperforms the reference method.

4   Discussion

Interpretation and evaluation: From the quantitative analysis and, particularly, the PSNR and LPIPS results, we observe an increase in image similarity of model outputs. This is further supported by the presented example reconstructions, showing enhanced reconstruction quality compared to the model inputs while preserving their key features. Hence, we can state that CycleGAN models can improve preregistration quality and should be considered for future work on end-to-end learnable reconstruction frameworks. The expert survey showed that the developed method is not yet on the level of specialized SVR reconstruction algorithms, which might be a result of observer bias and hidden confounders that need to be investigated in future work. Effects on downstream data analysis and diagnosis will also provide an intriguing direction for further work.

Outlook: A major limitation of this work is the generated training data for the model. Working with real data has the advantage of a realistic reconstruction setting. However, the absence of true HiRes data and the necessity to construct the target set Y from the output of another framework leaves us with an implicit upper bound of the method, which is predefined by the chosen method. Hence, we propose to carry on the presented work with HiRes volumes from acquisition with little or no fetal motion and introducing synthetic motion artefacts as in [5] to construct the LoRes set X. Additionally, a canonical atlas representation of the volumes in X could allow the translation model to transfer morphological details more precisely, as they would be spatially closer across the different volumes in the training set.

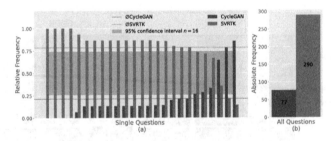

Fig. 4. In the expert survey, 19 out of 25 questions were answered significantly in SVRTK's favour. There are two edge cases where the CycleGAN model significantly outperforms SVRTK.

Acknowledgement. The authors gratefully acknowledge the HPC resources provided by (NHR@FAU ID PatRo-MRI). NHR funding is provided by federal and Bavarian state authorities. NHR@FAU hardware is partially funded by the German Research Foundation (DFG) – 440719683. Data had been provided by the iFind project, Wellcome Trust IEH 102431.

References

1. Gholipour A, et al. A normative spatiotemporal MRI atlas of the fetal brain for automatic segmentation and analysis of early brain growth. Sci Rep. 2017;7(1):476.
2. Kuklisova-Murgasova M, et al. Reconstruction of fetal brain MRI with intensity matching and complete outlier removal. Med Image Anal. 2012;16:1550–64.
3. Kainz B, et al. Fast volume reconstruction from motion corrupted stacks of 2D slices. IEEE Trans Med Imaging. 2015;34:1901–13.
4. Hou B, et al. 3-D reconstruction in canonical co-ordinate space from arbitrarily oriented 2-D images. IEEE Trans Med Imaging. 2018;37(8):1737–50.
5. Xu J, et al. SVoRT: iterative transformer for slice-to-volume registration in fetal brain MRI. International Conference on Medical Image Computing and Computer-Assisted Intervention. Springer. 2022:3–13.
6. Zhu JY, et al. Unpaired image-to-image translation using cycle-consistent adversarial networks. Proceedings of the IEEE international conference on computer vision. 2017:2223–32.
7. Kingma DP, et al. Adam: A method for stochastic optimization. CoRR. 2014;abs/1412.6980.
8. Zhang R, et al. The unreasonable effectiveness of deep features as a perceptual metric. Proceedings of the IEEE conference on computer vision and pattern recognition. 2018:586–95.

A Vesselsegmentation-based CycleGAN for Unpaired Multi-modal Retinal Image Synthesis

Aline Sindel, Andreas Maier, Vincent Christlein

Pattern Recognition Lab, FAU Erlangen-Nürnberg
aline.sindel@fau.de

Abstract. Unpaired image-to-image translation of retinal images can efficiently increase the training dataset for deep-learning-based multi-modal retinal registration methods. Our method integrates a vessel segmentation network into the image-to-image translation task by extending the CycleGAN framework. The segmentation network is inserted prior to a UNet vision transformer generator network and serves as a shared representation between both domains. We reformulate the original identity loss to learn the direct mapping between the vessel segmentation and the real image. Additionally, we add a segmentation loss term to ensure shared vessel locations between fake and real images. In the experiments, our method shows a visually realistic look and preserves the vessel structures, which is a prerequisite for generating multi-modal training data for image registration.

1 Introduction

Recent deep learning methods for multi-modal medical image registration require a large amount of training data. Since it is difficult and tedious to obtain precise ground truth from real data, image-to-image translation methods are effective means to synthetically augment multi-modal datasets. In ophthalmology, different imaging systems, such as color fundus (CF), fluorescein angiography (FA), and optical coherence tomography angiography (OCTA) are used for the diagnosis of retinal diseases. Our aim is to generate synthetic multi-modal pairs that can be used to train registration methods in a self-supervised manner. For that the position and shape of the vessels should be preserved by the image-to-image translation method, but the texture and style should be transferred to the other modality. Here, we concentrate on the image-to-image translation between CF and FA images. In CF the vessels are depicted in dark and in FA in light, but by both modalities the fovea is depicted in dark and the optic cup and disc are depicted in light, which needs to be considered by the translation methods.

Conditional generative adversarial networks (cGANs) were explored in literature for the image-to-image translation of CF and FA images. In case of aligned multi-modal images, Pix2Pix [1] based approaches can be used to learn a direct 1-to-1 mapping between both modalities. In this regard, VTGAN [2] is introduced for closely but not perfectly aligned CF-FA image pairs, which uses a coarse and a fine generator with attention blocks and a vision transformer as discriminator network. CycleGAN [3] based approaches learn a direct image-to-image translation for unpaired images. For the CF-FA translation task, Li et al. [4] enriches the CycleGAN with structure and appearance encoder networks which are inserted prior to the generator networks and Cai et al. [5]

extends the CycleGAN with multi-scale generator and discriminator networks and a quality-aware loss at feature level. In contrast, we extend the CycleGAN by including the vessel segmentation as a shared representation between both domains. There exist a bunch of approaches that generate CF images from extracted vessel segmentations. For instance, the cGAN by Liang et al. [6] adds a class feature loss for diabetic retinopathy grading and a retinal detail loss which is a combination of the reconstruction loss between real and fake image and perceptual loss using a specific layer from the pretrained VGG-19 network. Niu et al. [7] includes pathology specific descriptors into the cGAN to generate CF images with specific pathological features. The real and synthetic images are compared using perceptual and severity losses. By integrating the vessel segmentation into the CycleGAN, we tackle to reduce the domain gap of the vessels between both modalities.

In this paper, we propose VesselCycleGAN, a cGAN based approach for unpaired retinal image-to-image translation based on the vessel segmentation of CF and FA images using cycle consistency. We extend the CycleGAN pipeline by inserting a vessel segmentation UNet before the generator network, which we equip with a UNet vision transformer [8]. With the vessel segmentation network, we modify the identity loss to learn the translation from the vessel segmentation to the real image and we add a segmentation loss to preserve the same vessel structures in the real and generated images and apply our method to two datasets.

2 Materials and methods

2.1 VesselCycleGAN for unpaired retinal image-to-image translation

We incorporate a vessel segmentation network (V) into the CycleGAN [3] framework, as shown in Figure 1, which we place in front of the generator networks, such that

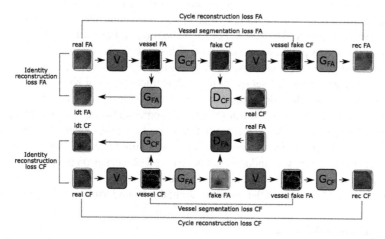

Fig. 1. Our unpaired image-to-image translation method based on the retinal vessel segmentation in multi-modal fundus images.

those do not learn the direct mapping between the two domains, but the mapping from the vessel segmentation to the particular domain. CycleGANs are conditional generative adversarial networks, consisting of two generator $G_{A/B}$ and two discriminator networks $D_{A/B}$, that learn the image-to-image translation between unpaired images from two domains A/B by using adversarial loss, cycle-consistency and identity-consistency losses [3]. The cycle-consistency loss $\mathcal{L}_{\text{cycA}}$ minimizes the difference between the real image A and its reconstruction $\hat{A}$ after passing through the cycle of applying both G_B and G_A, and here in our case V, G_B, V, and G_A

$$\mathcal{L}_{\text{cycA}}(A) = \lambda_A ||A - G_A(V(G_B(V(A))))||_1 \tag{1}$$

Using the identity-consistency loss $\mathcal{L}_{\text{idtA}}$, G_A originally learns the identity mapping of $G_A(A) \stackrel{!}{=} A$, however, in our modified CycleGAN this becomes

$$\mathcal{L}_{\text{idtA}}(A) = \lambda_A \lambda_{idt} ||A - G_A(V(A))||_1 \tag{2}$$

where G_A learns the aligned one-way image translation task of vessel segmentation A to real A. Additionally, we compute the Dice loss between the segmentation of the real A and fake B. The role of $D_{A/B}$ is as in the normal CycleGAN to distinguish unpaired real images A/B from fake images $\tilde{A}/\tilde{B}$ generated using $G_A(V(B))$ or $G_B(V(A))$. As generator network we employ the UNet-ViT [8] which is a four layer UNet ($D = 48$) with a pixel-wise vision transformer bottleneck (with 12 transform encoder blocks). As discriminator network we use the PatchGAN [1] and for the vessel segmentation network a four layer UNet ($D = 16$), which we pretrained for the vessel segmentation task.

2.2 Retinal datasets

We train and test our synthesis method using the CF-FA dataset [9] which consists of 59 pairs of color fundus (CF, 576×720) and fluorescein angiography (FA, 576×720) images from controls (29 image pairs) and from patients with diabetic retinopathy (30 pairs). We split the image pairs into train: 35, val: 10, and test: 14, with equally distributed healthy and non-healthy eyes. For each training image, we extract nine 512×512 patches, which are randomly cropped to 448 × 448. For the validation and test set, we directly extract up to nine 448 × 448 patches for each image. This results per modality into train: 315, val: 90 and test: 120 image patches. Since the original image pairs are not aligned, we register the images of the test set (prior to patch extraction) using KPVSA-Net [10].

Secondly, we use the HR fundus dataset [11] which consists of CF images and manual vessel segmentations. To train the vessel segmentation UNet, we use the color and green channel of the fundus images in two resolutions: the center 768 × 768 region and a downsized version by a factor of 4 to have a similar image size as the CF-FA dataset. During training, we randomly extract 512 × 512 patches on the fly from the 108 training and 36 validation images. For the image translation task, we use 81 484 × 484 patches from the CF images of the test set without the ground truth vessel segmentations.

2.3 Experimental details

Prior to the training of our retinal synthesis network, we train the vessel segmentation UNet on the augmented HR fundus dataset by using equally weighted binary cross-entropy and Dice loss for 800 epochs with early stopping, Adam optimizer, a learning rate $\eta = 2 \cdot 10^{-4}$, linear decay of η after 50 epochs, and batch size of 2. Then, we train the generator and discriminator networks of our retina synthesis GAN using Adam solver with a learning rate of $\eta = 2 \cdot 10^{-4}$ for 600 epochs with early stopping, a batch size of 1, $\lambda_{A/B} = 100$, $\lambda_{idt} = 1$, $\lambda_{seg} = 1$. For both tasks, we use online data augmentation (color jittering, horizontal flipping, rotation, and cropping). We compare our method with CycleGAN [3] and Pix2Pix [1] (both: G using ResNet encoder with 9 blocks with instance normalization), and with the VTGAN [2]. Pix2Pix and VTGAN require aligned training data, hence we registered our training and validation image pairs using KPVSA-Net [10]. For our method and CycleGAN, we use unaligned data with randomly sampled patches within the same class (healthy/unhealthy).

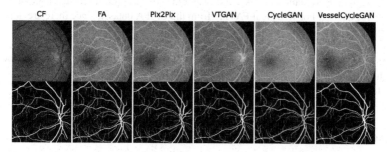

Fig. 2. FA synthesis results and vessel segmentation overlays (vessels segmented by our UNet).

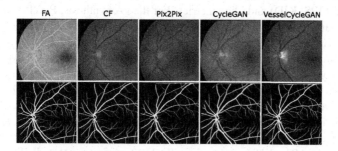

Fig. 3. CF synthesis results and vessel segmentation overlays (vessels segmented by our UNet).

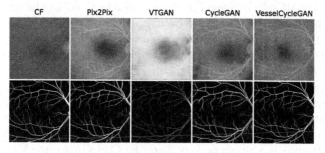

Fig. 4. FA synthesis results of the HRF dataset (vessels segmented by our UNet).

Tab. 1. Quantitative evaluation for FA and CF synthesis using the CF-FA test images. LPIPS and KID are computed between fake B and registered real B; Dice between the vessels of fake B and real A. Methods with * were trained using registered images.

A-to-B	CF-to-FA			FA-to-CF		
Metrics	LPIPS ↓	KID ↓	Dice ↑	LPIPS ↓	KID ↓	Dice ↑
Pix2Pix* (ResNet9)	0.3478	0.0104	0.7615	0.3371	0.0227	0.7264
VTGAN	0.3731	0.0383	0.8035	-	-	-
CycleGAN (ResNet9)	0.4296	0.0388	0.2471	0.3511	0.0182	0.3550
VesselCycleGAN (ResNet9 w/o seg)	0.3893	0.0322	0.8798	0.3507	0.0211	0.8458
VesselCycleGAN (w/o seg)	0.3652	0.0158	0.8471	0.3503	0.0227	0.8567
VesselCycleGAN	0.3685	0.0163	0.9534	0.3329	0.0148	0.9419

Tab. 2. Quantitative evaluation for FA synthesis for the HRF test images using the models trained on the CF-FA dataset. For KID, real FAs are from the CF-FA dataset, since there are none in the HRF dataset. Methods with * are trained using registered CF-FA images.

Metrics	Pix2Pix*	VTGAN*	CycleGAN	VesselCycleGAN
KID ↓ (unaligned fake - real FA)	0.0295	0.2010	0.0580	0.0515
Dice ↑ (fake FA - real CF)	0.6943	0.3211	0.2502	0.9439

3   Results

Table 1 summarizes the quantitative results for the CF-to-FA and FA-to-CF task using similarity (LPIPS, KID) and Dice metrics. For the FA synthesis, Pix2Pix obtained the best LPIPS and KID scores, but has only a relatively low Dice score of 0.76. Our VesselCycleGAN achieves a bit lower similarity scores, but the highest Dice score of 0.95 and is superior to VTGAN and the default CycleGAN. For the CF synthesis task, our VessselCycleGAN achieves the best LPIPS, KID, and Dice scores. Pix2Pix here only achieves the second best LPIPS score. For both synthesis tasks, the Dice scores of CycleGAN are very low, indicating that the vessel positions have not been preserved in the synthetic image. Moreover, we tested different settings for our VesselCycleGAN to show the advantage of adding the segmentation loss (gain of up to 10 % Dice score) and by using the UNet-ViT instead of the ResNet9 generator network. The qualitative results in Figure 2 and 3 reflect the findings. The structures in the synthetic images generated by VesselCycleGAN and Pix2Pix demonstrate visual similar structures to the real images. In the vessel segmentation overlays, deviating vessels between the content and generated image are marked in red (missed vessels) and cyan (added vessels). Our VesselCycleGAN has the highest overlap in the vessel structure with the content image. Pix2Pix and VTGAN show some small misalignment in the vessel details, as they learn a direct mapping between the domains from the registered data, which can show some small deformations in the vessel structure. Further, we tested the transferability of the trained models for CF images of the HRF dataset, where no ground truth FA images exist. In Figure 4, the synthetic image of VesselCycleGAN depicts the fine structures, the result of Pix2Pix is a bit blurry, very blurry for CycleGAN while VTGAN was not able to obtain a realistic result. Numerically, the KID between the FA images from the

CF-FA dataset and the generated FA images of the CF HRF images in Table 2, was best for Pix2Pix and second best for VesselCycleGAN. The Dice score for VesselCycleGAN is close the CF-FA dataset, while the competing methods have lower or very low results.

4 Discussion

We relax the unpaired image-to-image translation of multi-modal fundus images to direct mappings from the vessel segmentation to the other modality within the CycleGAN pipeline. Our method, which is trained with unpaired images, learns the modality specific visual patterns and preserves the vessel locations, and thus can be used to augment training data for multi-modal retinal registration methods. As future work, our vessel-based approach could be extended by also including optical disc segmentations and further methods to control the synthesis of pathological structures could be investigated.

References

1. Isola P, Zhu JY, Zhou T, Efros AA. Image-to-image translation with conditional adversarial networks. Proc IEEE CVPR 2017. 2017.
2. Kamran SA, Hossain KF, Tavakkoli A, Zuckerbrod SL, Baker SA. VTGAN: semi-supervised retinal image synthesis and disease prediction using vision transformers. 2021 IEEE/CVF ICCVW. 2021:3228–38.
3. Zhu JY, Park T, Isola P, Efros AA. Unpaired image-to-image translation using cycle-consistent adversarial networks. Proc IEEE ICCV 2017. 2017:2242–51.
4. Li K, Yu L, Wang S, Heng PA. Unsupervised retina image synthesis via disentangled representation learning. SASHIMI 2019. 2019:32–41.
5. Cai Z, Xin J, Wu J, Liu S, Zuo W, Zheng N. Triple multi-scale adversarial learning with self-attention and quality loss for unpaired fundus fluorescein angiography synthesis. IEEE EMBC 2020. 2020:1592–5.
6. Liang N, Yuan L, Wen X, Xu H, Wang J. End-to-end retina image synthesis based on CGAN using class feature loss and improved retinal detail loss. IEEE Access. 2022;10:83125–37.
7. Niu Y, Gu L, Zhao Y, Lu F. Explainable diabetic retinopathy detection and retinal image generation. IEEE J Biomed Health Inform. 2022;26(1):44–55.
8. Torbunov D, Huang Y, Yu H, Huang J, Yoo S, Lin M et al. UVCGAN: UNet vision transformer cycle-consistent GAN for unpaired image-to-image translation. Proc IEEE/CVF WACV 2023. 2023:702–12.
9. Hajeb Mohammad Alipour S, Rabbani H, Akhlaghi MR. Diabetic retinopathy grading by digital curvelet transform. Comput Math Methods Med. 2012;2021:761901.
10. Sindel A, Hohberger B, Maier A, Christlein V. Multi-modal retinal image registration using a keypoint-based vessel structure aligning network. MICCAI 2022. 2022:108–18.
11. Budai A, Bock R, Maier A, Hornegger J, Michelson G. Robust vessel segmentation in fundus images. Int J Biomed Imaging. 2013.

Enhancing Medical Image Segmentation with Anatomy-aware Label Dependency

Francesca De Benetti[1], Robin Frasch[1], Luis F. Rodríguez Venegas[1], Kuangyu Shi[1,2], Nassir Navab[1], Thomas Wendler[1,3]

[1] Chair for Computer Aided Medical Procedures and Augmented Reality, Technical University of Munich, Garching, Germany
[2] Department of Nuclear Medicine, Inselspital, Bern University Hospital, University of Bern, Bern, Switzerland
[3] SurgicEye GmbH & ScintHealth GmbH, Munich, Germany
francesca.de-benetti@tum.de

Abstract. Most Neural Networks for organ segmentation are trained to recognize the appearance of the organ, without considering the location of the organ in the body. However, a medical expert would include in their reasoning also the context around the organ. In this work, we propose reproducing this human behavior by enhancing the conventional multi-class segmentation pipeline with additional anatomical information. We apply this concept to a ventral organ segmentation model having a vertebrae label map as additional input, and to a vertebrae segmentation model enhanced by ventral organ information. In both cases, our proposed label dependency approach improved the performance of the baseline models: the dice score (DS) of the ventral organ segmentation improved by more than 3.5 % and the vertebrae identification rate by 1.8%.

1 Introduction

In recent years, deep learning has been proven to be a powerful tool for segmenting structures in the human body. However, neural networks (NNs) are often trained to recognize the appearance of the organ [1], without considering the context, namely the location of the organ in the body. On the other hand, a medical expert would include in their reasoning also the surroundings and the area of the body under examination. In this work, we propose reproducing this human behavior by introducing anatomical context information in our NN baseline. We tested this approach in two configurations: the first is ventral organ segmentation with vertebrae information as additional input, and the second is vertebrae segmentation with ventral organ information. In this perspective, the conventional multi-class segmentation pipeline can be enhanced with anatomical context information exploiting the relative position of the ventral organs with respect to the vertebral levels [2].

Data fusion consists in merging data from different sources to extract complementary and more accurate information than what would be possible using a single source. In medical applications, the different sources can be different imaging modalities [3] or other types of additional information (such as patient characteristics or history, biomarkers, symptoms, etc.) [4]. Here, label maps of surrounding anatomical structures are fused with the input image to exploit the co-existence of these input labels and the ones to be predicted. Since the dependency is derived from anatomy, we speak of *anatomy-aware label dependency*.

The main contributions of this work are:

1. Introducing complementary label maps as anatomical context for segmenting multiple organs along bigger regions of the body (*label dependency*).
2. Evaluating the impact of anatomy-aware label dependency in two applications and their respective network architectures.
3. Evaluating different data fusion approaches in both applications/architectures.

2 Materials and methods

2.1 Dataset acquisition and preprocessing

We built our dataset combining the VerSe19 and VerSe20 datasets [5] and the CT-ORG dataset [6]. VerSe includes (i) 374 CT volumes, (ii) the 3D coordinates of the vertebral centroids and (iii) the voxel-wise labeling of each vertebra (sacrum excluded) [5]. CT-ORG consists of 140 CT volumes, with voxel-wise annotations of lungs, liver, kidneys, bladder, brain, and bones (the last two being were discarded here) [6]. In both datasets the field of view and the spacing were variable.

To apply this approach, all the used volumes should include annotation of both ventral organs and vertebrae. To achieve this:

1. The publicly available Anduin pipeline [5] was applied to get vertebrae labels and centroids for CT-ORG.
2. A CNN with the CT-ORG data was trained, and used to infer ventral organ labels of VerSe.
3. Both VerSe and CT-ORG were extended by labels for the heart using a 3D UNet-based trained on in-house data [7].

After discarding low-quality volumes, the dataset included 94 volumes with labels of individual vertebrae, lungs, heart, liver, kidneys, and bladder. These masks were finally corrected manually by an experienced reader.

2.2 Configuration 1: ventral organ segmentation with vertebrae labels

2.2.1 Dataset adjustment. In addition to the pre-processing explained above, the sacrum was manually annotated, to provide a reference vertebra for the bladder. After that, the volumes were resampled to [3, 3, 3] mm. This configuration employed a 2.5D network (Section 2.2.2), therefore, one input sample was composed of 3 adjacent CT slices, and the ground truth was composed of the corresponding 3 slices in the ventral organ label map. Samples, where the organ of interests were not visible, were included in the dataset. A careful selection of the patient split ensured that all the vertebrae labels contained in the test set were also in the training set. We applied standard data augmentation techniques (rotation in [-10, 10]°, translation in [-10, 10] pixels, and scaling in [0.95, 1.05]).

The input context anatomy contained information about the shape and label of the vertebra (C1-7, T1-12, L1-5, sacrum), and was encoded in three ways. Encoding 1 (E1) used the original annotation to keep both the shape and label information. In Encoding 2 (E2), the vertebra label were encoded by setting to 1 the corresponding channel in a tensor with 25 channels (with the height and width of the CT slice). The last encoding method (E3) is similar to E2, but in this case, the channel is set to the label value starting from C1 (1) to sacrum (25).

2.2.2 Network architecture. The baseline model was a 2.5D UNet (inspired by [7]) with 5 layers, 3-channels input (3 adjacent slices), and 6-channels output (one per organ).

The early fusion model was the same as the baseline model, but the input CT and the encoded vertebra information (3 adjacent slices) were concatenated and fed to the network as a 6-channels input. In the intermediate fusion model, the two modalities (CT and context label map) are processed by two separate standard-UNet encoders. Then, the two latent spaces were concatenated and fed to a standard-UNet decoder. In the late fusion model, the encoded vertebra information was concatenated with the output of the decoder, and one last convolution layer was added to return the final segmentation.

To deal with the class imbalance, the loss function consisted of a weighted dice loss (wDL), in which dice scores (DS) for the single classes are weighted using inverse-frequency class weighting.

$$\text{wDL} = \sum_{i=1}^{\text{organs}} w_i(1 - DS_i) \tag{1}$$

where w_i is the inverse of the number of voxels of class i in the training dataset. To maintain the interpretability of the DS, the inverse weights are normalized [8].

Each organ was evaluated using the binary DS.

2.3 Configuration 2: vertebrae segmentation with ventral organ labels

2.3.1 Dataset adjustment. All the volumes were resampled to [0.775, 0.775, 1] mm, and the same dataset split ratio at the patient level and data augmentation techniques as in the first configuration were used.

The data fusion was implemented in a 2D network (Section 2.3.2), therefore the information stored in the 3D label map was converted to five 2D images, in one-hot-encoding fashion (i.e. one for each ventral organ - Fig. 1).

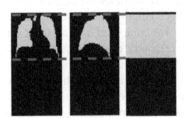

Fig. 1. Configuration 2: ventral organ label encoding (depicted in this case for the label map of the lungs); left coronal view, middle sagittal view, right resulting label encoding for network 2.

2.3.2 Network architecture. The baseline model was the Anduin pipeline [5], which consists of three separate stages (spine detection, vertebrae labeling, and vertebrae segmentation), each of those implemented with a different NN. Among these, the data fusion approach was introduced only in the vertebrae labeling stage because it is the least robust one. The vertebrae labeling stage was based on the Btrfly Net [9], a 2D architecture employing a coronal and a sagittal maximum intensity projection (MIP) of the CT of a spine as inputs. Two encoder branches, one per MIP, were concatenated before the bottleneck. Finally, the two decoder branches returned the outputs, in the form of a pair of 24-class heatmaps (one for each vertebrae from C1 to L5), one for each MIP. The location of the maximum of each of the 24 heatmaps was defined as centroids.

In the early fusion network, we concatenated the 5-channels tensor encoding of the organ information with each of the MIPs, before feeding them to the baseline architecture. In the intermediate fusion model (Fig. 2a), the 5-channels encoded organ information is passed to an additional branch, designed as the two used in the baseline. Its latent space is then concatenated with the other two in the bottleneck of Btrfly Net. For the late fusion model (Fig. 2b), the 5-channel encoded organ information is used as input to an additional network, with one-branch encoder and a two-branches decoder. The outputs of each of the decoder branches are then concatenated with the output of the corresponding branch of the baseline model.

The mean squared error (MSE) between the predicted heatmap and the ground truth was used as loss function. The identification rate (ID) of each vertebra with a 20 mm threshold [9] served as evaluation metric.

	Early	Intermediate	Late
E1	79.1 ± 22.4 %	88.3 ± 8.0 %	75.4 ± 20.1 %
E2	90.2 ± 6.3 %	70.5 ± 22.3 %	89.9 ± 4.3 %
E3	87.7 ± 6.2 %	80.6 ± 19.0 %	90.4 ± 6.0 %

Tab. 1. Configuration 1: DS (mean ± std) with the baseline model and all the combinations of data fusion approaches and encoding modalities.

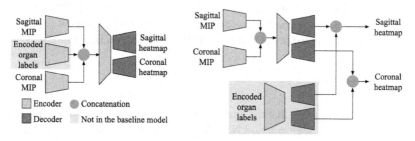

(a) Btrfly Net with intermediate fusion. (b) Btrfly Net with late fusion.

Fig. 2. Configuration 2 - data fusion approaches in the Btrfly Net.

Tab. 2. Configuration 1: DS per organ with the baseline model and the three best combinations of data fusion approach and encoding modality (mean ± std).

Organ	Baseline	Early+E2	Intermediate+E1	Late+E3
Background	99.2 ± 0.6	99.3 ± 0.5	99.4 ± 0.5	99.4 ± 0.5
Liver	78.5 ± 31.6	82.1 ± 31.1	85.9 ± 24.6	*91.4 ± 15.3*
Bladder	79.0 ± 26.8	*85.5 ± 25.9*	79.9 ± 29.6	82.0 ± 30.1
Lungs	82.0 ± 31.5	87.9 ± 26.7	77.4 ± 35.9	*90.4 ± 21.4*
Kidneys	86.8 ± 28.0	88.8 ± 25.4	*89.2 ± 24.7*	84.2 ± 29.9
Heart	94.0 ± 18.9	*97.7 ± 5.0*	96.4 ± 12.0	95.2 ± 16.1

	Early	Intermediate	Late
E1	79.1 ± 22.4 %	*88.3 ± 8.0 %*	75.4 ± 20.1 %
E2	*90.2 ± 6.3 %*	70.5 ± 22.3 %	89.9 ± 4.3 %
E3	87.7 ± 6.2 %	80.6 ± 19.0 %	*90.4 ± 6.0 %*

Tab. 3. Configuration 1: DS (mean ± std) with the baseline model and all the combinations of data fusion approaches and encoding modalities.

Model	ID rate
Baseline	82.3 ± 12.5
Early fusion	**84.1 ± 11.3**
Intermediate fusion	81.3 ± 14.3
Late fusion	82.2 ± 13.4

Tab. 4. Configuration 2: evaluation of vertebrae labelling stage, with and without data fusion, in terms of identification rate (ID) (mean ± std).

3 Results

The 2.5D baseline model in configuration 1 achieved an average DS of 86.6 ± 7.7 %. While our baseline model for configuration 2 (Tab. 4) yielded an ID rate = 82.3 ± 12.5%. In both configurations, the proposed label dependency approach improved the performance of the baseline models: +3.81 % DS in the first configuration (late fusion strategy with the encoding modality E3) and +1.8% ID rate in the second (late fusion).

However, in configuration 1, there is no agreement on which encoding modality is the best performing one (Tab. 3). Depending on the model, choosing the correct encoding modality can improve the performance by up to 15 %. The DS of the best three combinations of data fusion strategy and encoding modality are similar ($\in [88, 90.5]\%$), and this is also reflected in the corresponding detailed organ DS (Tab. 2).

4 Discussion

In this work, we showed that the anatomy-based label dependency is useful to improve the performance of segmentation NNs. We proved this for two configurations, namely the segmentation of heart, lung, liver, kidneys, and bladder using vertebrae information, and also, the vertebrae identification using the same five ventral organs as context anatomy. Interestingly, in both cases, the networks learned the label dependency without supervision, i.e. without explicitly telling it, e.g., that the lungs are normally located between T1 and T12, or that L1 is commonly at the same level as the kidneys. To our knowledge, such an anatomy-based approach has not been presented yet in the literature.

Our evaluations also provide insight into the way of encoding and combining the inputs. In particular, for the 5-organ segmentation (configuration 1), the choice of the encoding modality has a great impact on the performance of the data fusion approach. We can notice that the intermediate fusion model is significantly better when the vertebrae information is only weakly encoded. E3 works best for late fusion as it plays a role as postprocessing masking, while E2 does the opposite.

In the case of configuration 2, the early fusion provided the best results. This may be related to the fact that again the encoding proposed plays a role as preprocessing step which simplifies the learning process.

In contrast to [10], the attention of the network focusses on the location of the organ to be segmented, the proposed network needs additional information (the label map), but is able to handle many organs at the same time, even when they are overlapping.

This work is meant to first analyze the feasibility of using anatomy-based label dependency for multiorgan segmentation. Follow-up studies should include iterative approaches such that no input labels are needed as input, but rather where complementary configurations as the two presented here help each other towards high-performance anatomy-aware segmentation.

Acknowledgement. This work was partially funded by the German Ministry of Education and Research (BMBF, grant BiTSPro 13GW0357 A-C) and the German Research Foundation (DFG, grant NA 620/51-1).

References

1. Salahuddin Z, Woodruff HC, Chatterjee A, Lambin P. Transparency of deep neural networks for medical image analysis: a review of interpretability methods. Comput Biol Med. 2022;140:105111.
2. Cramer G, Darby S. Clinical Anatomy of the Spine, Spinal Cord, and ANS. 2013:1–672.
3. Wang G, Li W, Ourselin S, Vercauteren T. Automatic brain tumor segmentation using cascaded anisotropic convolutional neural networks. International MICCAI brain lesion workshop. Springer. 2017:178–90.
4. Venugopalan J, Tong L, Hassanzadeh HR, Wang MD. Multimodal deep learning models for early detection of alzheimer's disease stage. Sci Rep. 2021;11(1):1–13.
5. Sekuboyina A, Husseini ME, Bayat A, Löffler M, Liebl H, Li H et al. VerSe: a Vertebrae labelling and segmentation benchmark for multi-detector CT images. Med Image Anal. 2021;73:102166.
6. Rister B, Yi D, Shivakumar K, Nobashi T, Rubin DL. CT-ORG, a new dataset for multiple organ segmentation in computed tomography. Sci Data. 2020;7(1):1–9.
7. Çiçek Ö, Abdulkadir A, Lienkamp SS, Brox T, Ronneberger O. 3D U-Net: learning dense volumetric segmentation from sparse annotation. International conference on medical image computing and computer-assisted intervention (MICCAI). Springer. 2016:424–32.
8. Sugino T, Kawase T, Onogi S, Kin T, Saito N, Nakajima Y. Loss weightings for improving imbalanced brain structure segmentation using fully convolutional networks. Healthcare. Vol. 9. (8). MDPI. 2021:938.

9. Sekuboyina A, Rempfler M, Kukačka J, Tetteh G, Valentinitsch A, Kirschke JS et al. Btrfly net: vertebrae labelling with energy-based adversarial learning of local spine prior. International Conference on Medical Image Computing and Computer-Assisted Intervention (MICCAI). Springer. 2018:649–57.

10. Oktay O, Schlemper J, Folgoc LL, Lee M, Heinrich M, Misawa K et al. Attention u-net: learning where to look for the pancreas. arXiv preprint arXiv:1804.03999. 2018.

Double Grad-CAM Guidance for Improved MRI-based Pseudo-CT Synthesis

Gurbandurdy Dovletov[1], Stefan Lörcks[1], Josef Pauli[1], Marcel Gratz[2,3], Harald H. Quick[2,3]

[1]Intelligent Systems Group, Faculty of Engineering, University of Duisburg-Essen, Duisburg, Germany
[2]High-Field and Hybrid MR Imaging, University Hospital Essen, University of Duisburg-Essen, Essen, Germany
[3]Erwin L. Hahn Institute for MR Imaging, University of Duisburg-Essen, Essen, Germany
gurbandurdy.dovletov@uni-due.de

Abstract. Deep learning approaches are capable of learning the mapping function from MR to CT images and thus allow synthesizing pseudo-CTs. However, due to the lack of visual information in the source MRI domain, they often fail to generate bone regions accurately. To address this issue, we propose a double Grad-CAM guidance for U-Net (DGCG U-Net), which indirectly forces the network to focus more on bone structures. More specifically, we first train a Grad-CAM guided classification model in such a way that it distinguishes MR and CT images based solely on bone regions. After that, we utilize this pre-trained classifier and again use Grad-CAM technique to guide our U-Net model by forcing it to focus on bone regions. The performance of the proposed approach is evaluated on the publicly available RIRE data set. The results demonstrate that our model, compared to the baseline GCG U-Net, generates more accurate pseudo-CTs, resulting in approximately 2.5% and 5.1% improvement for MAE and MSE in the bone regions, respectively. The corresponding Grad-CAM guided classifier achieved an accuracy of 99%.

1 Introduction

Computer tomography (CT) has proven to be an essential imaging technique for many medical applications. In addition to high bone-tissue contrast, another principal advantage of CT is that its representation in Hounsfield Units (HU) can be directly mapped to electron densities. Therefore, CT is essential for radiotherapy planning and attenuation correction of positron emission tomography (PET) images. One main limitation, however, is that it introduces unwanted radiation exposure for patients.

With the rise of the deep learning era, one possible solution to overcome this limitation is synthesizing pseudo-CT (pCT) images from radiation-free modalities such as Magnetic Resonance Imaging (MRI) and utilizing them instead. To this end, Han [1] propose to adapt the U-Net [2] in such a way that its encoder part mimics the backbone of the VGG-16 model. Wolterink et al. [3] suggest using a state-of-the-art generative adversarial network (GAN) and its cyclic extension (cycleGAN) to achieve more realistic image synthesis. Although deep learning models can learn a mapping function from the MRI to the CT domain, they still fail to produce bone structures accurately. The main

T. M. Deserno et al. (Hrsg.), *Bildverarbeitung für die Medizin 2023*,
Informatik aktuell, https://doi.org/10.1007/978-3-658-41657-7_13

reason for such inaccuracies is the lack of information in the source domain since no signal from bones can be captured when using standard clinical MRI sequences. To tackle this problem, Leynes et al. [4] propose to capture more bone information by utilizing a Zero-Echo-Time (ZTE) sequence in addition to 2-echo Dixon MRI. Alternatively, Torrado-Carvajal et al. [5] suggest feeding U-Net with four images by explicitly adding fat- and water-only images to two Dixon images. Qi et al. [6] went further and propose using multiple MRI sequences and contrasts (T1, T2, T1C, and T1DixonC-Water) to train U-Net/GAN-based models. The main limitation of the methods in [4–6] is that they require additional image acquisitions and thus introduce additional costs. On the contrary, Dovletov et al. [7] suggest relying on a single MRI image sequence by utilizing additional Grad-CAM [8] guidance to focus their U-Net network on bone regions.

1.1 Contribution

This paper presents an improvement of the Grad-CAM guided U-Net approach from [7]. Our main contribution is the revision, and the subsequent extension of this approach by utilizing the Grad-CAM [8] guidance twice. We demonstrate that using the Grad-CAM for both image classification and image synthesis can reduce errors within bone regions.

2 Materials and methods

This section describes the data set used for the experiments, followed by the details regarding image registration and preprocessing. After that, the proposed approach and the training details are described. Lastly, we outline the utilized evaluation strategy and metrics.

2.1 Data

We assessed the proposed approach on the publicly available RIRE [9] data set with T1-weighted MR and CT head scans for 16 patients. Since images in the data set are not aligned with each other, and the ground truth transformation matrices are not provided, we registered MR and CT volumes using the mutual-information-based multi-resolution algorithm [10]. Because of its higher spatial resolution, the CT image (512×512) was chosen as a fixed modality, while the corresponding MR image (256×256) was deformed and linearly interpolated. We optimized the mutual information using gradient descent and set the learning rate to 0.01. After the registration was complete, we brought all volumes to the homogeneous voxel spacing (in spatial directions) and corrected the difference in the field of view. Lastly, we excluded image slices without valid counterparts and resized them to the resolution of 256×256 pixel. Thus, we utilized 553 2D image pairs in total for our experiments.

2.2 Double grad-CAM guidance

The recently published Grad-CAM guided U-Net (GCG U-Net) [7] approach serves as our entry point to an extended variant, namely the Double Grad-CAM Guided

U-Net (DGCG U-Net), which is proposed in the following. The main idea of the GCG U-Net is to guide the image-to-image translational network (U-Net) using an auxiliary pre-trained classifier and the Grad-CAM [8] technique. Its training procedure consists of two separate steps. First, a Convolutional Neural Network (CNN) is trained to distinguish between MR ($c = 0$) and CT ($c = 1$) images. After that, the knowledge of this classifier is utilized to guide U-Net to generate more accurate pseudo-CTs from the given MR images. Specifically, CT-class-specific ($c = 1$) Heat Maps (HM) for CT and pseudo-CT images are generated by means of the Grad-CAM approach and compared. Thus, these $HM_{pCT}^{c=1}$ and $HM_{CT}^{c=1}$ heat maps serve as an additional indirect similarity measure between the synthesized pseudo-CT and its corresponding ground truth CT image. Although Grad-CAM can provide explanations for CTs classified as "CT"class, the produced heat maps dependent heavily on the internal representation of the CT domain, learned by the classifier. As a result, the corresponding activation maps may be noisy and, therefore, may be distributed along the entire image space. Thus, Grad-CAM on its own cannot guarantee that $HM_{CT}^{c=1}$ heat maps would highlight the bone structures and thus would provide the best desirable guidance for U-Net. To mitigate this, we propose to extend GCG U-Net in such a manner that it utilizes Grad-CAM technique not only during the second stage (training of the U-Net) but also for the first stage when the MR-CT classification model is trained. More specifically, we propose to guide the classifier to focus on critical task-specific regions, such as bone areas. Thus, we set an additional constraint on the Grad-CAM heat maps for CT classifications generated during the training and force them to look similar to the ground truth bone segmentation maps. Our total objective to train the classifier can be formulated as follows

$$\mathcal{L}_{classifier} = \mathcal{L}_{CE} + \lambda_{KL}\mathcal{L}_{KL} \tag{1}$$

where $\mathcal{L}_{CE}$ is the standard cross-entropy (CE) classification term, and $\mathcal{L}_{KL}$ and λ_{KL} are Kullback-Leibler (KL) divergence loss and its weighting factor, correspondingly. We propose to calculate the KL divergence as follows

$$\mathcal{L}_{KL} = \sum_{i=1}^{M'} \sum_{j=1}^{N'} \text{softmax}(Seg)(i,j) \cdot \log \frac{\text{softmax}(Seg)(i,j)}{\text{softmax}(HM_{MR/CT}^{c=1})(i,j)} \tag{2}$$

where $HM_{MR/CT}^{c=1}$ is the Grad-CAM heat map of size $M' \times N'$ for an MR or CT input image classified as "CT"class, and Seg is the desired ground truth (GT) bone segmentation map (of the same size). Since KL divergence measures the similarity between two distributions and thus expects to get distributions as inputs, we propose normalizing both inputs using the softmax function. Thus, while the CE loss term is responsible for correct classifications, the KL loss term ensures that these decisions are made based solely on the bone regions.

2.3 Training

The proposed Double Grad-CAM guided U-Net approach is built similarly to the GCG U-Net in [7]. We set λ_{KL} to 1 while training the Grad-CAM guided MR-CT classification model. The network was trained on input images scaled to the range of

Tab. 1. Results of pseudo-CT synthesis with respect to the entire images. Each metric is reported with its average value ± corresponding standard deviation.

Name	↓ MAE [HU]	Entire Image ↓ MSE [HU^2]	↑ PSNR [dB]	↑ SSIM [%]
U-Net	101±35	69139±27664	24.3±1.9	79.6±6.8
GCG U-Net [7]	96±34	61072±27413	25.0±2.1	80.6±6.7
DGCG U-Net	99±34	62038±27434	24.9±2.1	80.5±6.6

[-1,1] for 25 epochs using the Adam optimizer and L2 regularization with a learning rate set to 0.0001. We increased image appearance variability using data augmentation (±7.5 degrees rotation; scaling with factors in [1; 1.15]; horizontal flipping with 50% chance).

2.4 Evaluation

Four-fold cross-validation is performed for evaluation, with four patients used for testing. We chose to use mean absolute error (MAE), mean squared error (MSE), peak-signal-to-noise ratio (PSNR), and structural similarity index measure (SSIM) as quantitative evaluation metrics. For better analysis and comparison of models, we also calculated MAE and MSE values for head and bone regions only. We generated head masks from MR images using Otsu's thresholding algorithm and (if necessary) manually corrected them. Bone masks, on the contrary, were generated from CT images using a threshold-based segmentation approach with a threshold value set to 350 HU (similar as in [7]). We also calculated the Dice Similarity Coefficient (DSC) between the bone segmentation from pseudo-CT and CT images.

3   Results

The averaged evaluation results are summarized in two tables. Table 1 reflects the performance considering the entire image, while Table 2 represents results for head and

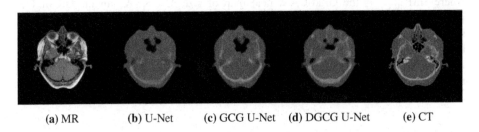

    (a) MR   (b) U-Net   (c) GCG U-Net (d) DGCG U-Net   (e) CT

Fig. 1. Example of pseudo-CT synthesis. (a) Input MR image; (b-d) Synthesized pseudo-CTs from U-Net, Grad-CAM guided U-Net (GCG U-Net), and Double Grad-CAM guided U-Net (DGCG U-Net); (e) Corresponding ground truth CT image. Note the improved synthesis of bone structures from (b) to (d).

Tab. 2. Results of pseudo-CT synthesis with respect to head and bone areas. Each metric is reported with its average value ± corresponding standard deviation.

| Name | Head Area | | Bone Area | | |
	↓ MAE	↓ MSE	↓ MAE	↓ MSE	↑ DSC [%]
U-Net	180±30	131393±38343	595±120	532695±198331	60.2±9.4
GCG U-Net [7]	169±32	116398±35502	477±106	372435±141401	66.7±9.0
DGCG U-Net	176±32	119198±35202	465±98	353391±127713	66.8±8.4

bone areas separately. When comparing MAE and MSE values on the entire images, the proposed approach performed similarly to the baseline GCG U-Net model. The PSNR (24.9±2.1 dB) and SSIM (80.5±6.6 %) values also did not improve or degrade and thus are in the same range. A similar tendency holds for MAE and MSE errors when considering only the head regions. The proposed DGCG U-Net, however, outperformed the baseline GCG U-Net when considering errors in the bone areas. Compared to GCG U-Net's MAE of 477±106 HU and MSE of 372435±141401 HU^2, we report 465±98 HU and 353391±127713 HU^2, respectively. Thus, this corresponds to an error reduction of approximately 2.5% for MAE and 5.1% for MSE. Figure 1 shows pseudo-CT synthesis results for all evaluated models. Regarding the classification performance, the proposed improved Grad-CAM guided classification model achieved an accuracy of 99% compared to 94% reported in [7], which represents 5% gain. For a better comparison of U-Net's guidance (in GCG U-Net and DGCG U-Net), in Figure 2, we visualize ground truth heat maps (for CTs classified as "CT"class) and heat maps for pseudo-CTs synthesized by corresponding U-Nets (also classified as "CT"class).

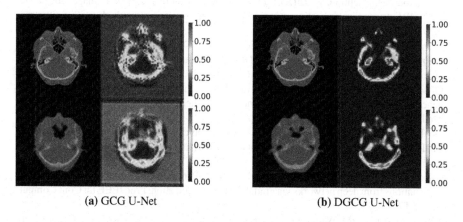

      (a) GCG U-Net   **(b)** DGCG U-Net

Fig. 2. Grad-CAM heat maps ($HM_{CT}^{c=1}$ and $HM_{pCT}^{c=1}$) for ground truth CTs and synthesized pseudo-CTs (both classified as "CT"class) from (a) GCG U-Net and (b) DGCG U-Net. The improved GT heat map in (b) (top image) is tailored towards the bone regions and is less noisy (zeros everywhere except for the bone areas).

4 Discussion

In this work, we present a double Grad-CAM guided U-Net (DGCG U-Net) for MRI-based pseudo-CT synthesis. By comparing the proposed approach to its predecessor (GCG U-Net), we demonstrate that utilizing Grad-CAM for both classification and image synthesis can even further reduce an error for the bone regions. Such improved synthesis of bone structures can be attributed to the superior performance of the classification model and better underlying reasoning (better heat maps) while making classification decisions. We support this conclusion by visually inspecting and comparing the ground truth heat maps (for CTs classified as "CT"class) in Figure 2 (top images). It can be noticed that the utilization of Grad-CAM for the classification model allows producing less noisy heat maps with zeros everywhere except for bone areas. Moreover, these heat maps more accurately cover the bone regions. This led to better guidance of the U-Net while learning to synthesize pseudo-CTs from MR images. Thus, as a result, more accurate pseudo-CTs (Fig. 1) were generated during the inference.

References

1. Han X. MR-based synthetic CT generation using a deep convolutional neural network method. Med Phys. 2017;44(4):1408–19.
2. Ronneberger O, Fischer P, Brox T. U-Net: convolutional networks for biomedical image segmentation. Med Image Comput Comput Assist Interv. Springer. 2015:234–41.
3. Wolterink JM, Dinkla AM, Savenije MH, Seevinck PR, Berg CA van den, Išgum I. Deep MR to CT synthesis using unpaired data. Simul Synth Med Imaging. Springer. 2017:14–23.
4. Leynes AP, Yang J, Wiesinger F, Kaushik SS, Shanbhag DD, Seo Y et al. Zero-echo-time and dixon deep pseudo-CT (ZeDD CT): direct generation of pseudo-CT images for pelvic PET/MRI attenuation correction using deep convolutional neural networks with multiparametric MRI. J Nucl Med. 2018;59(5):852–8.
5. Torrado-Carvajal A, Vera-Olmos J, Izquierdo-Garcia D, Catalano OA, Morales MA, Margolin J et al. Dixon-VIBE deep learning (DIVIDE) pseudo-CT synthesis for pelvis PET/MR attenuation correction. J Nucl Med. 2019;60(3):429–35.
6. Qi M, Li Y, Wu A, Jia Q, Li B, Sun W et al. Multi-sequence MR image-based synthetic CT generation using a generative adversarial network for head and neck MRI-only radiotherapy. Med Phys. 2020;47(4):1880–94.
7. Dovletov G, Pham DD, Lörcks S, Pauli J, Gratz M, Quick HH. Grad-CAM guided U-Net for MRI-based pseudo-CT synthesis. Annu Int Conf IEEE Eng Med Biol Soc. IEEE. 2022:2071–5.
8. Selvaraju RR, Cogswell M, Das A, Vedantam R, Parikh D, Batra D. Grad-cam: visual explanations from deep networks via gradient-based localization. Proc IEEE Int Conf Comput Vis. 2017:618–26.
9. West J, Fitzpatrick JM, Wang MY, Dawant BM, Maurer Jr CR, Kessler RM et al. Comparison and evaluation of retrospective intermodality brain image registration techniques. J Comput Assist Tomogr. 1997;21(4):554–68.
10. Mattes D, Haynor DR, Vesselle H, Lewellen TK, Eubank W. PET-CT image registration in the chest using free-form deformations. IEEE Trans Med Imaging. 2003;22(1):120–8.

Planning of Spherical Volumes for Treating Renal Tumors by Thermal Ablation with Tissue Shrinkage Estimation

Ayman Ahmed[1], Alfred M. Franz[1,2], Hans-Ulrich Kauczor[3], Philippe Pereira[4], Christof M. Sommer[3,5]

[1]Institute for Medical Engineering and Mechatronics, Ulm University of Applied Sciences, Ulm, Germany
[2]Institute for Computer Science, Ulm University of Applied Sciences, Ulm, Germany
[3]Clinic of Diagnostic and Interventional Radiology, Heidelberg University Hospital, Heidelberg, Germany
[4]Clinic for Radiology, Minimally-invasive Therapies and Nuclear Medicine, SLK Kliniken GmbH, Heilbronn, Germany
[5]Clinic for Neuroradiology - Interventional Neuroradiology Unit, Stuttgart Clinics, Katharinenhospital, Stuttgart, Germany
alfred.franz@thu.de

Abstract. Percutaneous thermal ablation techniques represent viable alternatives and minimally-invasive treatment methods for renal tumors. For treating larger tumors, multiple overlapping ablations are imperative. Currently, there is limited software available that incorporates tissue shrinkage into planning for ablation therapy while predicting the lowest number of ablation zones with complete tumor coverage. In this work, a time-power-dependent model to automatically estimate the microwave heating-induced tissue shrinkage is presented. The ablation extent of two commercially available microwave ablation (MWA) systems is modeled as a mathematical function of time and power, too. These models were implemented in a planning software to simulate the process of MWA more realistically and thus, enhance treatment planning. Seven clinical renal T1a, T1b and T2a tumors were tested with and without integrated models, and the proposed ablation plans of which were compared to manual plans of an experienced physician. In the case of built-in models, the software achieved improved planning proposals for all tumors in terms of zone number and total time of ablation.

1 Introduction

In Germany, with 17.336 cases in 2020, kidney cancer is the seventh most frequently diagnosed cancer in men and the tenth in women. While this type of cancer is one of the less common tumors, it is associated with a high mortality rate, accounting for 179.368 deaths worldwide in 2020. [1] Percutaneous ablation technique is an alternative method to treat tumors in addition to the conventional treatment approaches, where the tip of a needle-shaped instrument is punctured through the skin and inserted into the tumor to heat or cool it. The temperature change is concentrated to a focal zone, leading to a complete destruction of the tissue inside the zone. During ablation, tissue undergoes structural modifications in the dielectric and thermal properties, owing to tissue dehydration, protein denaturation and water vaporization. These temperature-dependent modifications induce a change of electromagnetic power deposition and lead

T. M. Deserno et al. (Hrsg.), *Bildverarbeitung für die Medizin 2023*,
Informatik aktuell, https://doi.org/10.1007/978-3-658-41657-7_14

to contraction in the tissue to be ablated. [2] In an ex vivo study, Sommer et al. [3] showed that tissue volumes shrink by 26%-42% during kidney ablation at 90 W for 5-10 min. Beside this study, Rossmann et al. [4] confirmed that relative shrinkage increased with increasing time and power of exposure. Consequently, the dimension of the ablated tissue, evaluated at the end of ablation procedure, could underestimate the actual treated tissue, thus affecting the treatment outcome.

Ablations on larger tumors present greater difficulty since multiple overlapping ablation zones are required. Based on medical imaging, such as computed tomography (CT), interventional radiologists must mentally plan and estimate the ablation procedure outcomes due to limited software available. Franz et al. [5] presented an open-source software tool for a planning approach based on an automatic random calculation of zone distribution for a given tumor considering two uncertainty parameters: tolerance of non-ablated tumor volume and tissue shrinkage. To date, however, there is no adapted model to estimate the concrete shrinkage for specific MWA devices, which can be used directly for the ablation therapy planning.

In this work, a time-power-dependent model to automatically estimate the microwave heating-induced tissue shrinkage is presented. The ablation extent of two commercial MWA systems is modeled as a mathematical function of time and power, too. These models were implemented in the planning software presented by Franz et al. [5] to simulate the process of MWA more realistically and thus, enhance the treatment planning.

2   Materials and methods

2.1   Shrinkage modelling

To estimate the effective ablated zone in the preoperative image and to compensate the underestimation of the pre-treatment dimension from post-treatment visualized zone, a shrinkage model will be necessary. The data used for modelling was obtained from two research groups [6, 7], who characterized the radial tissue shrinkage during the microwave ablation at different time and power settings based on ex vivo bovine liver models (Fig. 1a). Using Matlab Curve Fitting Toolbox, an 8-parameter logistic equation of t [sec] and p [W] was used to model the relative radial (transverse to the antenna) tissue shrinkage ξ [%], which was curve fit to data shown in Fig. 1a and the coefficients of which were determined after least squares fitting

$$\xi(t, p) = \frac{0.1829 + 50.2p}{(1 + \frac{t}{520.3 + 132.4^2 e^{-0.146p}})^{0.01371p - 1.514}} - 0.3421 \tag{1}$$

2.2   Modelling the performance of two MWA systems

Dophi™ M150E (Surgnova, Beijing, China) and Emprint™ (Medtronic, Dublin, Ireland) MWA devices were considered in this work due to their ability to create spherical ablations. Therefore, mathematical functions of time and power were developed for both systems based on manufacturer's data of ex vivo experiments carried out on bovine liver models to predict the radial extent of visualized coagulation in postoperative image. For

Dophi™ and Emprint™, a 5-parameter degree 2 polynomial function and a 7-parameter logistic equation representing the best fit models were used for data fitting, respectively

$$r_{\text{Dophi,vis}}(t, p) = 4.312 + 0.007297t + 0.1p + 1.015 \cdot 10^{-5}t^2 + 6.11 \cdot 10^{-19}tp \quad (2)$$

$$r_{\text{Emprint,vis}}(t, p) = \frac{0.2582p - 154.8}{4.063 + \left(\frac{t}{11.55^2 + e^{-p}}\right)^{0.001693p + 0.7686}} + 36.71 \quad (3)$$

2.3 Radius predictive model

The shrinkage model can be combined with the performance model of each ablation device resulting in a radius predictive model that predicts the actual system performance. Shrinkage of effective zone radius R from visualized one r is calculated assuming that the effective radius is 100%

$$\xi = \left(1 - \frac{r}{R}\right) \cdot 100\% \quad (4)$$

Effective data is calculated according to equation 4. To model the effective performance of Dophi™ and Emprint™, a degree 3 polynomial and a sigmoidal function were curve fit to the data of effective radius, respectively

$$r_{\text{Dophi,eff}}(t, p) = 3.339 - 0.00437t + 0.1864p + 1.961 \cdot 10^{-5}t^2 + 0.00064tp - \\ 0.002p^2 - 1.02 \cdot 10^{-7}t^2p - 4.39 \cdot 10^{-6}tp^2 + 2.218 \cdot 10^{-5}p^3 \quad (5)$$

$$r_{\text{Emprint,eff}}(t, p) = \frac{0.1905p - 58.52}{1 + \left(0.8733 + \frac{t}{33.08^2 + e^{-p}}\right)^{0.044p + 2}} + 34.71 \quad (6)$$

Shrinkage and effective performance models were implemented in the software prototype presented by Franz et al. [5] as functions of time and power to replace the uncertainty parameter of tissue shrinkage and estimate the actual zone radius.

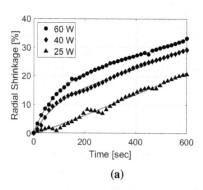
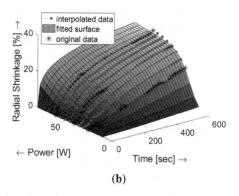

Fig. 1. Mean radial shrinkage at powers 25, 40 and 60 W (a) and shrinkage surface fit passes through original (black stars), as well as interpolated data points (red dots) (b).

3   Experiments

The same CT data of seven renal tumors used by Franz et al. [5] was used in this work to test the influence of built-in models and compare their proposed plans to the old software version based on two experiments:

- Experiment 1: planning of one-sized zones (∅:30 mm).
- Experiment 2: planning of zones with variation in their sizes (∅:30-40 mm). As the software from [5] only supported static ablation zone sizes, we used an extension (version 2021.12-preAlpha, available under `https://osf.io/r7f5d/`) that includes variable zone sizes, but static shrinkage.

For both experiments, the parameters were chosen as follows: safety margin: 5 mm; tolerance of non-ablated tumor volume: 3%; number of iterations: 50-100, depending on runtime. For each tumor in each experiment, five ablation plans were proposed by the software prototype.

4   Results

In the Open Science Framework, an installer of the software prototype with the integrated models is provided (page `https://osf.io/r7f5d/`). The number of ablation zones required and the total ablation time of all zones for the seven renal tumors are shown in Fig. 2. For all tumors in both experiments, the new software version suggested improved ablation plans in terms of number of zones and total ablation time compared to the previous static shrinkage model. Fig. 2b shows reduced zone numbers for both versions due to the variation in zone sizes. For the most cases, Dophi™ system had better performance compared to Emprint™. Manual plans were proposed by an experienced physician assuming a real-world scenario, i.e., ablation zones of different sizes were considered.

In the first experiment (Fig. 2a), ablation devices required 4.53 ± 0.31 (T1a), 8.66 ± 0.36 (T1b) and 16 ± 0.57 (T2a) zones, while last study reported 6.11 ± 0.47 (T1a), 10.77 ± 0.47 (T1b) and 21 ± 1 (T2a) zones. The physician estimated 6.66 ± 1.24 (T1a), 9.66 ± 3.68 (T1b) and 18 ± 0 (T2a) zones. Varying the zone sizes (Fig. 2b) reduces zone numbers by 2.37 ± 0.15 / 4.9 ± 0.02 / 8.7 ± 0.26 and 2.91 ± 0.01 / 3.77 ± 0.16 / 8.4 ± 0.46 zones for devices and static shrinkage model, respectively. A strong positive correlation was found between the continuous variables zone number and total ablation time. The (Bravias-)Pearson correlation coefficient for this relationship was significant 0.99 ($p < 0.05$).

5   Discussion

The uncertainty parameter tissue shrinkage in the software prototype presented by Franz et al. [5] was replaced in this work by a time-power-dependent shrinkage model. For more realistic clinical outcome, the performance of two commercial MWA devices was modeled as a function of time and power. The same seven clinical data sets from [5] were used to test the influence of the integrated models on the planning proposals and resulted in comparable zone numbers to reference plans of a physician within the first experiment (c.f. Fig. 2). Planning of ablations with different sizes using the algorithm with built-in models showed reduced zone numbers and ablation durations for all tumors.

Lee et al. [8] calculated a relative radial tissue shrinkage of 34.87% ± 7.41% at 65 W for an ablation time of 10 min in ex vivo bovine liver models after MWA. A comparable value of 32.3% is achieved using the developed shrinkage model (equation 1). Another research group [9] applied 65 W for 7 min and achieved approx. 30%, a close value to that from our model with small relative error (< 1.3%). Sommer et al. [3] described a similar tissue shrinkage and dehydration caused by MWA, noting an approx. 30% underestimation of effective coagulation in kidneys.

Using Dophi™ device, Habert et al. [10] performed in vivo experiments on swine livers. At lower powers, they achieved comparable results to our model (equation 2). The

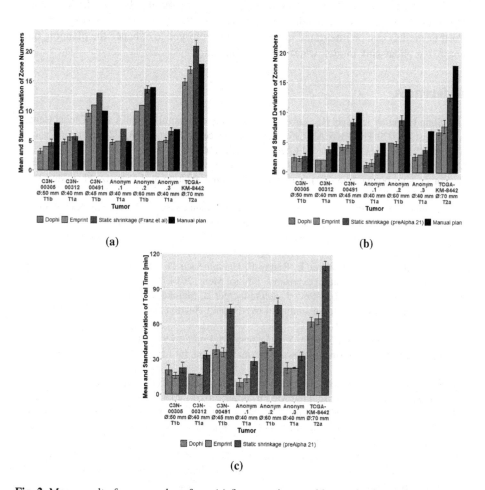

Fig. 2. Mean result of zone numbers from (a) first experiment with one-sized zones (∅:30 mm), (b) second experiment with variation in zone sizes (∅:30-40 mm) and (c) total ablation time from second experiment.

difference can be noticed at higher powers, up to 5 mm difference in radius at 100 W. The reason could be the heat-sink effect, i.e., the presence of blood vessels and perfusion.

However, there were certain limitations to this study. First, the mathematical models were developed based on ex vivo experimental studies and should be demonstrated by clinical in vivo studies. This might lead the developed models to overestimate the actual results when performing in vivo experiments. Second, the MWA devices used to investigate the extent of tissue shrinkage differ from the two systems modelled in this work. Third, the studies from which the experimental data was obtained performed the experiments on dead, non-tumorous liver, not kidney, animal tissues. Only few studies considered the shrinking of kidney tissue and the results of which were not helpful for modelling. It's noteworthy that liver tissue might have different dielectric and thermal properties compared to kidney tissue and thus a different response to microwave heating.

Complementary to this work, a follow-up study is recommended, in which the automated planning proposals from the software are evaluated based on ex vivo experiments. Further models can be integrated in the software prototype to enhance the planning outcome, e.g., heat-sink model, water evaporation, etc.

References

1. Sung H, Ferlay J, Siegel RL, Laversanne M, Soerjomataram I, Jemal A et al. Global Cancer Statistics 2020: GLOBOCAN Estimates of Incidence and Mortality Worldwide for 36 Cancers in 185 Countries. CA Cancer J Clin. 2021;71(3):209–49.
2. Lopresto V, Pinto R, Lovisolo GA, Cavagnaro M. Changes in the dielectric properties of ex vivo bovine liver during microwave thermal ablation at 2.45 GHz. Phys Med Biol. 2012;57(8):2309–27.
3. Sommer CM, Sommer SA, Mokry T, Gockner T, Gnutzmann D, Bellemann N et al. Quantification of tissue shrinkage and dehydration caused by microwave ablation: experimental study in kidneys for the estimation of effective coagulation volume. J Vasc Interv Radiol. 2013;24(8):1241–8.
4. Rossmann C, Garrett-Mayer E, Rattay F, Haemmerich D. Dynamics of tissue shrinkage during ablative temperature exposures. Physiol Meas. 2014;35(1):55–67.
5. Franz AM, Mittmann BJ, Röser J, Schmidberger B, Meinke M, Pereira PL et al. An open-source tool for automated planning of overlapping ablation zones. Proc BVM (2020):328–34.
6. Farina L, Weiss N, Nissenbaum Y, Cavagnaro M, Lopresto V, Pinto R et al. Characterisation of tissue shrinkage during microwave thermal ablation. Int J Hyperthermia. 2014;30(7):419–28.
7. Liu D, Brace CL. Numerical simulation of microwave ablation incorporating tissue contraction based on thermal dose. Phys Med Biol. 2017;62(6):2070–86.
8. Lee J, Rhim H, Lee MW, Kang TW, Song KD, Lee JK. Direction of tissue contraction after microwave ablation: a comparative experimental study in ex vivo bovine liver. Korean J Radiol. 2022;23(1):42–51.
9. Brace CL, Diaz TA, Hinshaw JL, Lee FT. Tissue contraction caused by radiofrequency and microwave ablation: a laboratory study in liver and lung. J Vasc Interv Radiol. 2010;21(8):1280–6.
10. Habert P, Di Bisceglie M, Hak JF, Brige P, Chopinet S, Mancini J et al. Percutaneous lung and liver CT-guided ablation on swine model using microwave ablation to determine ablation size for clinical practice. Int J Hyperthermia. 2021;38(1):1140–8.

Cerebral Vessel Tree Estimation from Non-contrast CT using Deep Learning Methods

Jonas Schauer[1,2], Florian Thamm[1,2], Oliver Taubmann[2], Andreas Maier[1]

[1]Pattern Recognition Lab, Friedrich-Alexander-Universität, Erlangen-Nürnberg, Germany
[2]Computed Tomography, Siemens Healthineers AG, Forchheim, Germany
`oliver.taubmann@siemens-healthineers.com`

Abstract. Non-contrast computed tomography (NCCT) is the primary first-line neuroimaging technique in the clinical workflow for patients with suspected ischemic stroke. We present a deep learning model to estimate the cerebral vessel tree from the NCCT instead of subsequently performed contrast-enhanced imaging techniques, e.g. computed tomography angiography (CTA). We employ a volumetric sliding window approach and feed the patches to a 3D U-Net. This U-Net has two outputs, a probability map that indicates vessel presence and a prediction of the corresponding CTA patch. The CTA regression target is used in addition to the supervised segmentation to optimize the 3D U-Net in a GAN-like manner in order to generate more realistic estimations for the vessel tree. Comparing our proposed model with the current state of the art for this task, a 2D U-Net operating on axial NCCT slices, we were able to slightly increase quantitative overlap metrics as well as achieve notably improved qualitative results w.r.t. spatial continuity of the segmented vessel tree.

1 Introduction

The World Health Organization classifies stroke as the second leading cause of death [1]. A stroke is defined as the damage or loss of brain cells as a result of a lack of oxygen that is caused by an interrupted blood supply of a part of the brain. This interruption can be caused by a blood clot blocking flow in cerebral vessel (ischemic) or by bleeding into the brain tissue (hemorrhagic). Non-contrast computed tomography (NCCT) is typically used to differentiate between these two. In case of an ischemic stroke, adequate treatment requires localization of the thrombus. A typical processing step in automatic detection of such occlusions is the segmentation of the cerebral vasculature, which is commonly performed in contrast-enhanced imaging modalities like computed tomography angiography (CTA). As time is a crucial factor for successful reperfusion a vessel estimation based on NCCT provides faster access to information about the patient's vasculature.

Various segmentation algorithms based on contrast-enhanced imaging techniques exist. For CTA in particular the VirtualDSA++ method of Thamm et al., which is based on a tracking principle using the connectivity in the vasculature, and the fully 3D end-to-end CNN OFF-eNet of Nazir et al. have been proposed [2, 3]. As for non-contrast imaging, Klimont et al. applied a 2D U-Net architecture for head artery segmentation in NCCT slices [4].

© Der/die Autor(en), exklusiv lizenziert an
Springer Fachmedien Wiesbaden GmbH, ein Teil von Springer Nature 2023
T. M. Deserno et al. (Hrsg.), *Bildverarbeitung für die Medizin 2023*,
Informatik aktuell, https://doi.org/10.1007/978-3-658-41657-7_15

In contrast to the slice-wise approach we apply a 3D U-Net that receives volumetric patches instead of slices in order to foster anatomical consistency of the vessels also in axial direction. In addition, an adversarial discriminator is employed to discourage unnatural gaps in the estimated cerebral vessel tree (CVT).

2   Materials and methods

2.1   Data

For the experiments a dataset consisting of the exams of 123 patients is used. For each patient a NCCT and CTA scan of the entire brain region is available. All scans were acquired at a single clinical site using a Somatom Definition AS+ (Siemens Healthineers, Forchheim, Germany). All patients suffered from ischemic strokes, 69% of which constituted large vessel occlusions (LVOs). The CTA scans are aligned to their NCCT counterparts by a nonrigid multimodal registration method [5]. The registered scans in NCCT space have a voxel size of 0.5 mm×0.5 mm×1 mm (x,y,z). All slices have a size of 512×512 voxels with an average of 183.7 slices in axial direction per scan.

A brain segmentation mask is used in order to exclude bone structures in the training process of our model. VirtualDSA++ is applied to the registered CTA to generate the reference segmentation of the cerebral vessel tree. As expected of thin vessel structures, this binary GT segmentation is very sparse; there are more than 150 times more background than vessel voxels. As a further preprocessing step, the HU values of the NCCT and CTA scans were clipped to the range between -100 HU to 300 HU and globally normalized to the range [0, 1].

Volumetric patches of size 64×64×32, hereafter considered as our samples, are extracted with a sliding window technique with an overlap of 12.5% from the complete scans. Besides the translational augmentation introduced by overlapping patches in their generation process, patches are flipped horizontally with a frequency of 50% and rotated around the z-axis with the same probability and a random angle up to 10% in either direction.

2.2   3D U-Net

These patches are then fed into a 3D U-Net with 5 levels [6]. The 2D U-Net as described for the task at hand by Klimont et al. serves as a baseline in our experiments [4]. We obtain a comparable 3D U-Net by replacing the 2D operations of this model with their 3D counterparts. The introduction of a third spatial dimension leads to an increased model capacity. In order to preserve comparability, the number of feature channels for each stage are thus reduced accordingly for the 3D U-Net. This leads to 544 feature channels of size 4×4×2 on the deepest level compared to 1024 channels of size 32×32×1 for the 2D U-Net.

Due to the sparse vessel labels, we choose the generalized dice loss (GDL) as it was shown to outperform other conventional loss functions for comparable tasks with imbalanced classes [7]. GDL introduces the squared reciprocal of the *a-priori* relative frequency as a weight for each class. We calculate the loss $\mathbb{L}_{GDL}(\hat{y}_{Seg}, y_{Seg})$ between a predicted batch $\hat{y}_{Seg} = G_{Seg}(x)$ and its corresponding ground truth labels y_{Seg}.

2.3 Auxiliary discriminator

As an auxiliary component, we investigate the use of an adversarial discriminator that is hypothesized to enhance the connectivity of the estimated vasculature by learning to distinguish between predicted CVTs, which often exhibit unnatural gaps due to lack of contrast, and the reference CVTs. Applying the discriminator directly to the probabilistic segmentation output $\hat{y}_{Seg}$ and the binarized reference leads to mode collapse. Therefore we use an additional model output that is trained to regress the corresponding CTA path in a supervised manner. The predicted CTA $\hat{y}_{CTA} = G_{CTA}(x)$ is obtained by predicting the residual between CTA and NCCT and then adding this prediction to the input NCCT. The residual prediction corresponds to an additional output channel of the 3D U-Net, here referred to as generator G, which receives the NCCT patch x. Due to their similarity, both tasks—segmentation and CTA regression—are expected to benefit from joint training as they share the same U-Net backbone.

We follow a related approach presented by Thamm et al. for domain transfer from CTA to NCCT [8]. In contrast to using a discriminator that outputs a scalar value indicating real or fake, a so-called PatchGAN is implemented [9]. To this end, we use a fully convolutional network that receives CTA patches as input and returns downsampled patches indicating for each voxel whether its neighborhood is likely to be part of a fake CTA (tending to 0) or a real CTA (tending to 1). For optimization of the discriminator D, the MSE loss of the probabilistic discriminator output is computed, denoted as $\mathbb{L}_{Dis}(\hat{y}_{CTA}, y_{CTA})$.

The discriminator loss alone does not result in reasonable performance for transferring the NCCT patch into CTA domain. It has to be stabilized by using an additional supervised CTA regression loss. We applied a supervised L1 loss for this purpose. The proposed model architecture is shown in Fig. 1.

The overall generator loss $\mathbb{L}_G$ for a NCCT patch x and its corresponding ground truth patches for segmentation y_{Seg} and CTA y_{CTA} is given as

$$\mathbb{L}_G(x, y_{Seg}, y_{CTA}) = \mathbb{L}_{GDL}(\hat{y}_{Seg}, y_{Seg}) + \mathbb{L}_{Dis}(\hat{y}_{CTA}, y_{CTA}) + \mathbb{L}_{L1}(\hat{y}_{CTA}, y_{CTA}) \quad (1)$$

2.4 Experimental setup

The dataset is split into training, validation and testing data for the experiments. The test data consists of the scans and segmentations of 13 patients, 11 patients are used for

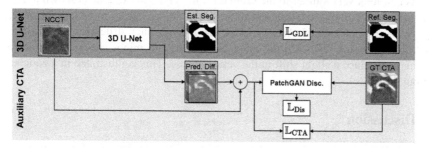

Fig. 1. 3D U-Net with additional discriminator for the auxiliary CTA prediction.

Tab. 1. Quantitative results for examined models.

Model	DSC	clDice
2D U-Net	0.590 (± 0.057)	0.543 (± 0.055)
3D U-Net (plain)	0.601 (± 0.062)	0.573 (± 0.071)
3D U-Net + aux. task	0.603 (± 0.061)	0.577 (± 0.069)

validation and the remaining 99 patients make up the training set. Minibatch stochastic gradient descent is used for optimization of the proposed model. Each batch consists of 16 training samples, which was the maximum feasible size in terms of GPU RAM capacity for the 2D U-Net architecture in our setup. For the sake of comparability the same batch size is used for the 3D U-Net variants. A learning rate of 10^{-4} is chosen heuristically and the parameters are optimized with an Adam optimizer. The number of epochs is limited to 200, but in order to achieve better generalization and to avoid overly long training times, early stopping is used. The segmentation performance is evaluated based on the CVTs reconstructed from the predicted slices/patches. The optimal threshold for the binarization of the probabilistic output is evaluated based on the validation set. As evaluation metrics, both the Dice Similarity Coefficient (DSC) and the centerline Dice Similarity Coefficient (clDice) were used [10].

3 Results

The 2D U-Net by Klimont et al. is used as a baseline for our experiments and is compared to our proposed 3D U-Net and as well as the version with the additional discriminator. The quantitative results are listed in Tab. 1.

From a qualitative point of view the additional third spatial dimension in the model leads to an improved continuity of the vessels across the slices, which is demonstrated by the highlighted areas in Fig. 2. Between the plain 3D U-Net and its extended version the primary observable difference is that there are less unconnected false positives in the background of the predictions. Comparing the predictions to the original ground truth CVTs it seems that the central vessel structures, i.e. Circle of Willis (CoW), are indicated quite well whereas for smaller vessel structures our proposed models do not appear to lead to more reliable results.

Concerning the CTA predicted in the auxiliary task, the extended 3D U-Net yields results that look very similar to the ground truth CTAs. An example is shown in Fig. 3. The majority of relevant arteries near the CoW are visible in most test set patients, e.g. the Anterior Cerebral Artery (arrow "A"). Even finer structures are recognized sporadically (arrow "B"). On the other hand, there are minor checkerboard artifacts that may introduce a slight shift in the vessel course. This is illustrated in a zoomed-in cut-out, Fig. 3 (c).

4 Discussion

The goal of this work was to improve estimation of the CVT from NCCT scans by using a 3D U-Net instead of its 2D variant and extending it with an auxiliary task employing

Fig. 2. Rendering of segmentations predicted by the baseline 2D and the 3D U-Net for a patient from the test set.

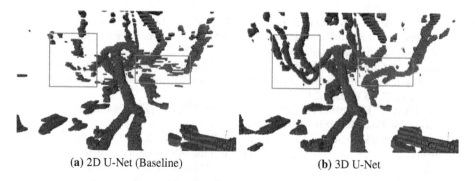

(a) 2D U-Net (Baseline)   (b) 3D U-Net

Fig. 3. Ground truth axial CTA slice in comparison with the slice predicted in the auxiliary task of an discriminator-extended 3D U-Net. On the right is a zoomed-in cut-out of the predicted slice to show the checkerboard artifact.

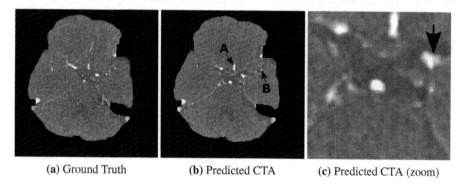

(a) Ground Truth   (b) Predicted CTA   (c) Predicted CTA (zoom)

an adversarial discriminator to obtain results that are more realistic and consistent with the actual anatomy. The plain 3D U-Net achieved a slight quantitative performance increase w.r.t. Dice and clDice metrics, which could just barely be improved upon by the discriminator variant. Qualitatively, however, both proposed models achieved noticeably improved continuity of the CVT (less artificial gaps), with the discriminator also being particularly helpful for reducing small false positive segmentations that are somewhat spatially removed from the larger vessels. On top of that, it enables domain transfer from NCCT to CTA with promising results.

References

1. World Health Organization. Global Health Estimates 2019: deaths by cause, age, sex, by country and by region, 2000-2019. Tech. rep. Geneva, 2020.

2. Thamm F, Jürgens M, Ditt H, Maier A. VirtualDSA++: automated segmentation, vessel labeling, occlusion detection and graph search on CT-Angiography data. The Eurographics Association, 2020.

3. Nazir A, Cheema MN, Sheng B, Li H, Li P, Yang P et al. OFF-eNET: an optimally fused fully end-to-end network for automatic dense volumetric 3D intracranial blood vessels segmentation. IEEE Trans Image Process. 2020;29:7192–202.

4. Klimont M, Oronowicz-Jaśkowiak A, Flieger M, Rzeszutek J, Juszkat R, Jończyk-Potoczna K. Deep learning for cerebral angiography segmentation from non-contrast computed tomography. PLOS ONE. 2020.

5. Chefd'hotel C, Hermosillo G, Faugeras O. Flows of diffeomorphisms for multimodal image registration. Proc IEEE ISBI. 2002:753–6.

6. Çiçek Ö, Abdulkadir A, Lienkamp SS, Brox T, Ronneberger O. 3D U-Net: learning dense volumetric segmentation from sparse annotation. Proc MICCAI. Cham, 2016:424–32.

7. Sudre CH, Li W, Vercauteren T, Ourselin S, Jorge Cardoso M. Generalised dice overlap as a deep learning loss function for highly unbalanced segmentations. Deep Learning in Medical Image Analysis and Multimodal Learning for Clinical Decision Support. Ed. by Cardoso MJ, Arbel T, Carneiro G, Syeda-Mahmood T, Tavares JMR, Moradi M et al. Cham: Springer International Publishing, 2017:240–8.

8. Thamm F, Taubmann O, Denzinger F, Jürgens M, Ditt H, Maier A. SyNCCT: synthetic non-contrast images of the brain from single-energy computed tomography angiography. Proc MICCAI. Cham: Springer International Publishing, 2021:681–90.

9. Isola P, Zhu JY, Zhou T, Efros AA. Image-To-Image Translation With Conditional Adversarial Networks. Proc CVPR IEEE. 2017.

10. Shit S, Paetzold JC, Sekuboyina A, Ezhov I, Unger A, Zhylka A et al. clDice - a novel topology-preserving loss function for tubular structure segmentation. Proc CVPR IEEE. 2021:16560–9.

Abstract: Trainable Joint Bilateral Filters for Enhanced Prediction Stability in Low-dose CT

Fabian Wagner[1], Mareike Thies[1], Felix Denzinger[1,2], Mingxuan Gu[1],
Mayank Patwari[1], Stefan Ploner[1], Noah Maul[1,2], Laura Pfaff[1,2], Yixing Huang[1],
Andreas Maier[1]

[1]Pattern Recognition Lab, Friedrich-Alexander-Universität Erlangen-Nürnberg, Germany
[2]Siemens Healthcare GmbH, Erlangen, Germany
fabian.wagner@fau.de

Low-dose computed tomography (CT) denoising algorithms aim to enable reduced patient dose in routine CT acquisitions while maintaining high image quality. Recently, deep learning (DL)-based methods were introduced, outperforming conventional denoising algorithms on this task due to their high model capacity. However, for the transition of DL-based denoising to clinical practice, these data-driven approaches must generalize robustly beyond the seen training data. We, therefore, propose a hybrid denoising approach consisting of a set of trainable joint bilateral filters (JBFs) combined with a convolutional DL-based denoising network to predict the guidance image. Our proposed denoising pipeline combines the high model capacity enabled by DL-based feature extraction with the reliability of the conventional JBF. The pipeline's ability to generalize is demonstrated by training on abdomen CT scans without metal implants and testing on abdomen scans with metal implants as well as on head CT data. When embedding RED-CNN/QAE, two well-established DL-based denoisers in our pipeline, the denoising performance is improved by 10 %/82 % (RMSE) and 3 %/81 % (PSNR) in regions containing metal and by 6 %/78 % (RMSE) and 2 %/4 % (PSNR) on head CT data, compared to the respective vanilla model. Concluding, the proposed trainable JBFs limit the error bound of deep neural networks to facilitate the applicability of DL-based denoisers in low-dose CT pipelines. We made our trainable bilateral filter layer package (PyTorch, GPU accelerated) publicly available [1, 2].

References

1. Wagner F, Thies M, Denzinger F, Gu M, Patwari M, Ploner S et al. Trainable joint bilateral filters for enhanced prediction stability in low-dose CT. Sci Rep. 2022;12(1):1–9.
2. Wagner F, Thies M, Denzinger F, Gu M, Patwari M, Ploner S et al. Trainable joint bilateral filter layer (PyTorch). https://github.com/faebstn96/trainable-joint-bilateral-filter-source. Accessed: 9 Dec 2022.

Improved Tractography by Means of DL-based DWI Image Enhancement

Marc Balle Sánchez[1], Maria Ávila González[1], Francesca De Benetti[1],
Aldana Lizarraga[2], Igor Yakushev[2], Nassir Navab[1], Thomas Wendler[1,3]

[1]Chair for Computer Aided Medical Procedures and Augmented Reality, Technical University of Munich, Garching, Germany
[2]Department of Nuclear Medicine, Klinikum Recths der Isar, Munich, Germany
[3]SurgicEye GmbH & ScintHealth GmbH, Munich, Germany
aldana.lizarraga@tum.de

Abstract. Diffusion weighted imaging (DWI)-based tractography estimates white matter (WM) fibers in the living brain. This tool enables studying brain connectivity between brain regions and planning operations on the brain. XTRACT is a recently developed program for automatically delineating 42 major WM tracts in high-quality DWI data. However, acquiring such data is time-consuming, limiting its clinical application. In this work, we propose using a deep neural network to enhance low-quality DWI data, representative of clinical imaging protocols. We hypothesized that such image enhancement would lead to a substantially more accurate tractography with XTRACT. Our results show that the method increases the correlation of tracts extracted from a clinical dataset with the ones extracted from a high-quality one from 64% to 83%. Clinically, this implies that both more tracts are detected and that the details of detected tracts are higher.

1 Introduction

Tractography is defined as the 3D virtual reconstruction of white matter (WM) tracts of the brain using data collected by diffusion weighted imaging (DWI). DWI is a Magnetic Resonance Imaging (MRI) technique sensitive to the random motion of water molecules. In WM, this motion occurs preferentially along the axons, due to the presence of cell membranes and myelin sheaths that restrict the movement across them. This makes DWI a popular imaging technique for non-invasive estimation of the WM fiber orientation. Tractography is routinely used, e.g., in surgical planning of tumor resection and studies of brain connectivity [1]. The signal measured in DWI depends on two main acquisition parameters of the image: (i) The b-value indicates how strong the diffusion-weighted images are and relates to the intensity and duration of the diffusion gradients. (ii) The b-vectors correspond to the directions in which the diffusion gradients are applied. To characterize the diffusion in each voxel, several mathematical models can be used, from the simplest, diffusion tensor imaging (DTI), to more complex models like "Balls and Sticks" which requires more diffusion data [2].

In conventional tractography, an expert defines a starting and ending points of a tract. This requires previous anatomical knowledge and is extremely time-consuming, making it almost unfeasible for clinical practice. Thus, efforts have been made to develop automatic tractography methods. To that end, the FMRIB Software Library (FSL) released the XTRACT [3] tool in March 2020. This command line tool automatizes tractography protocols for 42 major WM tracts. So far, however, XTRACT has only been tested on two high-quality datasets, namely, the Human Connectome Project [4], and the UK Biobank [5]. These databases are not representative of the clinical DWI data.

Recent studies tried to improve the quality of tractography outcomes by removing noise present DWI images. Cheng et al. [6] used a 1D-convolutional neural network (CNN) to reduce the rectified noise floor. This can derive from modern imaging techniques like parallel imaging and simultaneous multi-slice acquisition (SMS) where images with a low signal-to-noise ratio (SNR) are obtained. Similarly, Sagawa et al. [7] proposed a deep learning (DL)-based reconstruction approach to denoise DWI images obtained using SMS technology. An alternative to image denoising is directly inferring diffusion metric maps and fiber tractography using DL approaches, thus skipping the model fitting step [8]. Yet, the performance of the latter method is not sufficient for clinical use. Following the work of Tian et al. [9], we propose using a multi-channel 3D-CNN to increase the quality of a clinical dataset and thus improve XTRACT tractography.

The main contributions of this work are:

1. We propose a method to convert high-quality DWI images to low-quality ones resulting from a clinical image acquisition protocol and thus generate paired images for denoising methods.
2. We introduce a multiple-channel 3D-CNN for DWI image enhancement trained with the generated low-quality images and high-quality images as ground truth.
3. We investigate the contribution of adding high-level information, namely the b-vectors to the image enhancement network.
4. We analyze the proposed architectures in terms of image enhancement metrics, as well as, the quality improvement of the extracted tracts using XTRACT.

2 Materials and methods

2.1 Dataset description

2.1.1 The HCP dataset. The Human Connectome Project (HCP) dataset includes 100 subjects (age 28.6 ± 3.7 years). It was a multi-shell dataset containing three different b-values per subject: 1000, 2000 and 3000 s/mm^2. For each b-value, it contained 90 b-vectors, each of those resulting in a 3D volume, as well as 18 B0 images. In a B0 image, no diffusion gradients are applied. Besides diffusion data, each subject presents T1 and T2 images.

2.1.2 The in-house dataset. It includes 59 subjects (age 61.1 ± 4.09 years). It is a single shell dataset with a single b-value of 800 s/mm^2, 30 b-vectors, and one B0 image per subject. Each subject has also T1 and T2 images.

2.2 Image enhancement with a CNN

2.2.1 Dataset preparation. For noise reduction, we propose using a supervised CNN model trained on the HCP high-quality data (ground truth) and synthetically degraded images resembling clinical ones. Here, the degraded input data was targeted to be as similar as possible to our in-house data. In all input and ground truth images the skull was removed using BET [10].

To generate the low-quality input images, first, we chose the closest HCP b-value to our in-house dataset (1000 s/mm^2). In the same way, we picked the 30 closest HCP b-vectors using the Hungarian algorithm. The B0 (ground truth) image was obtained by averaging the 18 B0 present in the HCP dataset.

Since the b-vectors of the HCP and the clinical dataset do not match, we created a high-quality ground truth dataset. For those means, we fit the "Ball and Sticks" diffusion model using the original HCP amount of data (18 B0 and 90 DWI volumes). Once the model parameters were known, we synthetically generated DWI volumes using a b-value of 1000 s/mm^2 and the same b-vectors as the input.

2.2.2 Network architecture. We used a CNN model consisting of 10 layers of 3D convolution, batch normalization, and ReLU as activation function. We trained the model using a learning rate of 10^{-4}, an ADAM optimizer, and computing the L2 loss.

Two different models with the same architecture were trained for B0 images and DWI images. We used patches of size $64 \times 64 \times 64$ voxels. Each B0 and DWI patch was concatenated with the corresponding T1 and T2 patches.

Following the approach of Tian et al. [9], the model's output was defined to be the residuals between the input and the ground truth. Therefore, the final predicted images were obtained by subtracting the predicted residuals from the input.

We also trained an additional DWI model, incorporating the information from b-vectors. These 3D vectors were processed by a fully connected layer and concatenated to the feature map in the bottleneck of the CNN.

2.2.3 Training set-up. The data was split into 80% training, 20% validation and 20% testing. To determine the impact of the inclusion of the b-vectors in training, we performed a 5-fold cross-validation with and without the b-vectors.

2.2.4 Evaluation metric. To assess the quality of the predicted images we used the Structural Similarity Index Measure (SSIM) and the Peak Signal-to-Noise Ratio (PSNR). We also conducted a paired t-test to assess the statistical difference when incorporating the b-vectors.

2.3 XTRACT analysis

The main input for XTRACT is the difussion information resulting from the Ball and Sticks model. The main output is a NIfTI file for each tract containing the fiber probability distribution normalized by the total number of valid streamlines (Fig. 2).

Tab. 1. SSIM and PSNR values for the cross-validation of the models with and without b-vectors. The values correspond to the validation group. In brackets are shown the metric values between the input and the ground truth.

Fold	With b-vectors		Without b-vectors	
	SSIM [input]	PSNR [input]	SSIM [input]	PNSR [input]
1	0.9639 [0.9083]	33.1270 [29.8635]	0.9646 [0.9093]	33.3667 [30.0302]
2	0.9612 [0.9050]	32.6435 [29.6742]	0.9615 [0.9052]	32.9813 [29.8477]
3	0.9646 [0.9065]	33.4785 [29.9439]	0.9644 [0.9065]	33.2410 [29.9440]
4	0.9636 [0.9040]	33.3631 [29.9563]	0.9646 [0.9054]	33.7814 [30.1910]
5	0.9644 [0.9070]	32.8430 [29.6764]	0.9650 [0.9084]	33.3040 [29.9268]

2.3.1 Data preprocessing. Prior to run XTRACT, the Ball and Sticks diffusion model is fitted using Bedpostx [2] and a transformation from the standardized "MNI" (Montreal Neurological Institute) space to each subject space is calculated.

2.3.2 Atlas generation. To perform a comparison between results, an atlas must be generated for each group of data (HCP and in-house). To obtain these atlases, we followed the method proposed in Warrington et al. [3]. Thus, the subject-specific MNI-transformed tracts were normalized in the range [0, 1], binarized at a threshold of 0.001, and subsequently averaged across subjects.

2.4 Evaluation

Since the aim of this work is to improve the tractography, we evaluated the performance of our CNN by comparing the tracts that can be extracted from the ground-truth data with the ones extracted from the predicted data with the following metrics:

- We computed the Pearson's correlation (r) between each tract in the HCP atlas and the corresponding tract in the predicted noise-free in-house data.
- We compared the volumes of the tracts in both atlases.
- We evaluated the within-subject correlation (test/retest reproducibility) by computing the Pearson's correlation between the tracts extracted from images of the same patients. This was possible only for the 10 patients with two consecutive DWI scans.

All these steps were performed using the predicted images from the CNN with and without b-vectors.

3 Results

3.1 Image enhancement with CNN

Tab. 1 shows the values of the SSIM and PSNR for the validation group for all five folds with and without b-vectors. The models which do not incorporate b-vectors yielded better metric values, which was significant however only for the PNSR.

3.2 XTRACT

Fig. 1a shows the comparison between the correlation of the tracts of noisy and denoised images with HCP. The average correlation across tracts from the HCP and non-enhanced images was 0.6402 ± 0.2239, while the enhanced images 0.8324 ± 0.0528 using b-vectors and 0.8398 ± 0.0502 without them. The difference in correlation with HCP dataset from both configurations is significant (Wilcoxon test).

Regarding the volume of the tract atlases obtained, we observed that the tracts of the HCP atlas tend to be bigger than our atlas. Nonetheless, and following the trend of the correlation outcomes, this difference is $\approx 30\%$ smaller when the images are denoised.

To assess the reproducibility of XTRACT, we measured the within-subject correlation of ten subjects with two consecutive scans. For this, ten subjects, the reproducibility of XTRACT was significantly better (Wilcoxon test) in the original images with an average correlation across tracts of 0.6093 ± 0.2553 against 0.5140 ± 0.2213 of the enhanced images with b-vectors and 0.4987 ± 0.2213 without them.

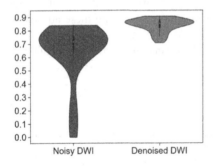 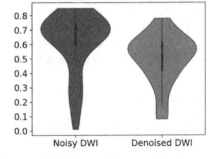

(a) Correlation with HCP atlas. (b) Within subject correlation (test-retest).

Fig. 1. Analysis performed to validate XTRACT in low quality and denoised data. Denoised DWI were obtained with the proposed NN and without b-vectors.

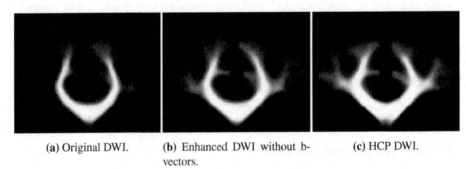

(a) Original DWI. (b) Enhanced DWI without b-vectors. (c) HCP DWI.

Fig. 2. The *fmi* tract atlas computed by XTRACT. The intensity value of a voxel is proportional to the number of streamlines crossing the voxel. With the original DWI, XTRACT is capable to detect only the main part of the tract, losing track of secondary branches.

4 Discussion

In this paper, we explored the possibility of improving tractography results from XTRACT by removing noise present in clinical DWI using a multi-channel 3D-CNN. Our results show that DL-based image enhancement increases the correlation of tracts extracted from a clinical dataset with the ones extracted from a high-quality one from 64% to 83%. Clinically, this implies that both more tracts are detected, and that the details of detected tracks are higher, which contributes to the clinical feasibility of XTRACT. We also tested XTRACT in terms of reproducibility using 10 subjects with two DWI consecutive scans. Denoised images did not improve reproducibility. We think that this could be due to a more detailed delineation of the tracts in the enhanced images, which leads to higher variability in the fine-grained details between scans. We also explored the impact of adding meta-information on the DWI in the training process, namely the b-vectors which did not yield any significant improvement. However, we believe that further work on evaluating different ways of fusing the b-vectors or processing them before adding them into the CNN can lead to a better performance of the model.

References

1. Sammartino F, Krishna V, King NKK, Lozano AM, Schwartz ML, Huang Y et al. Tractography-based ventral intermediate nucleus targeting: novel methodology and intra-operative validation. Movement Disord. 2016;31(8).
2. Behrens TE, Berg HJ, Jbabdi S, Rushworth MF, Woolrich MW. Probabilistic diffusion tractography with multiple fibre orientations: what can we gain? Neuroimage. 2007;34(1).
3. Warrington S, Bryant KL, Khrapitchev AA, Sallet J, Charquero-Ballester M, Douaud G et al. XTRACT-Standardised protocols for automated tractography in the human and macaque brain. Neuroimage. 2020;217.
4. Van Essen DC, Smith SM, Barch DM, Behrens TE, Yacoub E, Ugurbil K et al. The WU-Minn human connectome project: an overview. Neuroimage. 2013;80.
5. Miller KL, Alfaro-Almagro F, Bangerter NK, Thomas DL, Yacoub E, Xu J et al. Multi-modal population brain imaging in the UK Biobank prospective epidemiological study. Nat Neurosci. 2016;19(11).
6. Cheng H, Vinci-Booher S, Wang J, Caron B, Wen Q, Newman S et al. Denoising diffusion weighted imaging data using convolutional neural networks. bioRxiv. 2022.
7. Sagawa H, Fushimi Y, Nakajima S, Fujimoto K, Miyake KK, Numamoto H et al. Deep learning-based noise reduction for fast volume diffusion tensor imaging: assessing the noise reduction effect and reliability of diffusion metrics. Magn Reson Med Sci. 2021;20(4).
8. Li H, Liang Z, Zhang C, Liu R, Li J, Zhang W et al. SuperDTI: ultrafast DTI and fiber tractography with deep learning. Magn Reson Med. 2021;86(6).
9. Tian Q, Bilgic B, Fan Q, Liao C, Ngamsombat C, Hu Y et al. DeepDTI: high-fidelity six-direction diffusion tensor imaging using deep learning. Neuroimage. 2020;219.
10. Smith SM. Fast robust automated brain extraction. Hum Brain Mapp. 2002;17(3).

Deep Learning Approaches for Contrast Removal from Contrast-enhanced CT

Streamlining Personalized Internal Dosimetry

Marcel Ganß[1], Francesca De Benetti[1], Julia Brosch-Lenz[2], Carlos Uribe[3,4,5], Kuangyu Shi[1,6], Matthias Eiber[2], Nassir Navab[1], Thomas Wendler[1,7]

[1]Chair for Computer Aided Medical Procedures and Augmented Reality, Technical University Munich, Garching, Germany
[2]Department of Nuclear Medicine, Technical University of Munich, Germany
[3]Department of Integrative Oncology, BC Cancer Research Institute, Vancouver, BC, Canada
[4]Department of Radiology, University of British Columbia, Vancouver, BC, Canada
[5]Department of Functional Imaging, BC Cancer Research Institute, Vancouver, BC, Canada
[6]Department of Nuclear Medicine, Inselspital, Bern University Hospital, University of Bern, Bern, Switzerland
[7]SurgicEye GmbH & ScintHealth GmbH, Munich, Germany
marcel.ganss@tum.de

Abstract. In internal radiation therapy, dosimetry is essential to predict its efficacy and potential side effects. Contrast enhanced computed tomography (ceCT) is most commonly used as starting point for planning. However, native CT (nCT) is required for accurate dosimetry computations. In this work, we propose an in-silico method to remove the contrast agent from ceCT images so that the Hounsfield Units (HU) would be similar to those in nCT. Two approaches, one paired-image neural network (NN) and one un-paired NN, were applied to ceCT/nCT image pairs for contrast removal. We evaluated their performance in terms of HU values, and performed dosimetry calculations on the original nCT and ceCT, and on the in-silico nCTs to evaluate the impact on the dose rate. The two approaches yielded good results both in terms of HU reduction (more than 30%) and in the difference of dose rate against the original nCT (less than 1.38% vs. 4.76%).

1 Introduction

The use of internal radiation therapy is becoming increasingly more important in the treatment of different cancers. Yet its full potential is rolled out when personalized dosimetry calculations are used to optimize it. One of the requirements for dosimetry is the availability of native CT images (nCT), due to the correlation of its Hounsfield Units (HU) with the density and the chemical composition of the tissue. However, CTs with contrast enhancement (ceCT) are acquired in the clinical routine as starting point of therapy planning. With the injection of iodinated contrast agent, the contrast in soft tissues is increased to enable to answer diagnostics questions, but this increases the HU of soft tissue and thus hinders the ability to use the images for dosimetry. We propose to use image-to-image translation to remove the contrast agent in ceCT images in-silico, so that the dosimetry calculations can be performed without an additional nCT. This reduces the radiation burden and simplifies the clinical workflow.

© Der/die Autor(en), exklusiv lizenziert an
Springer Fachmedien Wiesbaden GmbH, ein Teil von Springer Nature 2023
T. M. Deserno et al. (Hrsg.), *Bildverarbeitung für die Medizin 2023*,
Informatik aktuell, https://doi.org/10.1007/978-3-658-41657-7_18

Image-to-image translation approaches for similar tasks were used by Liugang et al. [1] and Jakubicek et al. [2], who trained a supervised 2D U-Net based on a registered set of non-public ceCT and Virtual-Non-Contrast CT image pairs. Jakubicek et al. used also a conditional generative adversarial network (GAN). Song et al. [3] and Sandfort et al. [4] proposed a 2D CycleGAN optimization pipeline to translate ceCT to nCT for data augmentation purposes. Yet, none of these works compared the performance of paired and non-paired approaches, nor quantified their impact on internal dosimetry.

The main contributions of this work are:

1. Proposing and evaluating two image-to-image translation networks from ceCT to nCT in 3D, namely a paired (supervised) and an unpaired (unsupervised) approach.
2. Analysing the proposed approaches in terms of HU and also its relative importance in terms of absorbed dose for internal dosimetry.

2 Materials and methods

2.1 Dataset description

We retrospectively analyzed paired ceCT/nCT of patients treated at Klinikum Rechts der Isar (Munich) using SIRT (selective internal radiation therapy of the liver using ^{90}Y-spheres) and ^{177}Lu-PSMA (prostate-specific membrane antigen) radioligand therapy.

The SIRT dataset consists of 35 patients (33-86y) with different liver malignancies treated with ^{90}Y microspheres. Each patient has a ^{99m}Tc-MAA SPECT/CT that was acquired for planning the SIRT. Its CT was native and low-dose with 2.5 mm slice thickness and pixel spacing of 0.74-0.98 mm in x and y. In addition, a high-dose ceCT was acquired to perform therapy planning, with 0.9 to 5 mm slice thickness and voxel spacing of 0.68-1.52 mm in x and y. The field of view is variable, with the upper abdomen always included in the images.

The PSMA dataset includes 19 patients (59-77y), treated with ^{177}Lu-PSMA-I&T. Each patient had at least one full-body high-dose ceCT and 2 to 5 low-dose nCTs. The field of view is variable, with the thorax and abdomen always contained in it. In total, the PSMA dataset consisted of 23 ceCT and 65 nCT volumes, with pixel spacing <1 mm in x and y and 1.2-5 mm slice thickness.

In both datasets the ceCT and nCT were acquired in two different imaging sessions (with a 7-10 days interval).

2.2 Preprocessing

We used SimpleITK to set up a registration pipeline, consisting of an initialization using the center of mass and at most 100 rigid and 20 deformable transformation (B-spline) iterations using mean squared error (MSE) as similarity metric. Then we cropped the intersection of both images, to get two equally sized images with the same field of view. We included in our paired dataset 7 SIRT and 19 PSMA patients, which had good results in the registration at visual inspection by an expert reviewer.

For all the volumes in the dataset, we generated the masks of liver, spleen, kidneys, aorta, and esophagus ("target organs") using a version of nnUNet [5] which was pre-trained on the Multi-Atlas Labeling Beyond the Cranial Vault dataset. The label maps were then manually corrected by an expert reviewer.

All volumes were resampled to an isotropic spacing of 2 mm. In the CTs, the HU values were clamped to $[-511, 512]$ and then normalized to $[0, 1]$. We applied data augmentation (translation in $[0, 32]$ voxels and rotation in $[0, 180]°$).

2.3 Networks architectures

We implemented a paired NN ("Paired Network", PN) and an un-paired one ("Cycle-GAN", cGAN), which were built combining generator and discriminator models. The generator model is a 3D U-Net [6] with 4 layers and sigmoid as final activation. The architecture of the discriminator is the same as the encoder of the generator architecture, followed by a 3D average pooling layer and a flatten operation to a 1D vector.

2.4 Training pipeline

A 5-fold cross-validation (5f-CV) was set up with the 26 paired patients. It was used in all the steps of the training pipeline. At each epoch one patch of size $(128,64,128)$ voxels is randomly extracted from the input CT. During inference the patches were extracted following a grid, to ensure all the regions in the body were included.

Image Context Restoration approach [7] was used as unsupervised pre-training strategy, to learn semantic knowledge about the human anatomy and to bootstrap the learning process of the image translation task. The generator network was trained to correct $N = 32$ swapped cubes of size $(16,16,16)$ voxels, which were randomly selected in each input image at each training iteration. We trained each fold of our 5f-CV set-up for 1500 epochs. The pre-trained weights were used to initialize the generators (PN and cGAN), while the pre-trained encoder was used to initialize the cGAN discriminator.

2.4.1 Training: paired network. The PN consisted of one generator network, which predicted nCT from ceCT. It was trained on registered images only with the 5f-CV, for at most 150 epochs. We defined a joint loss, which required a ground truth (GT) image Y_i, a predicted image $\hat{Y}_i$ and their masked versions using the label map previously defined (S_i and $\hat{S}_i$) for each organ i

$$\mathcal{L}_{\text{PN}}(\hat{Y}_i, Y_i) = \alpha * L2(\hat{S}_i, S_i) + \beta * L2(\hat{Y}_i, Y_i) \tag{1}$$

where $\alpha = 0.9$ and $\beta = 0.1$ were selected empirically. $\mathcal{L}_{\text{PN}}$ encourages the network to focus on the segmented areas, while learning useful information about the surroundings.

2.4.2 Training: CycleGAN. The cGAN pipeline [8] included two generator (ceCT $\mapsto$ nCT and nCT $\mapsto$ ceCT) and two discriminator networks. The cGAN was trained with the 5f-CV set-up plus 19 ceCT and 18 nCT, which were not included in the paired dataset. We used MSE as the adversarial loss, L1 as cycle-consistency and identity losses, and MSE as discrimination loss with an equal weighting of GAN-generated and real images.

2.4.3 Inference. All predicted patches were aggregated to avoid artifacts due to over-lapping. The prediction domain was mapped back to the HU range $[-511, 512]$.

2.5 Dosimetry

We simulated the 3D dose rate map with the GATE Monte Carlo simulation platform for medical physics simulation [9]. The inputs of the calculations were the PET (PSMA patients) or the SPECT (SIRT patients) to define the source, and one CT scan to define the geometry. Each voxel in the geometry was assigned to a density and chemical composition using conventional approaches [10]. We simulated a ^{90}Y source with the built-in ion source of GATE and 10^8 primaries. We computed the dose rate in six patients (3x PSMA, 3x SIRT). For each, we ran four dosimetry simulations, one per CT type (namely: original nCT, original ceCT, cGAN-nCT and PN-nCT). The total organ dose was computed for liver, spleen, left and right kidneys (separately) and aorta, using the label map of the original ceCT. Even though the dose in the aorta is not relevant from a dosimetric perspective, it was interesting to test our contrast removal approach in pure blood areas containing high amounts of contrast media.

3 Results

The registration method was evaluated by computing the Dice Score (DS) between corresponding organs in nCT and ceCT. Relatively flexible organs, such as the aorta and the esophagus, had a DS of 0.77 ± 0.18 and 0.50 ± 0.21, respectively. Whereas it was 0.91 ± 0.04 for the liver, 0.82 ± 0.10 for the spleen and 0.82 ± 0.12 for the kidneys.

We evaluated the HU reduction computing the L2 difference between the HU ($RMSE_{HU}$) of original nCT, and the HU of the PN-nCT or the cGAN-nCT in all 26 image pairs (Fig. 2). The HU predicted by the PN are more similar to the HU of the original nCT (6.52 ± 0.87 HU), than those from cGAN (7.82 ± 0.99 HU). Indeed, the reduction of $RMSE_{HU}$ in the PN is 45.16%, whereas it is 34.32% in the cGAN. The initial $RMSE_{HU}$, defined as the RMSE between the original nCT and the original ceCT, was 11.89 ± 2.65 HU.

We further compared the Cumulative Distribution Functions of the HU values (CDF_{HU}) of the predicted nCTs and the original nCT/ceCT (Fig. 3). The CDF is defined

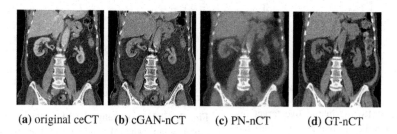

(a) original ceCT   (b) cGAN-nCT   (c) PN-nCT   (d) GT-nCT

Fig. 1. Comparison of (a) original ceCT, (b) cGAN prediction (cGAN-nCT), (c) Paired network prediction (PN-nCT), and (d) original nCT (GT-nCT); patient of the PSMA dataset.

as the probability a HU value of the image x is below T: $P(x < T)$. Both networks are able to approximate the CDF of the original nCT, however the higher HU intensities (i.e., the bones) are slightly overreduced.

We evaluated the dose rate per organ in terms of percentage difference against the dose rate calculated based on the original nCT. The average percentage dose difference (PD) in the 6 patients in the five organ of interest is: $PD_{ceCT} = 4.76$ % (range: [3.49, 5.51]%), whereas it drops to $PD_{cGAN} = 0.83\%$ (range: [-0.31, 1.95]%) and $PD_{PN} = 1.38\%$ (range: [-0.03, 2.02]%). The largest reduction in the dose, defined as $|PD_i - PD_{ceCT}|$, is in the aorta for cGAN-nCT: 4.75%. The difference between PD_{cGAN} and PD_{ceCT} is stastistically significant (p<0.01), as well as, between PD_{PN} and PD_{ceCT}.

4   Discussion

We propose two in-silico approaches for contrast removal of ceCTs in internal dosimetry. To the best of our knowledge this is the first paper addressing this problem in 3D and evaluating it quantitatively in terms of HU and change in deposited dose. Both image-to-image translation approaches are able to improve the input images in terms of HU reduction (more than 30%), as well as, minimization of PD (less than 1.38% vs. 4.76%) given GT images for five organs of interest in radioisotope therapies.

Converting ceCT to nCT may also be of interest in the field of attenuation correction in PET and SPECT also towards dose-reduction. An evaluation of our approaches for that application are out of the scope of this work, but is worth evaluating in future.

Since nCT and ceCT cannot be acquired simultaneously, the registration procedure was indispensable to generate a paired dataset for the PN training and to gain quantitative evaluation criteria. However, registration of different CT modalities (low/high dose, nCT/ceCT) is non-trivial and even small registration errors may lead to errors in the ground truth. The same problem arises in the PN were results tend to be blurry. Moreover,

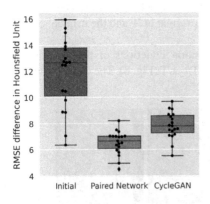

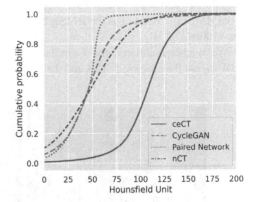

Fig. 2. RMSE$_{HU}$ in the five target organs when the original nCT is compared with the original ceCT (left), the PN-nCT (middle) and cGAN-nCT (right).

Fig. 3. CDF$_{HU}$ in range [0,200] HU in the five target organs when the original nCT is compared with the original ceCT, the PN-nCT and cGAN-nCT; exemplary patient of the PSMA dataset.

the PN suffers more than the cGAN from imperfect segmentation masks, because they are utilized in optimization of the model. Yet, the PN provides the best results in generating a nCT from a ceCT in terms of HU reduction.

In the cGAN, the cycle-consistency loss encouraged the model to balance between the reduction of the contrast agent and the removal of meaningful anatomical structures, allowing for sharper and more detailed predictions (Fig. 1). Due to several interdependent models the cGAN pipeline is more complex to train, but it can easily be scaled by additional unpaired data, free from registration and segmentation preprocessing. Moreover, it provides the highest level of PD reduction in our test set. Further studies with bigger training sets are worth pursuing as follow-up for this work.

Despite being limited to six patients, the dosimetry evaluation shows that avoiding an additional nCT is feasible using our in-silico generated nCT. This enables more precise quantification of the effect of the therapy and thus better personalization of it.

Acknowledgement. This work was partially funded by the German Ministry of Education and Research (BMBF, grant BiTSPro 13GW0357 A-C) and the German Research Foundation (DFG, grant NA 620/51-1).

References

1. Liugang G, Kai X, Chunying L, Zhengda L, Jianfeng S, Tao L et al. Generation of virtual non-contrast CT from intravenous enhanced CT in radiotherapy using convolutional neural networks. Front Oncol. 2020;10.
2. Jakubicek R, Vicar T, Chmelik J, Ourednicek P, Jan J. Deep-learning based prediction of virtual non-contrast CT images. 2021 International Symposium on Electrical, Electronics and Information Engineering. Seoul (Republic of Korea), 2021.
3. Song C, He B, Chen H, Jia S, Chen X, Jia F. Non-contrast CT liver segmentation using CycleGAN data augmentation from contrast enhanced CT. Interpretable and Annotation-Efficient Learning for Medical Image Computing. Ed. by Cardoso J, Van Nguyen H, Heller N, Henriques Abreu P, Isgum I, Silva W et al. (Lecture Notes in Computer Science). Cham, 2020.
4. Sandfort V, Yan K, Pickhardt PJ, Summers RM. Data augmentation using generative adversarial networks (CycleGAN) to improve generalizability in CT segmentation tasks. Sci Rep. 2019;9(1).
5. Isensee F, Petersen J, Klein A, Zimmerer D, Jaeger PF, Kohl S et al. nnU-Net: self-adapting Framework for U-Net-Based Medical Image Segmentation. arXiv:1809.10486 [cs]. 2018.
6. Falk T, Mai D, Bensch R, Çiçek Ö, Abdulkadir A, Marrakchi Y et al. U-Net: deep learning for cell counting, detection, and morphometry. Nat Methods. 2019;16(1).
7. Chen L, Bentley P, Mori K, Misawa K, Fujiwara M, Rueckert D. Self-supervised learning for medical image analysis using image context restoration. Med Image Anal. 2019;58.
8. Zhu JY, Park T, Isola P, Efros AA. Unpaired image-to-image translation using cycle-consistent adversarial networks. IEEE International Conference on Computer Vision. 2017.
9. Papadimitroulas P. Dosimetry applications in GATE Monte Carlo toolkit. Phys Medica. 2017;41.
10. Schneider W, Bortfeld T, Schlegel W. Correlation between CT numbers and tissue parameters needed for Monte Carlo simulations of clinical dose distributions. Phys Med Biol. 2000;45(2).

Unsupervised Super Resolution in X-ray Microscopy using a Cycle-consistent Generative Model

Adarsh Raghunath[1], Fabian Wagner[1], Mareike Thies[1], Mingxuan Gu[1], Sabrina Pechmann[2], Oliver Aust[3], Daniela Weidner[3], Georgiana Neag[3], Georg Schett[3], Silke Christiansen[2], Stefan Uderhardt[3], Andreas Maier[1]

[1]Pattern Recognition Lab, FAU Erlangen-Nürnberg, Germany
[2]Fraunhofer Institute for Ceramic Technologies and Systems IKTS, Germany
[3]Department of Rheumatology and Immunology, FAU Erlangen-Nürnberg, Germany
adarsh.raghunath@fau.de

Abstract. X-ray microscopy (XRM) is a tomographic imaging modality that has gained interest in the context of understanding bone-related diseases on the micro scale due to its high spatial resolution and strong bone to soft tissue contrast. Although in-vivo imaging of bone structures on the micro scale is desired from a medical perspective, high radiation dose so-far prohibits imaging living animals. Research has been focused on generating high-quality reconstructions while maintaining a low X-ray dosage. However, low dose acquisitions result in noisy images with a lower resolution. This study focuses on using an unsupervised deep-learning approach to accurately reconstruct high-resolution (HR) XRM images from their noisy low-resolution (LR) counterparts. We consider an unsupervised approach in a general case where paired data (low-/high resolution pairs) are unavailable. We propose the use of a cycle-consistent generative adversarial network (GAN) for this super resolution task which is to learn the mapping from noisy LR to HR images. Quantitative and qualitative assessments show that our method produces accurate high-resolution XRM reconstructions from their noisy low-resolution counterparts, increasing the peak signal-to-noise ratio (PSNR)/structural similarity index (SSIM) from 18.15/0.52 (baseline) to 31.94/0.73 (proposed method). We believe that our proposed XRM super resolution pipeline provides a valuable tool toward high-resolution in-vivo XRM imaging.

1 Introduction

CT is used for a wide variety of applications and has become one of the most popular medical imaging modalities. Since it relies on X-rays for imaging, acquiring CT scans can cause stochastic, damaging effects in living tissue [1]. Therefore, the dosage at the time of acquisition plays an important role. CT image quality, as in most imaging, is described in terms of contrast, spatial resolution, image noise, and artifacts. Low-dosage CT acquisitions can result in having a decreased optical resolution, which can affect feature detection during analysis [2]. Producing high resolution (HR) CT images when maintaining a minimal radiation dose has therefore been a major motivation for the recent development of super resolution (SR) algorithms.

Compared to hardware-based methods, image-based super resolution algorithms are easier to apply as they only require access to the measured data. Here conventional model-based and learning-based methods can be distinguished. Model-based SR algorithms model the image degradation process and regularize the up sampling SR reconstruction process using various priors [3]. Learning-based SR algorithms learn a nonlinear mapping from a training data set consisting of paired LR and HR images to recover missing high-frequency details. However the success of such supervised learning algorithms in practice is highly limited by the availability of paired data. This motivates us to explore unsupervised learning strategies where paired data are not available. Among deep learning-based unsupervised super-resolution methods for medical images, GANs trained in a cyclic manner has been a popular approach [4]. We introduce a cycle-consistent GAN network with fewer parameters compared to existing methods, which takes on an unsupervised approach (using unpaired images) to denoise and super resolve low-resolution XRM images up to 4 times to obtain HR XRM images. SRGAN is used as the baseline model which uses a deep residual network with skip-connections [5]. Inspired by the recent success of CycleGAN, our model uses two pairs of generator-discriminator blocks to enforce a 'cycle consistency' between the two domains (LR and HR), for unpaired image-to-image translation [6].

2 Materials and methods

The conventional imaging forward model [7] can be formulated as

$$x = SHy + \epsilon \tag{1}$$

where SH denotes the down-sampling and blurring system matrix, and ϵ the introduced noise. In this work, we develop a neural network model to perform adversarial learning in a cyclic manner to invert Eq. 3322-srproblem and estimate a high-resolution image $\hat{y}$ from the low-resolution XRM measurement x. We focus on reconstructing 2D high-resolution XRM scans from their low-resolution counterparts using a cycle-consistent generative model. We draw inspiration from the popular SRGAN [5] for building our model. The difference between our model and SRGAN apart from architectural aspects is that we train our model in an unsupervised setting whereas SRGAN is trained in a supervised manner.

2.1 Cycle-consistent generative model

In order to enforce cycle-consistency between the two domains(Y –> HR and X –> LR), we use two generators, G and F, and two discriminators, D_X and D_Y. Generator G is used to learn the mapping between the LR image from domain X and its corresponding HR image in domain Y, and generator F translates an image from domain Y to domain X. Discriminator D_X distinguishes between the image generated by generator F and the domain X, whereas discriminator D_Y distinguishes between the image generated by generator G and the domain Y.

The generators G and F share a similar architecture. We use 32 identical residual blocks in both generators as compared to SRGAN which uses 16. Each block consists of a 3×3 convolution with 64 filters, batch normalization, parametric ReLU, a second 2D convolution function, and a second batch normalization. Two convolution layers with 3

×3 kernels follow before and after the residual blocks. Finally, there is a pixel shuffling block which uses a scaling factor s. The only difference between G and F is that the scale factor for F is the reciprocal of G (F down-samples the image as compared to G). The architecture we follow is illustrated in Fig. 1.

Our study requires a strong discriminator as compared to the one proposed in SRGAN. We use two discriminators D_X and D_Y with the architecture (Fig. 2). It contains ten convolution layers with the number of channels doubling in each layer starting from 64 to 1024. Each convolution layer is followed by a batch normalization and a leaky ReLU activation layer ($\alpha = 0.2$). As compared to SRGAN, we add two more blocks of convolution layers to extract more abstract features. Strided convolutions are used to reduce the image resolution each time the number of features is doubled.

2.2   Loss function

A combination of several loss terms is used to formulate our overall objective function. The overall objective function combines to

$$\mathcal{L}(G, F, D_X, D_Y) = \lambda_1 \mathcal{L}_{\text{GAN}}(G, F, D_X, D_Y, X, Y) + \lambda_2 \mathcal{L}_{\text{CYC}}(G, F) + \\ \lambda_3 \mathcal{L}_{\text{PER}}(G, F, X, Y) \quad (2)$$

2.2.1   Adversarial loss. Adversarial loss is used for both the mapping functions G and F. For the function $G : X \rightarrow Y$ along with its discriminator D_Y, the objective function is given as

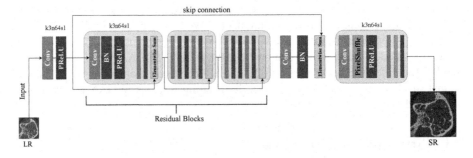

Fig. 1. The generator comprises of feature extraction and up-scaling layers. It consists of 32 residual blocks with skip connections. The number of feature maps used are denoted by n, kernel size by k and the stride used by s.

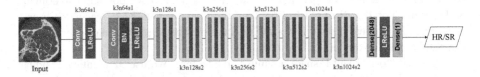

Fig. 2. Architecture of the discriminator. Kernel size used for convolution is denoted by k, number of feature maps by n and stride by s.

$$\mathcal{L}_{\text{GAN}}(G, D_Y, X, Y) = \mathbb{E}_y[\log D_Y(y)] + \mathbb{E}_y[\log(1 - D_Y(G(x)))] \tag{3}$$

Based on the $min_G max_D$ loss function, G tries to minimize the objective against an adversary D which tries to maximize it. Similarly, we use an adversarial term for the mapping function $F : Y \rightarrow X$ and discriminator D_X, which is given as $\mathcal{L}_{\text{GAN}}(F, D_X, Y, X)$.

2.2.2 Cycle consistency loss. Cycle consistency loss is introduced to reduce the space of possible mapping functions between the input distribution and the desired output distribution [6]. To enforce cycle-consistency, we make use of a forward cycle consistency loss ($x \rightarrow G(x) \rightarrow F(G(x)) \rightarrow x$) and a backward cycle consistency loss ($y \rightarrow F(y) \rightarrow G(F(y)) \rightarrow y$). The combined objective function is given as

$$\mathcal{L}_{\text{CYC}} = \mathbb{E}_x[||F(G(x)) - x||_1] + \mathbb{E}_y[||G(F(y)) - y||_1] \tag{4}$$

2.2.3 Perceptual loss. We follow in the steps of SRGAN and add a perceptual loss to our objective function. For this purpose, we use a VGG19 network and the loss is based on the ReLU activations of the pre-trained network. ϕ respresents the features from a particular layer of the network. The loss describes the Euclidean distance between $\phi(G(X))$ and the reference image $\phi(Y)$ as well as between $\phi(F(Y))$ and its corresponding $\phi(X)$. The objective function is given as

$$\mathcal{L}_{\text{PER}} = \mathbb{E}_x[||\phi(x) - \phi(F(G(x)))||_2^2] + \mathbb{E}_y[||\phi(y) - \phi(G(F(y)))||_2^2] \tag{5}$$

2.3 Dataset and training details

In our study, we aim to super resolve ex-vivo XRM scans of mouse tibia bones. The bones contain small cavities with few-micrometer diameter that contain osteocyte cells which are heavily involved in the remodeling of the tissue [8]. Understanding the bone metabolism is crucial for developing treatments for bone-related diseases. XRM images are reconstructed using the CT reconstruction pipeline of Thies et al. [9]. Each high-resolution XRM slice contains 2048×2048 pixels from which random patches of size 256×256 were extracted which are used as HR ground truth images during training. These patches are further subject to a blur kernel and bicubic down-sampling to down-sample them to 64×64 (scale factor = 4) low resolution images. Both HR and LR images are then used in an unpaired setting to create our training data set. In the training process, we empirically set $\lambda_1, \lambda_2, \lambda_3$ to 0.01, 1.0 and 0.05. A learning rate of 0.0004 is used and is divided by 10 after half the number of epochs. The model was implemented in PyTorch and was run for 100 epochs on an NVIDIA A100 GPU.

Tab. 1. The average values of PSNR and SSIM for the different methods along with the standard deviation over the different test samples are shown.

Algorithm	PSNR (mean ± std)	SSIM (mean ± std)
Bicubic	18.15 ± 1.12	0.52 ± 0.02
SRGAN	28.09 ± 0.60	0.63 ± 0.07
Unsupervised (Ours)	31.94 ± 1.63	0.73 ± 0.03

3 Results

We compare our unsupervised cycle-consistent model with bicubic interpolation and supervised SRGAN. We create a low-resolution down-sampled test set of size 512×512 from the high-resolution XRM scans different from the ones used during training. To evaluate the performance, we calculate the average PSNR and SSIM metrics over 10 different samples in our custom test dataset. For further investigation we compare patches of size 256×256. Tab. 1 shows the average PSNR and SSIM values over the test data set. Our method performs better than bicubic and SRGAN in terms of both PSNR and SSIM. In contrast to SRGAN, our cyclic approach produces visually more appealing images with sharp edges and high contrast. The bicubic method blurs the small lacunae and vessel structures which are particularly interesting when investigating bone-related diseases. Fig. 3 shows example predictions of the compared methods.

4 Discussion

We have investigated the XRM low-resolution image restoration problem in an unsupervised setting where paired images are unavailable. For this purpose, we use a feed

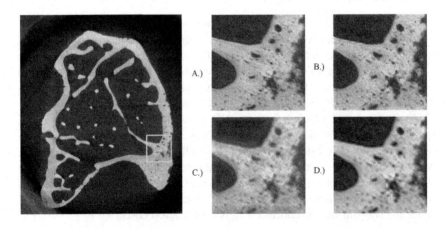

Fig. 3. Visual comparison of model evaluation on Bone CT data. A.) Ground truth image, B.) Ours (Unsupervised cycle-consistent model), C.) SRGAN(Supervised) and D.) Bicubic interpolation.

forward generative model which is trained in a cyclic manner using unpaired XRM data. The GAN model uses multiple residual blocks with skip connections. Both local and global features are cascaded through skip connections before being fed into the reconstruction network. Compared to existing methods, our method uses fewer parameters and produces sharper and visually appealing predictions. Our method improves PSNR over SRGAN by almost 4 db and SSIM by 0.1. In our study, we observed that using a deeper architecture for the discriminator compared to the existing SRGAN architecture can improve the quality of generated images. The context of pre-clinical osteoporosis research demands preserving and enhancing the minute lacunae and vessel structures in the bone to properly distinguish and quantify them. These structures are better captured by our method in comparison to SRGAN which produces noisy results and bicubic interpolation which produces blurred predictions. One of the biggest challenges that we faced in this study is the training of our model which is also a general issue while training GANs as they are difficult to converge to the desired distribution and can often collapse to a narrow distribution. We also observed that predicted XRM images can contain intensity range offsets compared to the ground truth images. Further research is required to stabilise the training process and reduce the training time.

In summary, the proposed method preserves fine anatomical details and produces sharp images while transforming from LR to HR. The results we presented in this work can be vital to advance the research on super-resolution of LR image data in the context of osteoporosis research.

References

1. Wagner F, Thies M, Karolczak M et al. Monte carlo dose simulation for in-vivo X-ray nanoscopy. Proc BVM. Springer, 2022:107–12.
2. Wagner F, Thies M, Gu M et al. Ultralow-parameter denoising: trainable bilateral filter layers in computed tomography. Med Phys. 2022.
3. Babacan SD, Molina R, Katsaggelos AK. Variational bayesian super resolution. IEEE Trans Image Proc. 2010;20(4):984–99.
4. You C, Li G, Zhang Y et al. CT super-resolution GAN constrained by the identical, residual, and cycle learning ensemble (GAN-CIRCLE). IEEE TMI. 2019;39(1):188–203.
5. Ledig C, Theis L, Huszár F et al. Photo-realistic single image super-resolution using a generative adversarial network. Proc CVPR. 2017:4681–90.
6. Zhu JY, Park T, Isola P et al. Unpaired image-to-image translation using cycle-consistent adversarial networks. Proc ICCV. 2017:2223–32.
7. Yang J, Wright J, Huang TS et al. Image super-resolution via sparse representation. IEEE Trans Image Proc. 2010;19(11):2861–73.
8. Grüneboom A, Kling L, Christiansen S et al. Next-generation imaging of the skeletal system and its blood supply. Nat Rev Rheumatol. 2019;15(9):533–49.
9. Thies M, Wagner F, Huang Y et al. Calibration by differentiation-self-supervised calibration for X-ray microscopy using a differentiable cone-beam reconstruction operator. J Microsc. 2022;287(2):81–92.

McLabel: A Local Thresholding Tool for Efficient Semi-Automatic Labelling of Cells in Fluorescence Microscopy

Jonas Utz[1], Maja Schlereth[1], Jingna Qiu[1], Mareike Thies[2], Fabian Wagner[2], Oumaima Ben Brahim[3], Mingxuan Gu[2], Stefan Uderhardt[3], Katharina Breininger[1]

[1]Department Artificial Intelligence in Biomedical Engineering, FAU Erlangen-Nürnberg
[2]Pattern Recognition Lab, FAU Erlangen-Nürnberg
[3]Department of Medicine 3 - Rheumatology and Immunology, FAU Erlangen-Nürnberg
jonas.utz@fau.de

Abstract. In this work, we present a semi-automatic labelling tool for the annotation of complex cellular structures such as macrophages in fluorescence microscopy images. We present McLabel, a napari plugin that allows users to label structures of interest by simply scribbling outlines around the area of interest, using the triangle thresholding method with post-processing to identify the desired structure. Additionally, manual adaption of the threshold allows for quick and fine-grained local correction of the segmentation. The tool is evaluated in a user study with five experts, who annotated images both with and without the tool. The results show that variability in annotations between experts is reduced when the labelling tool is used and annotation time is reduced by a factor of five on average. Our plugin is publicly available on https://github.com/jonasutz/mclabel.

1 Introduction

Segmentation is a critical step in the analysis of biomedical images, particularly in fluorescence microscopy. Segmentations are used to identify and differentiate structures or features within the image. This is an important pre-requisite for further analysis including identifying specific cell types or structures, quantifying the size and shape of cells or organelles, and studying the spatial organization of cells within tissues. However, obtaining segmentations manually is a laborious process. Deep neural networks have recently been used to automate single-cell segmentation [1]. To learn robust representation and improve the generalizability of the segmentation model, a large number of cells with high-quality annotations are required. Depending on the cells or structures of interest, manual annotation can be extremely time-consuming, laborious, and prone to high inter-rater variability.

As an example, resident tissue macrophages, immune cells responsible for disposing of pathogens and mediating immune response [2], can form dynamic, highly complex morphological structures (pseudopods) to examine the surrounding tissue for pathogens [3]. To better quantify their interaction with the tissue as well as immune response behavior, a pixel-exact annotation of their structures is of interest; however, this is extremely time-consuming due to their complex shape. A variety of different approaches for semi-automatic labelling exist, including seed-based approaches like the Random

---

The original version of this chapter was revised. The correction to this chapter is available at
https://doi.org/10.1007/978-3-658-41657-7_68

T. M. Deserno et al. (Hrsg.), *Bildverarbeitung für die Medizin 2023*,
Informatik aktuell, https://doi.org/10.1007/978-3-658-41657-7_20

Walker [4]; however, these approaches are sensitive to neighboring structures with similar intensity, which are frequently encountered in fluorescence images. We therefore select a different interaction strategy. In this paper, we propose a semi-automatic method that only requires a scribble around a cell as user input and supports fast and reliable cell boundary delineation. By searching the triangle threshold within the approximated outlined area (i.e. the scribble) followed by connected component detection, our method automatically refines the coarse annotation to fine-grained annotation. To validate the effectiveness of our tool, we conducted a user study, where five annotators labeled 12 macrophages with and without the tool. We calculated the pairwise agreement between individual annotations to assess the general rater concordance. We further evaluated the annotation efficiency by recording the annotation time. Our method, which is shipped as a plugin for the napari image viewer, can be easily integrated into python-based annotation and analysis frameworks.

2 Materials and methods

In this work, we present McLabel, a semi-automatic annotation tool for cellular structures such as macrophages in fluorescence microscopy. McLabel is implemented as a plugin for the open-source image viewer napari [5], which is widely used in the domain of biomedical imaging. Our tool aims to minimize the manual effort needed for obtaining fine-grained boundary annotation of a single cellular structure.

2.1 General setup

The steps to obtain the segmentation of a single cellular structure using McLabel are as follows (see also Fig. 1):

1. The user draws an outline around a structure of interest in the image. This outline can be an approximated contour enclosing the macrophage and does not need to be an exact delineation of the structure.
2. Based on the outline, a local image bounding box (i.e., a rectangular image patch) is extracted. Pixels that are outside of the outline are set to 0.
3. An intensity histogram of the image patch with 64 bins is computed and used to determine a threshold using the triangle threshold finding algorithm [6].
4. On the thresholded patch, a connected component analysis is conducted.
5. A non-maximum suppression based on area is performed to remove connected components outside of the cellular structure.

The triangle threshold finding algorithm is used since it is designed to handle skewed histograms, which are often present in fluorescence microscopy images due to the black background. Since the threshold is selected on a per-cell basis-based approach, an individual threshold for each structure is obtained which takes into consideration the dynamic nature of microscopy images. If an annotator is not satisfied with the automatic computation of the threshold, a slider in the graphical user interface of McLabel allows individual adjustments of the threshold while still using the post-processing pipeline, i.e. connected component analysis with non-maximum suppression. The above pipeline can then be repeated for all structures of interest within the image, which allows to select per-cell/per-structure optimal threshold values.

2.2 Dataset

To evaluate our plugin, we use a dataset of 12 macrophages in different states and shapes. The macrophages are part of an in-vitro study and were stained with WGA-FITC for the cell membrane and DAPI for the nuclei. Images were obtained with a Zeiss LSM 880 confocal laser scanning microscope at the University Hospital Erlangen. We compute the maximum-intensity projection along the z-axis to obtain 2-D images since the cells are fixed to a petri dish in a cell culture and the third dimension is not required for segmentation. An example for a macrophage with cell protrusions can be found in Fig. 1.

2.3 User study

A user study with five annotators was performed to examine annotation speed and reliability. Annotations were performed in the open-source image viewer napari (version: 0.4.16) [5] using the McLabel plugin with the proposed functionality. To minimize rater variability across displays with limited dynamic range, the contrast of the images was limited from $[0, 255]$ to $[0, 75]$ using the built-in contrast limits in the napari software. Annotators were not allowed to change the contrast limits or other visualization parameters other than magnification during the annotation procedure. Annotators were first asked to annotate the macrophages manually using only the built-in tools of napari, i.e., a brush and a paint bucket. In a second run, annotators were asked to label the same macrophages with the help of our plugin McLabel. If the annotators were not content with the output by McLabel, manual adjustments using the threshold slider and the built-in tools of napari were allowed. Before the study, each annotator had the opportunity to familiarize themselves with napari and McLabel. For both rounds of annotation, the annotation time was recorded for each macrophage individually.

2.4 Evaluation metrics

To examine different aspects of annotator variability we consider three different evaluation metrics. Specifically, we computed the Dice score as an overlap-based metric, the

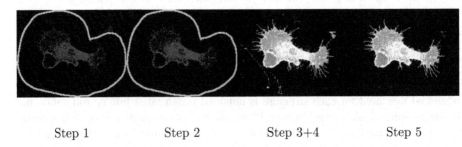

| Step 1 | Step 2 | Step 3+4 | Step 5 |

Fig. 1. Steps involved in computing the segmentation of a macrophage using McLabel.

adjusted mutual information as an information theoretic-based metric, and the Hausdorff distance as a spatial distance-based metric. Since these are widely applied metrics in medical image segmentation their derivation is kept brief here. For a detailed derivation of the metrics see [7]. Each metric is calculated pairwise for all macrophages among all annotators and reported with mean and standard deviation across all pairs of raters.

Dice similarity score. The Dice score [8] is the ratio of the area of overlap between two sets of segmented pixels U and V, e.g., the annotations of two raters. It is computed as

$$\text{Dice}(U, V) = \frac{2|U \cap V|}{|U| + |V|}. \tag{1}$$

The Dice score is 0 if there is no overlap between the two annotations, and is 1 if there is a perfect overlap between the two.

Mutual information. Mutual information (MI) can be used to measure the similarity between image segmentations [9]. The MI between two label assignments U and V is calculated as

$$\text{MI}(U, V) = \sum_{i=1}^{|U|} \sum_{j=1}^{|V|} P(i, j) \log\left(\frac{P(i, j)}{P(i)P'(j)}\right) \tag{2}$$

where $P(i) = |U_i|/N$ is the probability that a pixel picked at random from U falls into class U_i. Respectively, $P'(j) = |V_j|/N$ and the probability of a randomly picked pixel falling into both classes U_i and V_j is $P(i, j) = |U_i \cap V_j|/N$. The total number of pixels is denoted as N. For cellular instance segmentation, the number of classes equals the number of instances. We use the chance adjusted mutual information (AMI), which is defined as

$$\text{AMI} = \frac{\text{MI} - E[\text{MI}]}{\text{mean}(H(U), H(V)) - E[\text{MI}]} \tag{3}$$

where $E[\text{MI}]$ is the expected value of MI and $H(U)$ and $H(V)$ the entropy of U and V. If the AMI is close to zero, it means that the two label assignments are largely independent of each other. On the other hand, if the AMI is close to one, it indicates that there is a high level of agreement between the two label assignments. An AMI of exactly one indicates that the two label assignments are identical.

Hausdorff distance. The Hausdorff distance measures the maximum distance computed from all points in one set to their respective closest point in the second set and can be denoted as

$$\text{HD}(A, B) = max\left(\max_{a \in A} \min_{b \in B} \|a - b\|, \max_{b \in B} \min_{a \in A} \|b - a\|\right) \tag{4}$$

where A and B denote the contours of U and V, respectively. A Hausdorff distance of 0 indicates perfect overlap of both contours [7].

3 Results

3.1 Annotation duration

The total annotation duration for all five annotators performing fully manual annotations of all 12 macrophages varied from 2282 seconds to 3396 seconds. Using our semi-automatic annotation tool McLabel, the total annotation duration varied from 175 seconds up to 1466 seconds. The distribution of annotation duration among raters is depicted in a scatter plot in Figure 2. The average annotation duration for manual segmentation was 2820 seconds, and 584 seconds using McLabel. Among all raters, the average annotation duration was reduced to approximately one fifth of the time using McLabel, compared to fully manual annotations.

3.2 Inter-annotator comparison

The average Dice score of all pairwise combinations of raters is 0.91 ± 0.01 for fully manual annotation and 0.96 ± 0.01 for semi-automatic annotation using McLabel. This indicates that rater agreement was increased when annotations were obtained using McLabel. The mean inter-annotator Hausdorff distance was reduced to 44.5 ± 11 px using McLabel, compared to 79.7 ± 29 with fully manual annotation. The AMI increased to 0.88 ± 0.04 with McLabel compared to 0.74 ± 0.03 with fully manual annotation. All scores are reported in Table 1.

4 Discussion

We present McLabel, a semi-automatic tool for accelerating macrophage annotation in fluorescence microscopy images. With only a scribble around the macrophage as the

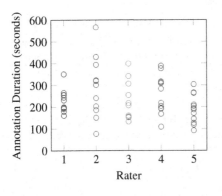

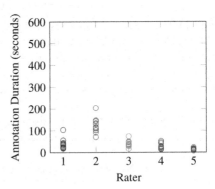

(a) Fully manual annotation

(b) Annotation using McLabel.

Fig. 2. Annotation time distribution for 5 annotators (a) without and (b) with McLabel, each circle represents a macrophage. When compared to fully manual annotation, the use of McLabel reduced manual annotation time by a factor of five on average.

Tab. 1. Inter-annotator comparison using Dice coefficient, Hausdorff distance, and adjusted mutual information. Reported are mean and standard deviation across pairwise comparisons for five raters.

	Dice Coefficient	Hausdorff Distance	Adjusted Mutual Information
w/o. McLabel	0.91 ±0.01	79.7 ± 29 px	0.74 ± 0.03
w. McLabel	0.96 ± 0.01	44.5 ± 11 px	0.88 ± 0.04

user input, our method automatically detects the cell structure. It further allows for local adaption of the segmentation threshold and manual editing to refine the segmentation in a semi-automatic manner. We show that the use of McLabel allows to significantly reduce the required time for annotation of cellular structures with a user study on an example dataset of 12 macrophages. This reduction in annotation time lowers the barrier to train domain specific neural networks and enables high-throughput cell analysis. Additionally, we show that the agreement among raters is increased when our tool is used. However, our study does not come without shortcomings. Similar to other (semi-)automatic labelling algorithms, McLabel potentially introduces a bias into the annotations as all other automatic annotation algorithms by providing a suggestion for the annotation - this bias was not part of the analysis in this work and will be studied in future work.

Acknowledgement. We gratefully acknowledge funding by the Deutsche Forschungs-gemeinschaft (DFG, German Research Foundation) - Projektnummer 405969122 (J. U., S. U., K. B.) and Dhip campus - Bavarian aim (K. B., M. S.,J. Q.).

References

1. Stringer C, Wang T, Michaelos M, Pachitariu M. Cellpose: a generalist algorithm for cellular segmentation. Nature Methods. 2020;18(1):100–6.
2. Mills C. M1 and M2 Macrophages: Oracles of Health and Disease. Critical Reviews in Immunology. 2012;32(6):463–88.
3. Uderhardt S, Martins AJ, Tsang JS, Lämmermann T, Germain RN. Resident Macrophages Cloak Tissue Microlesions to Prevent Neutrophil-Driven Inflammatory Damage. Cell. 2019;177(3):541–55.
4. Grady L. Random Walks for Image Segmentation. IEEE Transactions on Pattern Analysis and Machine Intelligence. 2006;28(11):1768–83.
5. Sofroniew N, Lambert T, Evans K, Nunez-Iglesias J, Bokota G, Winston P et al. napari: a multi-dimensional image viewer for Python. 2022.
6. Zack GW, Rogers WE, Latt SA. Automatic measurement of sister chromatid exchange frequency. Journal of Histochemistry & Cytochemistry. 1977;25(7). PMID: 70454:741–53.
7. Taha AA, Hanbury A. Metrics for evaluating 3D medical image segmentation: analysis, selection, and tool. BMC Medical Imaging. 2015;15(1).
8. Dice LR. Measures of the Amount of Ecologic Association Between Species. Ecology. 1945;26(3):297–302.
9. Russakoff DB, Tomasi C, Rohlfing T, Maurer CR. Image Similarity Using Mutual Information of Regions. Computer Vision - ECCV 2004. Ed. by Pajdla T, Matas J. Berlin, Heidelberg: Springer Berlin Heidelberg, 2004:596–607.

WEB-ANEULYSIS

A Web-based Application for the Analysis of Aneurysm Data

Rebecca Preßler[1], Monique Meuschke[2], Henrik Voigt[1], Kai Lawonn[1]

[1]Institute of Computer Science, University of Jena, Germany
[2]Department of Simulation and Graphics, University of Magdeburg, Germany
rebecca.debora.pressler@uni-jena.de

Abstract. The analysis and treatment of cerebral aneurysms are important in neuroradiology. To support physicians in these tasks a desktop application for the visual analysis of aneurysm data called ANEULYSIS was developed. Because desktop applications complicate collaborative data exploration by physicians working at different locations, we present WEB-ANEULYSIS, a web-based version of ANEULYSIS written with the THREE.js library. Especially the collaborative treatment planning is supported by our application. Therefore, WEB-ANEULYSIS provides features for calculating morphological descriptors, positioning landmarks on the vessel surface, and deploying medical implants inside the vessel. We used WEB-ANEULYSIS for the treatment planning of different cerebral aneurysm data sets and performed a qualitative evaluation together with two neuroradiologists.

1 Introduction

Cerebral aneurysms are pathological dilations of brain arteries. They bear the risk of rupture, which can be fatal for patients. To estimate the risk of rupture it is important to analyze morphological parameters, such as size and location, as well as hemodynamic parameters, such as blood flow velocity and wall shear stress [1]. A common method for the treatment of aneurysms is stenting. A stent is a tube-shaped vessel implant made of metal or synthetic fibers which prevents the aneurysm from rupturing.

In a previous work [2] an application called ANEULYSIS has been developed to visualize simulated aneurysm data and to help physicians access the aneurysm rupture risk. ANEULYSIS is a powerful desktop application consisting of five visualization modules. It is linked to an aneurysm database from which the user can select a specific aneurysm case for detailed analysis. For the selected case, morphological descriptors are calculated and numerous visualization methods are provided to analyze simulated scalar, vector, and tensor fields with respect to rupture risk.

In order to share results more easily with other experts working at other facilities, an additional web-based module [2] was integrated. It visualizes an exported aneurysm case from the desktop application including pre-computed morphological descriptors and user-defined landmarks as well as the most important hemodynamic information. However, this web-based module is heavily dependent on the previous analysis of a data set using the desktop application. Therefore, in this paper, we present a new web-based application, called WEB-ANEULYSIS, which has no dependencies on the desktop application. Moreover, we included new features that support aneurysm treatment planning which was also not possible with the previous web-based module.

© Der/die Autor(en), exklusiv lizenziert an
Springer Fachmedien Wiesbaden GmbH, ein Teil von Springer Nature 2023
T. M. Deserno et al. (Hrsg.), *Bildverarbeitung für die Medizin 2023*,
Informatik aktuell, https://doi.org/10.1007/978-3-658-41657-7_21

2   Methods and materials

In this section, we summarize the generation of the simulated aneurysm data that serve as input for WEB-ANEULYSIS. Afterwards, we give an overview of the technical implementation of WEB-ANEULYSIS. In addition, we describe the user interface of WEB-ANEULYSIS and explain new features compared to the previous web-based module of ANEULYSIS.

2.1   Input data

Similar to ANEULYSIS, WEB-ANEULYSIS uses simulated aneurysm data as input which are generated using computational fluid dynamics (CFD). In the following, we shortly summarize the data simulation and post-processing.

2.1.1   Extraction. First, a geometrical model of the aneurysm and parent vessel artery is reconstructed from clinical image data, comprising CTA, MRA, or DSA images. Therefore we follow the pipeline by Mönch et al. [3], using a threshold-based segmentation to separate the aneurysm and its parent vessel from surrounding tissue. Afterwards, a surface model is reconstructed with the Marching Cube algorithm. Moreover, artifacts of the reconstructed surface are manually corrected and the mesh quality is optimized.

2.1.2   CFD. In the next step, the extracted surface model is transformed into an unstructured volumetric grid [4], which is used as input for the CFD simulation to compute numerically patient-specific hemodynamics by solving the Navier-Strokes equation [5] (more details w.r.t. the performed CFD simulations are provided in [2]). The simulation results in time-dependent scalar and vector fields describing physical forces acting on the vessel wall and internal blood flow.

2.1.3   Post-processing. To support treatment planning in WEB-ANEULYSIS, the centerline of the 3D vascular surface model is needed. We calculate the centerline with the Vascular Modeling Toolkit [6], an open-source python library. Taking the 3D surface model as input, the program computes the centerline semi-automatically, which can be exported as a vtp file. In addition, blood flow-representing path lines are emitted at the ostium, the cross-sectional area between the aneurysm and the healthy parent vessel with an adaptive fifth-order Runge-Kutta method. The integration is performed every 0.01 s. Furthermore, we apply the aneurysm detection approach by Lawonn et al. [7]. With this, all parts of the vessel surface model that belong to an aneurysm are automatically detected. With this also multiple aneurysms can be detected. Finally, an id list is exported that specifies which vertices of the vessel surface belong to an aneurysm and which to the healthy vessel part. This id-list is used in WEB-ANEULYSIS to highlight aneurysms in different colors, where healthy parent vessel parts are colored grey.

2.2 Implementation

The previous web-based module [2] is written in HTML5 with JavaScript and WebGL (Web Graphics Library). WebGL is a JavaScript API that is used to render 2D and 3D graphics on the HTML canvas context. It provides important functions to handle vertex data, transfer them in buffers to the GPU (graphics processing unit), and allows the usage of vertex and fragment shaders written in the OpenGL shading language (GLSL). Nevertheless, WebGL has its limitations. However, applications implemented in WebGL require a high implementation effort, since WebGL does not provide modular algorithms that can be easily integrated into new applications.

To reduce the implementation effort, we developed a new web-based application to analyze aneurysm data using THREE.js. THREE.js is a JavaScript library based on WebGL and greatly simplifies its use. Due to the stronger modular character of THREE.js, numerous algorithms for image generation, analysis, manipulation, and visualization are provided without restricting WebGL in its original functionality. For example, generated objects can be colorized with predefined shaders, but it is still possible to write and define your own shaders. Also, the given ray casting feature and the possibility of adding predefined geometries are very helpful and greatly reduce the development effort for complex applications such as WEB-ANEULYSIS. This also results in easier expandability of the application, where we were able to design and integrate new features to better support treatment planning as in the previous web-based module of ANEULYSIS.

The user interface of WEB-ANEULYSIS looks similar to the previous web-based module [2]. The basic look with the intractable aneurysm model in the center, the container in the upper left corner, which shows the morphological descriptors, and a GUI from the Dat.GUI library on the right side are adopted. For the visual representation of two simulated scalar fields acting on the vessel wall a combination of color-encoding and an image-based hatching scheme [8] is used as in the previous web-based module. But the interface of WEB-ANEULYSIS has also two new elements: a header with clickable buttons and a second container for additional information. Both are needed for the new features, described in Section 2.3. With THREE.js we also improve the interaction with the vessel model. The rotation, zooming, and shifting of the model are much smoother and completely accessible with a mouse. Furthermore, the touch control, needed for tablets and smart devices, is now supported as well as the automatic window resizing.

2.3 New features of web-aneulysis

We conducted informal interviews with two neuroradiologists (16 and 18 years of work experience), where we showed them the previous web-based module of ANEULYSIS to determine whether important features are missing that would support aneurysm analysis. Both mentioned that treatment planning is an important use case, where it should be possible to discuss different treatment options with colleagues. Furthermore, patient education support was highlighted as an important use case. They want to be able to add, place and measure virtual implants and mark and annotate the aneurysm model. With this knowledge, we design and add the following features to WEB-ANEULYSIS.

3 Landmarks

By selecting the Landmark button in the header the landmark editing will be activated. Compared to the previous web-based module where just exported landmarks from the desktop application could be loaded, it is now possible to set, annotate, and remove landmarks on the vessel surface. The landmarks are displayed as yellow torus geometries, so the selected surface region, where a landmark should be placed, is highlighted but not covered by the landmark. By clicking the left mouse button, a landmark will be placed and by clicking the middle mouse button, the currently hovered landmark will be removed. Clicking the right mouse button on a landmark will open an additional window, where the user can enter or edit an annotation. If the user hovers above an annotated landmark, the written annotation will be displayed in the container in the lower left corner (Fig. 1a). If landmarks consist of a previously performed analysis, they will be loaded at the beginning of a session.

3.1 Morphological descriptors

The calculation function computes morphological descriptors, for example, the height, width, or diameter of the aneurysm. This feature was formerly only usable in the desktop application. As input for the computation of the morphological descriptors, the surface model and an id-list are taken, where the id-list results from the automatic aneurysm detection. After selecting the Calculation button the application starts the calculation of the morphological descriptors using the Math.js library [9]. Details regarding the computation of the descriptors can be found in [2]. The calculated values show up in the corresponding container on the left of the surface model. Depending on the model size and the number of vertices the calculation will take some minutes but is only necessary once. The result is saved in a txt file and reloaded by the application during a new analysis.

3.2 Stents

The stent deployment function is a new feature that gets the centerline as input. The user can click on two positions on the centerline, which define the beginning and end of

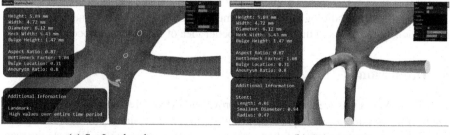

(a) Set Landmarks (b) Calculated Stent

Fig. 1. The landmark editing where an annotated landmark was placed on the vessel surface (a) and the stent function (b) with the visualization of a calculated stent and its size information.

the stent. Afterwards, we determine all points along the centerline that lay between the selected positions. Next, we compute the overall distance of these positions by summing up pairwise Euclidean distances. With this, we get the length of the stent. In the third step, we create an invisible orthogonal plane around every centerline point belonging to the stent. With the help of these planes, all intersection points with the vessel surface and their distances to the corresponding centerline point are computed and stored in a list. Afterwards, from these intersections, we determine the minimum distance between each centerline point belonging to the stent and the vessel surface. This results in the vessel radius at each centerline point, which is used as the local radius of the stent.

With this information, it is now possible to render a stent model inside the vessel surface. We use a predefined THREE.js function that takes all the centerline points belonging to the stent to define a curve. From this curve and corresponding radius information, we are able to create a tube geometry around the centerline which represents the stent. An example of a stent deployment can be seen in Figure 1b.

If the pointer hovers above the model the calculated stent information (length, diameter, and radius) are shown in the lower left container. By clicking the middle mouse button the currently hovered stent model will be removed.

4   Results

We conducted informal interviews with the two neuroradiologists to assess the added value of WEB-ANEULYSIS over the existing web-based module. The neuroradiologists are familiar with the diagnosis and treatment planning of cerebral aneurysms. They should assess if WEB-ANEULYSIS supports aneurysm treatment planning using stenting and whether it can be used to explain planned treatment to patients. For this purpose, they analyzed and stented multiple aneurysms using WEB-ANEULYSIS. The neuroradiologists described the definition of a stent as easy without having problems regarding the interaction to place stents in the vessel. This allowed them to assess the suitability of different stent configurations in the vessel, which would support decision-making in the clinical routine. However, they would have liked to be able to vary the mesh density of the placed stents and to be able to place multiple stents inside each other, which we will integrate in the future. Besides treatment planning, they used WEB-ANEULYSIS for patient education, where the deployment of a stent inside the extracted aneurysm of a patient was shown. Compared to previously manually created sketches used for patient education, the neuroradiologist could now much easier show what treatment is planned. In addition, patients stated that they had a better idea of the planned procedure.

5   Discussion

With WEB-ANEULYSIS we were able to improve and extend previous work. To meet the needs of the physicians we improved the aneurysm risk assessment and treatment planning. The direct computation of the morphological descriptors within WEB-ANEULYSIS is a start to transfer the desktop application into a web application. This is necessary to better support the collaborative aneurysm analysis, especially in the case of physicians working at different locations and does not have access to local data sets of the opposite clinic. The landmark functions are designed to visually support the discussion by different physicians, but they could also be used for explanations to patients. Treatment planning can benefit from features like the stent function since different stent configurations can be compared. In case that paper will be accepted, we will make WEB-ANEULYSIS freely available.

5.1 Limitations

It cannot be guaranteed that the extracted surface models and simulation results accurately reflect patient-specific situations and conditions. It is possible that the simulated blood flow differs from the actual patient-specific one due to necessary assumptions regarding the flow and boundary conditions for CFD. Landmarks and annotations are quite helpful, but it must be considered that especially if the physicians use this application asynchronously to work on a case over a distance, misunderstandings from annotations may arise. A short note can rarely replace a conversation. If a stent is placed in the model, the CFD simulations have to be recalculated to evaluate the effects of the stent on the forces acting on the vessel wall. However, this function is currently not included due to the time-consuming calculations of the CFD simulations.

5.2 Future work

We improved the web-based aneurysm analysis and treatment planning, but there is still room for further extensions and a detailed evaluation with physicians. Especially the communication between physicians and the possibility to work synchronously on the same data set can be further improved. For example a screen sharing or chat feature could be implemented. In addition, further functions of ANEUYLSIS should be integrated. For example, visualizations, such as the virtual DSA representation by Preßler et al. [10], mimic the look of real medical images with which physicians are familiar. Also, the centerline calculation and aneurysm detection currently requiring separate applications should be integrated into WEB-ANEULYSIS to further reduce the number of needed programs.

References

1. Cebral JR, Mut F, Weir J, Putman CM. Association of hemodynamic characteristics and cerebral aneurysm rupture. Am J Neuroradiol. 2011;32(2):264–70.
2. Meuschke M, Preim B, Lawonn K. ANEULYSIS: a system for the visual analysis of aneurysm data. Comput Graph. 2021;98:197–209.
3. Mönch T, Neugebauer M, Preim B. Optimization of vascular surface models for computational fluid dynamics and rapid prototyping. Proc of Second Int. Workshop on Digital Engineering. 2011:16–23.
4. Janiga G, Berg P, Beuing O, Neugebauer M, Gasteiger R, Preim B et al. Recommendations for accurate numerical blood flow simulations of stented intracranial aneurysms. Biomed Eng-Biomed Te. 2013;58(3):303–14.
5. Sanchez M, Ambard D, Costalat V, Mendez S, Jourdan F, Nicoud F. Biomechanical assessment of the individual risk of rupture of cerebral aneurysms: a proof of concept. Ann Biomed Eng. 2013;41(1):28–40.

6. Izzo R, Steinman D, Manini S, Antiga L. The vascular modeling toolkit: a Python library for the analysis of tubular structures in medical images. J Open Source Softw. 2018;3(25):745.

7. Lawonn K, Meuschke M, Wickenhöfer R, Preim B, Hildebrandt K. A geometric optimization approach for the detection and segmentation of multiple aneurysms. Comput Graph Forum. Vol. 38. (3). 2019:413–25.

8. Meuschke M, Voß S, Beuing O, Preim B, Lawonn K. Combined visualization of vessel deformation and hemodynamics in cerebral aneurysms. IEEE Trans Vis Comput Graph. 2017;23(1):761–70.

9. Jong J de, Mansfield E. Math.Js: an advanced mathematics library for JavaScript. Comput Sci Eng. 2018;20(1):20–32.

10. Preßler R, Lawonn K, Preim B, Meuschke M. Virtual DSA visualization of simulated blood flow data in cerebral aneurysms. Proc of BVM. Springer, 2022:241–6.

Towards Clinical Translation of Deep Learning-based Classification of DSA Image Sequences for Stroke Treatment

Timo Baumgärtner[1], Benjamin J. Mittmann[1], Till Malzacher[2], Johannes Roßkopf[2], Michael Braun[2], Bernd Schmitz[2], Alfred M. Franz[1]

[1]Department of Computer Science, Ulm University of Applied Sciences
[2]Neuroradiology Section, District Hospital Guenzburg
alfred.franz@thu.de

Abstract. In the event of stroke, a catheter-guided procedure (thrombectomy) is used to remove blood clots. Feasibility of machine learning based automatic classifications for thrombus detection on digital substraction angiography (DSA) sequences has been demonstrated. It was however not used live in the clinic, yet. We present an open-source tool for automatic thrombus classification and test it on three selected clinical cases regarding functionality and classification runtime. With our trained model all large vessel occlusions in the M1 segment were correctly classified. One small remaining M3 thrombus was not detected. Runtime was in the range from 1 to 10 seconds depending on the used hardware. We conclude that our open-source software tool enables clinical staff to classify DSA sequences in (close to) realtime and can be used for further studies in clinics.

1 Introduction

Worldwide, ischemic stroke, in which a blood clot blocks blood vessels in the brain, is one of the most common causes of death [1]. In addition to drug treatment (thrombolysis), removal of the blood clot using a catheter-guided procedure (thrombectomy) has now become widely accepted and has shown a significantly better outcome for patients [2]. However, there continue to be numerous challenges in performing thrombectomy, resulting in reperfusion of occluded vessels being achieved in only 70-80% of cases, with treatment remaining unsuccessful in the remaining patients [3].

Thrombectomy is usually performed under fluoroscopic guidance. Here, digital subtraction angiography (DSA) can be used to visualize the vascular tree in relation to the instruments. Vascular occlusions frequently occur in the middle cerebral artery (MCA), specifically in the M1 - M3 segments, with the MCA having a diameter of approximately 3 mm in the M1 segment immediately after the branch from the internal carotid artery, which then narrows further in the M2 segment and M3 segment. M3 occlusions are more difficult to detect and treat, but are also often less critical than, for example, M1 occlusions. One challenge for the physician is to quickly identify whether a blood clot is still present in the DSA sequence just acquired or whether it has already been successfully removed. Automatic classification of DSA sequences using machine learning methods has already been demonstrated in studies, for example by Nielsen et al. who used an EfficientNet-B0-based convolutional neural network (CNN) with gated recurrent units (GRU) to classify with respect to thrombolysis in cerebral infarction (TICI) and achieved an accuracy of 0.95 ± 0.03 [4]. Another work by Su et al. uses a multi-path CNN for automatic TICI classification with which they achieve an average area under the curve (AUC) value of 0.81 [5]. In a preliminary work of ours, we demonstrated that using an EfficientNetV2 architecture with GRU, DSA sequences can be classified into thrombus-free and non-thrombus-free, achieving an AUC of 0.94 [6].

While the feasibility of automatic classification has been demonstrated by the listed studies, to the best of our knowledge, the classifications were performed offline using dedicated computers and could not yet be used live in the clinic. With the work presented here, based on our preliminary work, we want to go one step further towards clinical translation: (1) we present an open-source application that can be installed together with the trained network on arbitrary computers and classify DICOM data there, (2) after performing a 5-fold cross-validation in the preliminary evaluation work [6], we re-train the network with all training data in this work, and (3) test the classification on new datasets acquired in the clinic with a different DSA system. The trained network and the classification tool are published.

2   Methods

2.1   Open-source application for classification

Focusing on enabling users from medical research in using the classification, we develop a prototypical graphical user interface. We envision to provide several functionalities, such as (1) Loading of DICOM and nifti image files, (2) Showing an one-image-preview of the loaded series, (3) Loading of any model that shall be used for classification, (4) Selection of the classification threshold based on statistical evaluation on the training data and displaying these statistics, (5) Classification of the loaded data and (6) Keeping the requirements of the application in terms of the hardware as low as possible with a classification result provided in less than 60 seconds.

In order to combine the graphical user interface (GUI) capabilities of the .NET framework using Windows presentation foundation (WPF) and the typical python-based PyTorch implementation for machine learning, we employ a classic client-server architecture. The python service can therefore be started as the server, providing an interface that the user application can query. These endpoints can provide functionality like model interference (e.g. classifying provided images) or image rendering, to employ the same image preprocessing as it is used for the model. We use the python package nibabel [1] to load the nifti-files. In case of DICOM data, we use the commandline tool plastimatch [2] to convert them into the nifti file format. In order to comply with the security of patient data and to keep loading times short, both the python service as well as the user application need to run on the same machine, sharing the same filesystem.

In order to make the model applicable for non-technical users such as clinical staff, we provide an interactive view, enabling to choose the threshold (e.g. the value at which the application labels a sample as positive/negative) and run the classification. Thereby,

---

[1](https://nipy.org/nibabel/)
[2](https://plastimatch.org/)

one can optimize different metrics (like the Matthews correlation coefficient MCC [7]) according to their needs. We initially provide an optimized threshold value of 0.57, which is found by optimizing the rates of false positives and true positives. We therefore adapt the proposed closest-point-criterion [8], which, when using FPR instead of $(1 - FPR)$ as abscissa, can be rewritten as

$$\text{threshold} = \arg \max_t \sqrt{(1 - FPR_t)^2 + TPR_t^2} \tag{1}$$

where FPR is the false positive rate and TPR is the true positive rate, found by evaluating the correctness of classification results utilizing threshold t on the training data.

2.2 Network architecture and model retraining

One network setup that yielded good results in [6] is EfficentNetV2+GRU. We employ this architecture for classification, as shown in Fig. 1a. We utilize two models, one that was trained for frontal sequences, and another that was trained for lateral sequences. The final classification is the mean of both predictions.

In [6], crossfold-validation was used to estimate the quality of the classification, since the amount of data samples was quite limited. In order to provide maximum performance of the model, we combined training and test dataset and trained one single model on all of it. We use the metrics of the crossfold-validation to estimate the models performance. However, we plan to continually assess the performance of our model with future data (Sec. 4).

2.3 Evaluation methods

The objective was to evaluate the software and the new trained model regarding (1) functionality, (2) classification correctness and (3) runtime on different systems. We were able to evaluate our system on three new cases that were generated with another angiography unit than the training data, namely a *Siemens ARTIS icono biplane* instead of a *Siemens ARTIS zee biplane*. These three cases were selected by physicians, consisting of two DSA sequences each: One before the treatment was started, inherently containing one or even multiple thrombi. The other one was taken after the treatment. The first case shows an M1 thrombus, all thrombi were removed. The second case initially shows an M1 thrombus which was removed, one small peripheral M3 thrombus was remaining. The third case shows a thrombus in the carotid terminus, all thrombi were successfully removed, however, the sequence shows flow reversal in the vessels, which might be mistaken for an occlusion by inexperienced observers.

We benchmarked several different hardware configurations, solely running on CPU or utilizing GPU, and both on various budget levels. For testing the CPU performance, we compare an Intel i7-7700K with 8 threads with an Intel i7-11700KF with 16 threads. Regarding the GPU, we evaluate a Nvidia GTX 1050Ti Mobile and a Nvidia RTX 3090. The tests were conducted under Python 3.10.8, PyTorch 1.18, CUDA 11.7.1 and Nvidia GPU driver 526.98, which were the most recent compatible versions at this time. We therefore benchmarked the three new cases, resulting in $n = 6$ datapoints, and took the mean of the timings. Since the classification time might deviate depending on the file size, we also calculated the standard deviation for these measurements.

Tab. 1. Details about the tested cases.

	Case 1		Case 2		Case 3	
	Pre	Post	Pre	Post	Pre	Post
Size in MB (Combined)	283	199	199	210	210	263
Raw Classification Output	0.77	0.24	0.70	0.25	0.79	0.49

3 Results

A screenshot of our developed application is shown in Fig. 1b. In order to support the concept of Open Science, we provide our application as well as the trained model to the community by making it open-source [3].

In all three cases, the first and second sequences were correctly classified as non-thrombus-free and thrombus-free. However, the small remaining M3 thrombus was not detected, a behavior that we already know from our previous study which needs discussion (Sec. 4). In case 3, the raw output (0.49) was close to the threshold of 0.57, but still below, which was due to a misleading flow reversal in the vessels, by which experienced physicians would not have been irritated. Table 1 shows the raw combined classification result for all three cases along with the respective file size of the frontal and lateral sequence combined.

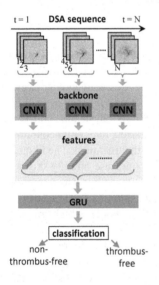

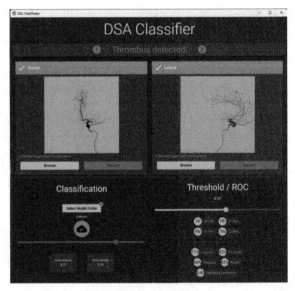

(a) Architecture of the neural network (adapted from [6]).

(b) Screenshot of the application.

Fig. 1. Details of the application.

[3](https://osf.io/n8k4r/)

Tab. 2. Required mean classification time in seconds with standard deviation (n=6).

Highend GPU	Basic GPU	Highend CPU	Basic CPU
Nvidia RTX 3090	Nvidia GTX 1050Ti	Intel i7-11700KF	Intel i7-7700K
24GB VRAM	4GB VRAM	32GB RAM	16GB RAM
1.1s ± 0.1	1.8s ± 0.1	4.8s ± 0.5	8.8s ± 0.9

The resulting benchmarks can be seen in Table 2. The timings were calculated using six datapoints, namely our three cases that each consisted of preinterventional and postinterventional sequences. We show the approximate time in seconds needed to classify one case, in order to estimate necessary hardware constraints. Preliminary steps are not included, but typically add less than 15 seconds for data conversion (if necessary) and 5 seconds for image loading along with preprocessing.

4 Discussion

Despite the new angiography system, our system was able to classify all sequences correctly for large vessel occlusions in the M1 segment. In the second case, our system was unable to detect the remaining small peripheral thrombus. As these kind of thrombi were not focus of the training process, we already expected this behavior. However though, as these cases would usually not be treated by thrombectomy, this was not part of the goals for the system ([6]). In the future, we plan to extend the training data and retrain the model to investigate if M2 and M3 thrombi can also be detected.

We conclude, that for our tool to be used, no highend hardware is needed. If necessary, the classification can be done on the CPU in still reasonable time, although we see that the maximum number of threads influences performance. However though, the system already greatly benefits from entry-level graphic cards. The use of high-end hardware in return does not yield great advances, when seen in relation to the costs. The classification time of up to approximately 10 seconds seems acceptable. In addition, the conversion of the DICOM data along with preprocessing is estimated in the experimental runs to take at most 30 seconds. Thus, the total duration also seems to be in an acceptable range, especially since the runtime can certainly still be optimized.

As the values of the various metrics will likely be different on unseen new data, the use of these values for estimating an optimal threshold should be treated carefully. We therefore propose to incorporate ways of obtaining user feedback concerning the correctness of the classification, to store this feedback along with the raw classification output, and to continually recompute and optimize the threshold using these values. Furthermore, more test cases are needed. We currently prepare a larger study that assesses the quality of our model.

We envision a system that provides physicians hints right in the moment of the thrombectomy with an additional safety. For this, we plan a watch-dog-system that runs in the background and only warns the physician if it detects remaining thrombi. Since the current system can only classify whole sequences into thrombus-free and non-thrombus-free, we are working on visualizing the parts of the sequence that lead to the classification. This will give clinicians more and deeper insight into the decision, which in turn will make the system more credible and the process more efficient.

It's important to note that this does not, at any time, replace the educated assessment of the physicians themselves, nor the ones of assisting staff. The goal is to provide an additional layer of assessment that solely provides a supplementary opinion that, in case of a warning, might motivate the physician to check for critical sections once more. By, in the best case, triggering a reassessment from the clinical staff, treatment quality will be at least the same as without the application.

We faced problems with the specific PACS system in the clinic, an *AGFA HealthCare IMPAX EE R20 XVIII SU1*, as it sometimes failed to export DICOM data correctly. We therefore currently investigate several possibilities for a realtime connection, such as the connection to the angiography system's manufacturer's API as well as the potential use of framegrabbers. In addition to converting DICOM data on import, the current prototype also allows nifti files to be imported directly, which are useful for demonstration, research and fallback purposes.

Whereas the path to a medical product is still long, we are confident that our application along with the planned study is a step in the right direction. Also, we may help radiologists test the classification in their clinical environment, even during ongoing procedures if ethically approved.

Acknowledgement. This work was funded by the Federal Ministry for Economic Affairs and Climate Action (BMWK, Funding Code: ZF4640301GR8)

References

1. Lopez AD, Mathers CD, Ezzati M, Jamison DT, Murray CJL. Global and regional burden of disease and risk factors, 2001: systematic analysis of population health data. Lancet. 2006;367(9524):1747–57.
2. Goyal M, Demchuk AM, Menon BK, Eesa M, Rempel JL, Thornton J et al. Randomized assessment of rapid endovascular treatment of ischemic stroke. N Engl J Med. 2015;372(11):1019–30.
3. Yoo AJ, Andersson T. Thrombectomy in acute ischemic stroke: challenges to procedural success. J Stroke. 2017;19(2):121–30.
4. Nielsen M, Waldmann M, Sentker T, Frölich A, Fiehler J, Werner R. Time matters: handling spatio-temporal perfusion information for automated TICI scoring. MICCAI 2020. 1st ed. Vol. 12266. (Lecture Notes in Computer Science (LNCS)). Springer Nature Switzerland, 2020:86–96.
5. Su R, Cornelissen SAP, van der Sluijs M, van Es ACGM, van Zwam WH, Dippel DWJ et al. autoTICI: automatic brain tissue reperfusion scoring on 2D DSA images of acute ischemic stroke patients. IEEE Trans Med Imaging. 2021;40(9):2380–91.
6. Mittmann BJ, Braun M, Runck F, Schmitz B, Tran TN, Yamlahi A et al. Deep learning-based classification of DSA image sequences of patients with acute ischemic stroke. Int J Comput Assist Radiol Surg. 2022;17(9):1633–41.
7. Chicco D, Jurman G. The advantages of the Matthews correlation coefficient (MCC) over F1 score and accuracy in binary classification evaluation. BMC genomics. 2020;21(1):6.

8. Perkins NJ, Schisterman EF. The inconsistency of "optimal" cutpoints obtained using two criteria based on the receiver operating characteristic curve. Am J Epidemiol. 2006;163(7):670–5.

Leveraging Semantic Information for Sonographic Wrist Fracture Assessment Within Children

Christoph Großbröhmer[1], Luisa Bartram[1], Corinna Rheinbay[1,2], Mattias P. Heinrich[1], Ludger Tüshaus[2]

[1]Institut für Medizinische Informatik, Universität zu Lübeck
[2]Klinik für Kinderchirurgie, Universitätsklinikum Schleswig-Holstein, Lübeck
c.grossbroehmer@uni-luebeck.de

Abstract. The use of ultrasound for the diagnosis of pediatric distal forearm fractures provides a radiation-free, rapid, and inexpensive alternative to radiography. Computer-aided examination and diagnosis support may contribute to the increasing popularity of fracture sonography. Although machine learning approaches are considered the tool of choice for medical image processing, the success of data-driven methods is highly dependent on the quality and quantity of image data. Both conditions are not necessarily met in the field of pediatric bone sonography, so supporting measures for the application of deep learning techniques are required. One possible solution is the incorporation of additional semantic information. In this work, we investigate to what extent the use of existing state-of-the-art frameworks together with segmentations of anatomical structures can increase the classification accuracy of the detection of distal forearm fractures in children using ultrasound.

1 Introduction

Distal forearm fractures are the most common fractures in growing-age children [1] and are diagnosed usually with a two-plane radiograph, which involves harmful ionizing radiation. One way to circumvent this is to examine the bones using ultrasound, which is a non-invasive, versatile, fast, cost-effective and less painful medical imaging technique. The examination, following the standardized clinical WRIST-SAFE algorithm [2], includes an image of 3 planes each of the ulna and radius and shows equal effectiveness compared to radiographic imaging [3]. In addition to avoiding ionizing radiation, this method offers an acceleration of the clinical workflow and wide applicability in practices without X-ray equipment. As part of the technical advancement of mobile ultrasound equipment, it is possible, especially in the emergency department setting, to perform point of care ultrasound (POCUS) directly on the patient at the bedside. Although fracture sonography offers multiple advantages over radiography, it is not yet widely used in clinical practice. Despite all the advantages mentioned, it should be noted that the actual performance and the results of bone ultrasound are very examiner- and experience-dependent. One way of promoting and facilitating this technique might be intelligent software that supports the medical practitioner during the examination by means of fracture classification or highlighting of anatomical structures. Image classification and segmentation are common tasks in medical informatics for which deep learning techniques have proven to be effective. However, learning in the ultrasound

© Der/die Autor(en), exklusiv lizenziert an
Springer Fachmedien Wiesbaden GmbH, ein Teil von Springer Nature 2023
T. M. Deserno et al. (Hrsg.), *Bildverarbeitung für die Medizin 2023*,
Informatik aktuell, https://doi.org/10.1007/978-3-658-41657-7_23

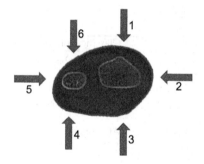

Fig. 1. Wrist SAFE Algrorithm, adopted from [2]. The captured planes are (1) Radius dorsal, (2) Radius radial, (3) Radius volar, (4) Ulna volar, (5) Ulna ulnar and (6) Ulna volar.

imaging domain has been proven to be challenging due to low imaging quality caused by noise and artefacts [4]. While there are several techniques to alleviate these challenges such as transfer learning or domain adaptation, the implementation of these methods is highly dependent on domain and task similarity and can be effortful and might not yield the best performance. Another approach is the utilisation of additional semantic information, such as segmentations of anatomical structures, typically as pretext learning tasks or by using them alongside the image as classification network input.

A more direct way is to use well-suited methods developed for this type of additional information as a proxy and subsequently derive the original query from its results. In this work, we investigate the employment of proxy segmentation and detection networks for a classification task. We train both a nnUNet and a Mask R-CNN with ultrasound images of the wrist and corresponding multi-class segmentation labels, and extract binary fracture classification from segmentation and detection results. Their performance is evaluated in terms of accuracy, sensitivity, specificity, precision and F1-Score.

1.1 Dataset

A total of 180 ultrasound images and diagnoses from 43 patients have been retrieved retrospectively from the clinic PACS-System in the context of a suspected fracture of the distal forearm. All images have been captured on a GE LOGIQ S7 device following the WRIST-SAFE-Algorithm (Fig. 1) and thus depict either the radius or ulna in dorsal, lateral or volar planes. The dataset includes a total of 79 positive fractures. In accordance with the clinical diagnosis, a maximum of 4 different target structures (fracture, bone, growth joint, ossification core) have been labelled by an experienced pediatric surgeon and two university students with backgrounds in medicine and medical informatics. Cases with missing labels (for growth joints and ossification cores) and heterogeneity of segmentation shape and thickness limit the application of machine-learning segmentation algorithms.

2   Materials and methods

All experiments have been conducted with a five-fold cross-testing with patient-level splits to prevent information bias. Each split consists of 148 training and 32 testing samples. Training data of the first split was used to select network hyperparameters,

Tab. 1. Overview of the classification pipelines.

Method	Training Input	Inference Output	Classification Decision
ResNet	Ultrasound Image	Softmax Scores $S_{positive}$, $S_{negative}$	$S_{positive} > S_{negative}$
nnUNet	Ultrasound Image + Semantic Segmentations	Segmentation Map	At least one pixel classified as fracture
Mask R-CNN	Ultrasound Image + Instance Segmentations + Instance Bounding Boxes	For each instance: • Segmentation • Bounding Box • Softmax $S_{instance}^{class}$	At least one $S_{instance}^{fracture} > \tau$

whereas testing data has only been used for computing metric scores. We seek to classify each image in the test set as "fracture" (positive) or "no fracture" (negative). An overview of the architectures and classification pipelines is presented in Table 1.

2.1 Classification network

As a baseline, we retrain an IMAGENET-pretrained Resnet18 [5] without any segmentation information for 50 epochs. We perform image augmentations by randomly shifting, cropping, rotating and vertical flipping. Experiments with larger backbones (e.g. ResNet50) early led to overfitting and were therefore discarded.

2.2 Segmentation network

We employ the popular nnUNet framework [6] to generate segmentations on our 2D image data. Although the framework has been developed for 3D images, it showed the best performance of all segmentation networks investigated. Augmentations include elastic deformations, scaling, rotations, brightness shifts and mirroring. As soon as a single pixel is segmented as a fracture by the nnUNet, we classify the image as positive.

2.3 Detection network

We further investigate the results of the detection and instance segmentation network Mask R-CNN. For each detected object, it returns a segmentation, a bounding box and an associated softmax score. We also train the detection network Mask R-CNN [7] with an IMAGENET-pretrained ResNet50 backbone for 30 epochs and employ random shifting, cropping and rotating as augmentations. We threshold found fracture instances by τ and only classify an image as positive if there is at least one fracture instance with a softmax score greater than τ. We report metrics for $\tau = 0$ (Mask R-CNN$_0$) and $\tau = 0.5$ (Mask R-CNN$_{0.5}$), which led to the top accuracy averaged on all folds.

Tab. 2. Mean classification results and standard deviation percent, referring to the 5-fold cross testing.

	Accuracy	Sensitivity	Specificity	Precision	F1 Score
ResNet	76.25 ± 5.08	69.69 ± 18.64	77.97 ± 5.36	70.02 ± 9.25	69.44 ± 13.86
nnUNet	80.00 ± 5.45	68.86 ± 13.39	87.38 ± 10.40	82.34 ± 9.77	73.86 ± 8.99
Mask R-CNN$_0$	78.12 ± 3.42	70.07 ± 9.21	84.17 ± 4.09	77.19 ± 6.29	72.92 ± 5.43
Mask R-CNN$_{0.5}$	81.25 ± 6.81	68.07 ± 7.81	90.39 ± 4.17	85.85 ± 0.93	75.66 ± 4.95

3 Results and discussion

The results presented in Table 2 show that the fracture classification benefits from leveraging segmentations. While the ResNet achieves the lowest values in all metrics, both the nnUNet and the Mask R-CNN can increase the accuracy, specificity, precision and F1 score of the classification. The only metric which leads to comparable results for all methods appears to be sensitivity. However, the standard deviation decreases significantly with the use of segmentations, which is also reflected in the decrease of F1 score standard deviation by 5-9%. This may indicate that both the nnUNet and the Mask R-CNN are more robust since the F1 score is defined as a harmonic mean between sensitivity and precision. This corresponds with the Mask R-CNN receiver operation characteristic curves shown in Figure 2. The mean area under the curve is 0.80 ± 0.04. The best results in terms of accuracy and F1 score are obtained by the Mask R-CNN$_{0.5}$ with 81.25% and 75.66% respectively.

Figure 3 shows qualitative results of the nnUNet and the Mask R-CNN. Both methods were able to correctly classify the fracture in the top example, while both failed to detect the fracture in the middle example. The ResNet baseline gave false negatives to both images. While the image in the bottom row has been classified negatively by the annotator and the other methods, the nnUNet labels a small region positively. The corresponding area depicts a blurry corticalis which can easily be interpreted as an ultrasound characteristic artefact. However, another plane of the same patient clearly

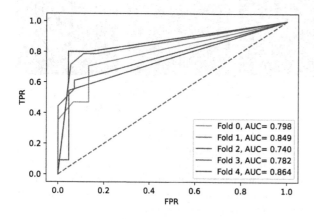

Fig. 2. Mask R-CNN Reciever Operation Characteristic Curves for all 5 folds. TPR and FPR denote True Positive Rate and False Positive Rate respectively.

shows a fracture, exemplifying the difficulties of ultrasound diagnosis and the possible benefits of highlighting regions of interest during examination. Further investigation should also address the possible benefit of combining classification results from different images for decision consensus. This assumption is also supported by the work of Zhang et al., who in a similar work were able to increase the accuracy of fracture classification by utilizing multiple 2D frames sampled from 3D sweeps [8]. Although it is outside the scope of this work and inconsistent labels make quantitative evaluation difficult, the relevant fractures appear to be well detected by both architectures.

While these results are not sufficient in terms of a medical application, they clearly indicate the large potential for improvement in machine learning in the ultrasound domain by the inclusion of additional data. Even with relatively little effort, we could boost classification performance substantially. A possible explanation for the low accuracy is the small size of the dataset. Additionally, some images are not located in the ideal slice, so bone boundaries, which are essential for diagnosis, are not sharply delineated. The next steps in further improving classification accuracy might include advanced

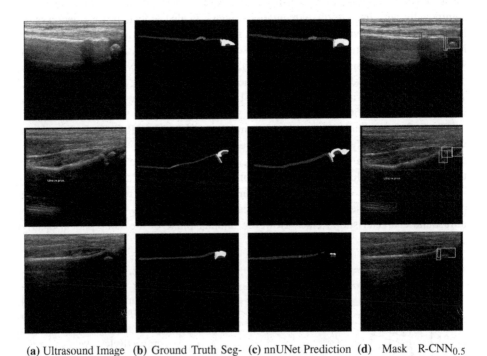

(a) Ultrasound Image (b) Ground Truth Seg- (c) nnUNet Prediction (d) Mask R-CNN$_{0.5}$
                        mentation   Prediction

Fig. 3. Three qualitative segmentation and bounding box prediction examples. The nnUNet (c) and Mark R-CNN (d) predictions correspond to the input ultrasound image (a), while (b) shows the ground truth segmentation. Label colors are defined as followed: Blue denotes the bone corticalis, green the growth joint and yellow the ossification. Possible fractures are depicted in red. Bounding box predictions (c) have been refined by non-maximum suppression to remove multiple instances of the same object. All images have been classified negatively by ResNet18.

pretaining, data augmentation schemes and leveraging the temporal domain by including video data in both classification and user guidance.

4 Conclusion

We demonstrated that the use of available segmentation and detection frameworks, without complicated adaptation of the methodology, is able to increase accuracy and robustness in the diagnosis of pediatric forearm fractures on ultrasound images. We obtained the best results with a Mask R-CNN, correctly detecting 81% of all fractures. Although this accuracy is not sufficient yet for medical practice, the results show that the direct inclusion of semantic information through proxy fractures can in principle lead to an improvement of classification accuracy of 5%. Further investigations should compare these results with other methods for the integration of semantic information.

References

1. Kraus R, Schneidmüller D, Röder C. Häufigkeit von Frakturen der langen Röhrenknochen im Wachstumsalter. Deutsches Ärzteblatt. 2005:5.
2. Ackermann O, ed. Fraktursonografie. Berlin, Heidelberg: Springer Berlin Heidelberg, 2019.
3. Ackermann O, Wojciechowski P, Dzierzega M, Grosser K, Schmitz-Franken A, Rudolf H et al. Sokrat II – an international, prospective, multicenter, phase IV diagnostic trial to evaluate the efficacy of the wrist SAFE algorithm in fracture sonography of distal forearm fractures in children. Ultraschall in Med. 2019;40(03):349–58.
4. Liu S, Wang Y, Yang X, Lei B, Liu L, Li SX et al. Deep learning in medical ultrasound analysis: a review. Engineering. 2019;5(2):261–75.
5. He K, Zhang X, Ren S, Sun J. Deep residual learning for image recognition. 2016:770–8.
6. Isensee F, Jaeger PF, Kohl SAA, et al. nnU-Net: a self-configuring method for deep learning-based biomedical image segmentation. Nat Methods. 2021;18(2):203–11.
7. He K, Gkioxari G, Dollár P, Girshick R. Mask R-CNN. Proc IEEE ICCV. IEEE, 2017:2980–8.
8. Zhang J, Boora N, Melendez S, Rakkunedeth Hareendranathan A, Jaremko J. Diagnostic accuracy of 3D ultrasound and artificial intelligence for detection of pediatric wrist injuries. Children. 2021;8(6):431.

Applicability of BI-RADS Criteria for Deep Learning-based Classification of Suspicious Masses in Sonograms

Christian Schmidt, Heinrich M. Overhoff

Westfälische Hochschule, University of Applied Sciences, Medical Engineering Laboratory, Gelsenkirchen, Germany
Christian.Schmidt@w-hs.de

Abstract. Breast ultrasound exams are often performed alongside mammograms for the detection and classification of suspicious masses. The breast imaging reporting and data system (BI-RADS) defines standardized terminology for describing such lesions and provides criteria to help radiologists classify them. In this work we investigate, which of these criteria are most pertinent for deep learning-based classification of breast masses in sonograms. For this purpose, we use a large, publicly available breast ultrasound dataset which contains sonograms of benign and malignant masses. We generate five versions of each sonogram, which display various regions and focus on several BI-RADS criteria of the displayed mass. Convolutional neural networks (CNNs), with much lower complexity than generally used in the literature, are trained for each image version set. We examined the classification accuracies and confidence of each model. The shape of the mass is the largest single contributor to classification success, this model achieved 89% accuracy. Passing the network additional information about the mass's margin and echo patterns further increased classification accuracy to 96%.

1 Introduction

Breast cancer is by far the most common cancer in women, accounting for a quarter of all new cancers in 2020 [1]. In adjunct with mammograms, ultrasound exams are commonly used as a supplementary screening tool. This is especially the case, if the patient has dense breast tissue, or if an anomaly was found during a previous mammogram or physical exam [2]. Suspicious masses found during an exam can be either benign (e.g., cysts, fibroadenomas) or malignant tumors.

With rising computational capabilities in recent years, many algorithms for automatic breast tumor classification have been proposed. Some studies focused on local features [3] of suspicious masses instead of the whole image. In these cases, classification was performed by means of statistical analysis of certain contour properties like circularity and contour irregularity. Most of the recent approaches are based on transfer learning and utilize very deep networks with high complexity [4–7], like VGG16, GoogLeNet and Darknet53. These models are between 11 and 53 layers deep and contain $10^7 - 10^8$ parameters. A gap between relatively low image data complexity and high network complexity leads to issues regarding generalizability [8]. Although many common measures, like data augmentation, dropout, and batch regularization are implemented to

Tab. 1. Image versions and their corresponding BI-RADS criteria ('×' indicates criterion is not visible in image, '✓' indicates criterion is visible, but not specifically emphasized, '✓✓' indicates this criterion is visible and emphasized).

Image type	Shape	Margin	Orientation	Echo pattern	Post. features
US	✓	✓	✓	✓	✓
CS	✓✓	×	✓✓	×	×
ROI	✓	✓	✓	✓✓	×
CGV	✓✓	✓✓	✓✓	×	×
MA	✓✓	✓✓	✓✓	✓✓	×

reduce overfitting, this remains an issue. Yu et al. [9] reviewed 86 studies, which used deep learning-based algorithms for radiologic diagnosis. Almost a quarter of reviewed classification algorithms underperformed in terms of accuracy by more than 0.1, when applied to an external dataset.

BI-RADS, which was developed and published by the American College of Radiology, is a quality assurance tool, that aims to assist the standardized reporting for breast imaging. It provides criteria to assess breast sonograms, and standardized terminology to describe findings. Using these criteria, suspicious masses are assigned to one of seven BI-RADS categories based on their probability of malignancy.

In this work we investigate which properties of masses in breast ultrasound images are important for deep learning-based classification into benign and malignant masses. This will be achieved by first automatically creating five different versions of ultrasound images, which highlight various criteria presented in BI-RADS reports. Subsequently, convolutional neural networks (CNNs) are trained to classify each image version. Furthermore, we hypothesize, that for appropriate image versions, highly accurate classifications are possible with a network structure of low complexity.

2 Materials and methods

2.1 Dataset

The data used in this work stems from the BUSI (breast ultrasound images) dataset [10]. It consists of 780 breast ultrasound images (437 benign, 210 malignant, 133 normal) of women aged 25-75. Expert ground truth segmentations are provided for each image. All state-of-the-art classification studies that we use as a comparison in the results section, only include benign and malignant masses in their data, therefore we decided to omit normal images from our consideration, to improve comparability. All images were resized to 128×128 pixels and gray values were normalized to a range of [0,1] prior to training.

2.2 BI-RADS criteria and relation to image versions

The BI-RADS atlas [11] describes five main criteria, which characterize the suspicious mass:

- Shape: Describes whether the general shape of the mass is oval, round, or irregular.
- Orientation: Indicates if the mass's long axis is parallel to the skin or not.
- Margin: Describes if the margin (contour) of the mass is circumscribed or not, meaning if the mass is well delimited from the surrounding healthy tissue.
- Echo pattern: Characterizes the echogenicity inside the mass. This helps identify the type of tissue that composes the mass (e.g., liquid, fat, or connective tissue).
- Posterior features: Attenuation of the sound waves posterior to (below) the mass. According to the BI-RADS atlas, this criterion offers little predictive value.

To evaluate the relevance of these criteria for deep learning models, we created five different versions of each sonogram (Fig. 1), which focus on different BI-RADS criteria. The first version, unprocessed sonograms (US), are taken directly from the BUSI dataset, without further preprocessing. We generate the second version, contour shape images (CS), by training a contour segmentation model (details on model architecture and training in section 2.3) on the US dataset. This model outputs images, which we use as CS images, where gray values represent a probability of belonging to the contour of the mass. Contour gray value images (CGV) are the third version. They use CS images as a mask and apply it to the US, to obtain the gray values in the margin area of the mass. The fourth version, mass area images (MA) use the whole area of the mass instead of just the contour, but are otherwise generated the same way as CGV. Finally, for region of interest

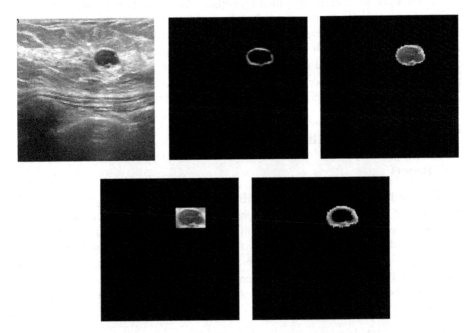

Fig. 1. Five different image versions. Top left: unprocessed sonogram (US), top middle: contour shape (CS), top right: mass area (MA), bottom left: region of interest (ROI) and bottom right: contour gray values (CGV).

images (ROI), a tight rectangular area is cropped around the mass area segmentation. Tab. 1 gives an overview of all image versions and their relation to BI-RADS criteria.

2.3 Segmentation and classification models

For both the segmentation and classification models, we use variations of the classic encoder-decoder-based 2D U-Net structure [12]. Our dataset was randomly split into training, validation, and test data at a 60 : 30 : 10 ratio for all experiments. Additionally, data augmentation in the form of horizontal flip and scaling was applied before training.

The *segmentation model* consists of seven convolutional layers (number of filters: 32, 64, 128, 256, 128, 64, 32; kernel size 3×3) each followed by a max-pooling and a dropout layer. It was trained for 50 epochs, using the mean squared error loss function, the Adam optimizer, and a learning rate of $\eta = 1 \cdot 10^{-4}$. We trained two segmentation models, one for the contour of the mass and one for the whole mass area. The *classification model* consists of five convolutional layers (number of filters: 32, 64, 128, 64, 32; kernel size 3×3) each followed by max-pooling and dropout layers. It was trained for 150 epochs, using the categorical cross-entropy loss, the Adam optimizer, and a learning rate of $\eta = 1 \cdot 10^{-4}$. Our segmentation model contains $2 \cdot 10^6$, the classification model $0.75 \cdot 10^6$ trainable parameters, for a total of $2.75 \cdot 10^6$ parameters. This is a small fraction of parameters, compared to commonly used transfer learning architectures like VGG16 ($138 \cdot 10^6$), YOLOv3 (Darknet53, $65 \cdot 10^6$) or GoogLeNet ($7 \cdot 10^6$). The code was implemented using Python 3.9 and Tensorflow 2.6. In the results section below we will evaluate the following metrics:

- *Accuracy*, which is the overall proportion of correctly classified images.
- *Sensitivity and specificity*, where sensitivity is the proportion of correctly classified true positives (malignant tumors) and vice versa.
- *Classification confidence score* (CCS) is the output of the network's final softmax layer and will give insight to the certainty of correct predictions. Note that this is not a direct equivalent to probabilities, since the network has not been calibrated according to [13], but will provide a relative indication, as to which model produces the most confident predictions.

3   Results

The five image versions (Fig. 1), which were automatically created using our segmentation models, are the basis of the classification experiments. Tab. 2 shows the quantitative results of these experiments. Out of our proposed models, the MA model performed best in terms of overall accuracy (accuracy = 0.96), while the US model performed worst (accuracy = 0.83). Both CGV and MA models showed very high sensitivities of up to 97%, meaning that nearly all malignant tumors were correctly identified by these models. In terms of average CCS (Fig. 2), CS model showed the worst performance ($CCS_{CS} = 0.845$), while the CGV model performed best ($CCS_{CGV} = 0.895$).

Tab. 2. Classification results (accuracy, sensitivity and specificity) for competing methods (top) and proposed method (bottom). [4, 6] used the BUSI dataset, [5, 7] used private datasets.

Method	Acc.	Sens.	Spec.	Model
Al Dhabyani et al. [4]	0.94	-	-	DAGAN data augmentation + NASNet
Chiao et al. [5]	0.85	-	-	Mask-R-CNN
Kalafi et al. [6]	0.93	0.96	0.90	VGG16
Han et al. [U]S	0.83	0.73	0.91	
CS	0.89	0.89	0.89	
ROI	0.89	0.92	0.86	
CGV	0.92	0.97	0.86	
MA	0.96	0.95	0.96	

4 Discussion

Our findings are in congruence with explanations found in the BI-RADS atlas. Shape of the suspicious mass (CS images, accuracy = 0.89) contains the most predictive information of any singular BI-RADS criterion and already results in higher classification accuracy than the full US (accuracy = 0.83). By additionally passing margin information to the network (CGV, accuracy = 0.92) and adding the echo pattern inside the mass (MA, accuracy = 0.96), we incrementally improved classification accuracy. Even though US contain the most amount of image data, their related classification results are inferior to those using a segmentation of the suspicious mass. We were able to achieve classification accuracies, which are in line with, or slightly better than presented in current literature, while employing a considerably smaller neural net than commonly

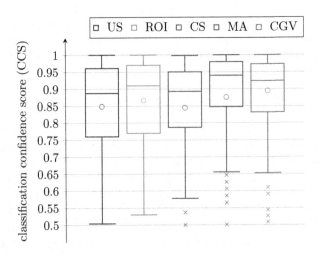

Fig. 2. Box plot of classification confidence scores of examined image versions. Circle inside the box indicates the mean value.

used for such tasks. Fig. 2 substantiates this hypothesis. Models showed significantly lower classification confidence scores, when they were given too much information not pertaining to the suspicious mass (CCS_{US} = 0.849 vs. CCS_{CGV} = 0.895, p = 0.01), but also when given too little pertinent information about echo patterns and margin of the mass (CCS_{CS} = 0.845 vs. CCS_{CGV} = 0.895, p = 0.02). Significance values p were determined with a two-sample Student's t-test.

Further research is required to determine if the differences in sensitivity and specificity observed in this work persist through other datasets. In addition, the hypothesis that our reduced net structure leads to improved external validity, also has to be confirmed in future work.

References

1. Worldwide cancer data, world cancer research fund international. https://www.wcrf.org/cancer-trends/worldwide-cancer-data/. Accessed: 2022-11-15.
2. Breast ultrasound, Johns Hopkins medicine. (https://www.hopkinsmedicine.org/health/treatment-tests-and-therapies/breast-ultrasound. Accessed: 2022-11-15.
3. Li H, Meng X, Wang T, Tang Y, Yin Y. Breast masses in mammography classification with local contour features. Biomed Eng Online. 2017;16:44.
4. Al-Dhabyani W, Gomaa M, Khaled H, Fahmy A. Deep learning approaches for data augmentation and classification of breast masses using ultrasound images. International Journal of Advanced Computer Science and Applications. 2019;10.
5. Chiao JY, Chen KY, Liao K, Hsieh I, Zhang G, Huang TC. Detection and classification the breast tumors using mask R-CNN on sonograms. Med(Baltim). 2019;98:e15200.
6. Kalafi E, Jodeiri A, Setarehdan K, Ng W, Rahmat K, Mohd Taib NA et al. Classification of breast cancer lesions in ultrasound images by using attention layer and loss ensemble in deep convolutional neural networks. Diagn. 2021;11:1859.
7. Han S, Kang HK, Jeong JY, Park MH, Kim W, Bang WC et al. A deep learning framework for supporting the classification of breast lesions in ultrasound images. Phys Med Biol. 2017;62.
8. Bejani MM, Ghatee M. A systematic review on overfitting control in shallow and deep neural networks. Artif Intell Rev. 2021;54:6391–438.
9. Yu AC, Mohajer B, Eng J. External validation of deep learning algorithms for radiologic diagnosis: a systematic review. Radiol: Artif Intell. 2022;4(3):e210064.
10. Al-Dhabyani W, Gomaa M, Khaled H, Fahmy A. Dataset of breast ultrasound images. Data Brief. 2019;28:104863.
11. Mendelson E, Böhm-Vélez M. ACR BI-RADS ultrasound. In: ACR BI-RADS atlas, breast imaging reporting and data system. Reston, VA, 2013.
12. Ronneberger O, Fischer P, Brox T. U-Net: convolutional networks for biomedical image segmentation. Vol. 9351. 2015:234–41.
13. Guo C, Pleiss G, Sun Y, Weinberger KQ. On calibration of modern neural networks. (ICML'17). JMLR.org, 2017:1321–30.

Abstract: Tattoo-Tomographie
Freihand-3D-Photoakustik und multimodale Bildfusion

Niklas Holzwarth[1], Melanie Schellenberg[1], Janek Gröhl[2], Kris Dreher[1],
Jan-Hinrich Nölke[1], Alexander Seitel[1], Minu D. Tizabi[1], Beat P. Müller-Stich[3],
Lena Maier-Hein[1]

[1]Abteilung Intelligente Medizinische Systeme, DKFZ, Heidelberg, DE
[2]Cancer Research UK Cambridge Institute, University of Cambridge, UK
[3]Allgemein-, Viszeral- und Transplantationschirurgie, Uniklinikum Heidelberg, DE
n.holzwarth@dkfz.de

Photoakustische Tomographie (PAT) ist eine neuartige Bildgebung, die es ermöglicht, morphologische und funktionelle Gewebeeigenschaften wie zum Beispiel die Sauerstoffsättigung in Echtzeit und räumlich aufgelöst darzustellen. Obwohl dies ein vielversprechender Ansatz für Diagnose, Therapie und Verlaufskontrolle verschiedener Erkrankungen ist, lassen aktuelle photakustische Sonden lediglich die Aufnahme im eingeschränkten Bereich der zweidimensionalen (2D) Bildebene zu. Wir stellen daher in den neuartigen Ansatz der Tattoo-Tomographie vor, welcher ohne externe Trackinghardware eine 3D-Rekonstruktion von PAT Bildern ermöglicht. Zentrales Element ist hierbei ein optisches Muster (Tattoo), welches vor der PAT-Messung auf der Haut oberhalb der Zielstruktur platziert wird. Das klar definierte Design des Musters ermöglicht es, die räumliche Lage der PAT-Sonde aus einzelnen Schnittbildern relativ zum Koordinatensystem des Musters zu bestimmen und daraus ein 3D-Volumen zu rekonstruieren. In einer Erweiterung kann das Tattoo-Konzept zudem zur Bildfusion von PAT mit anderen Bildgebungsverfahren, wie zum Beispiel CT und MRT, verwendet werden. Die Integration von entsprechenden Markern der gewünschten Fusionsmodalität in die Geometrie des optischen Musters ermöglicht hier die Bestimmung der Fusionstransformation. Der Tattoo-Ansatz wurde in Phantom- und in vivo Experimenten evaluiert. Die Ergebnisse zeigen, dass Tattoo-Tomographie eine präzise 3D-Rekonstruktion mit Submillimetergenauigkeit sowie eine Bildfusion zwischen PAT und CT/MRT mit einem Targetregistrierungsfehler < 3mm (Phantom) ermöglicht. Im Gegensatz zu bisherigen Verfahren kommt Tattoo-Tomographie ohne komplexe externe Hardware oder aufwändiges, maßgeschneidertes Training neuronaler Netze aus. Durch seine einfache Anwendbarkeit und Präzision hat der Ansatz somit das Potential, sich zu einem wertvollen Instrument für klinische 3D-Photoakustik zu entwickeln [1].

References

1. Holzwarth N, Schellenberg M, Gröhl J, Dreher K, Nölke JH, Seitel A et al. Tattoo tomography: Freehand 3D photoacoustic image reconstruction with an optical pattern. Int J Comput Assist Radiol Surg. 2021;16(7):1101–10.

© Der/die Autor(en), exklusiv lizenziert an
Springer Fachmedien Wiesbaden GmbH, ein Teil von Springer Nature 2023
T. M. Deserno et al. (Hrsg.), *Bildverarbeitung für die Medizin 2023*,
Informatik aktuell, https://doi.org/10.1007/978-3-658-41657-7_25

Abstract: the MIDOG Challenge 2021

Mitosis Domain Generalization in Histopathology Images

Marc Aubreville[1], Nikolas Stathonikos[2], Christof A. Bertram[3], Robert Klopfleisch[4],
Natalie ter Hoeve[2], Francesco Ciompi[5], Frauke Wilm[6], Christian Marzahl[6],
Taryn A. Donovan[7], Andreas Maier[6], Mitko Veta[8], Katharina Breininger[6],
and the MIDOG contributors

[1]Technische Hochschule Ingolstadt, Ingolstadt, Germany
[2]UMC Utrecht, Utrecht, The Netherlands
[3]University of Veterinary Medicine, Vienna, Austria
[4]Freie Universität Berlin, Berlin, Germany
[5]Radboud UMC, Nijmegen, The Netherlands
[6]Friedrich-Alexander-Universität Erlangen-Nürnberg, Erlangen, Germany
[7]Schwarzman Animal Medical Center, New York, USA
[8]TU Eindhoven, Eindhoven, The Netherlands
marc.aubreville@thi.de

The density of mitotic figures (MF) within tumor tissue is known to be highly correlated with tumor malignancy and thus is an important marker in tumor grading. Recognition of MF by pathologists is subject to a strong inter-rater bias, limiting its prognostic value. State-of-the-art deep learning methods can support experts but have been observed to strongly deteriorate in a different clinical environment. The variability caused by using different whole slide scanners has been identified as one decisive component in the underlying domain shift. The goal of the MICCAI MItosis DOmain Generalization (MIDOG) 2021 challenge was the creation of scanner-agnostic MF detection algorithms. It was the first challenge to be held on the topic of histology domain generalization. The challenge used a training set of 200 cases, split across four scanning systems. The test set comprised an additional 100 cases split across four scanning systems, including two previously unseen scanners. We evaluated and compared the approaches that were submitted to the challenge and identified methodological factors contributing to better performance. The winning algorithm yielded an F_1 score of 0.748 (CI95: 0.704-0.781). Additionally, we compared the performance of the algorithms to six pathologists. Irrespective of whether the original challenge ground or a newly generated object-level consensus of five experts was used as the basis for evaluation, we found that the best algorithms achieved higher performance levels than all experts. Further, the best algorithm reached the highest F_1 values on either definition of the ground truth, reaching values of 0.742 and 0.748 on the five-expert consensus and the original challenge ground truth, respectively [1].

References

1. Aubreville M, Stathonikos N et al. Mitosis domain generalization in histopathology images–The MIDOG challenge. Med Image Anal. 2023;84:102699.

© Der/die Autor(en), exklusiv lizenziert an
Springer Fachmedien Wiesbaden GmbH, ein Teil von Springer Nature 2023
T. M. Deserno et al. (Hrsg.), *Bildverarbeitung für die Medizin 2023*,
Informatik aktuell, https://doi.org/10.1007/978-3-658-41657-7_26

Limits of Human Expert Ensembles in Mitosis Multi-expert Ground Truth Generation

Ludwig M. Lausser[1], Christof A. Bertram[2], Robert Klopfleisch[3], Marc Aubreville[1]

[1]Technische Hochschule Ingolstadt, Ingolstadt, Germany
[2]Institute of Pathology, University of Veterinary Medicine, Vienna, Austria
[3]Institute of Veterinary Pathology, Freie Universität Berlin, Berlin, Germany
{ludwig.lausser,marc.aubreville}@thi.de

Abstract. Computer vision classification tasks rely on the availability of ground truth labels. Especially in medical imaging, these are typically given by experts and can be of differing quality. To reduce the expert bias influence on labels, commonly blinded multi-expert consensus labels are used as ground truth in machine learning. In this work, we approach the question of how good a multi-expert consensus can be for the example of mitotic figure (MF) identification, which is a relevant task in tumor malignancy assessment. For this, we provide an exhaustive evaluation of all possible majority ensembles of 23 pathologists who independently assessed MFs based on a preselected region of interest. We compared the ensemble against a immunohistochemistry-based ground truth. We found that there were upper bounds to the recognition of MFs by the experts, which were, in our dataset, an accuracy, sensitivity and specificity of 88%, 82%, and 100%, respectively. An analysis of our results revealed cells in prophase and blurry cells to be amongst the most challenging to recognize.

1 Introduction

Recent substantial enhancements in pattern recognition for pathology relied on the availability of large-scale datasets, including high-quality labels created by involving multiple independent experts. One task in the field of histopathology that has shown a particularly high potential for computer-aided diagnosis is the task of mitotic figure (MF) identification, which is a task known to be prone to a high discordance between experts [1, 2]. A high level of expert discordance severely impacts the definition of a ground truth, i.e. of annotation labels generated using the gold standard, which are expected to be of higher quality than the system under test [3]. This is especially true, since, besides potential (mean-free) label noise created by ambiguities in the visual representation or by fluctuations in attention and focus, there may be differences in the criteria and standards used by different pathologists to determine what constitutes a MF, which could also induce a non mean-free bias. This plays an important role when ensembling multiple expert opinions to create the ground truth for machine learning.

In this work, we aim to investigate the question of how statistically robust the ground truth can be expected to be, and how many experts are required to reach a saturation in expert consensus. For doing so, we provide an exhaustive overview on all potential majority vote ensembles of a MF recognition experiment, which allows us to provide tight upper bounds on the reachable accuracy, sensitivity and specificity.

© Der/die Autor(en), exklusiv lizenziert an
Springer Fachmedien Wiesbaden GmbH, ein Teil von Springer Nature 2023
T. M. Deserno et al. (Hrsg.), *Bildverarbeitung für die Medizin 2023*,
Informatik aktuell, https://doi.org/10.1007/978-3-658-41657-7_27

2 Material and methods

2.1 Dataset $\mathcal{D}$

Twenty-three expert pathologists, all of whom were board-certified, participated in our experiment[4]. They were requested to annotate all MF objects in 40 hematoxylin- and eosin (H&E)-stained digital histopathology images (representing 40 cases) of canine cutaneous mast cell tumor, scanned at a resolution of $0.25\frac{\mu m}{px}$. On each image, all experts annotated the same pre-defined mitotically most active region of the image, spanning a size of 2.37mm^2 and having an aspect ratio of 4 : 3.

To generate a immunohistochemistry (IHC)-based ground truth, we destained the H&E stain from the slides, and restained the same specimens with a stain against phosphohistone H3 (PHH3). Histone H3 is known to be phosphorylated in the mitotic phase of the cell cycle and the staining against PHH3 is known to be highly specific for MFs[5]. We registered both, the originally scanned H&E-stained slides and the newly PHH3-stained slides using the method by Jiang et al. [6] and provided the registered pairs to a pathologist with a high experience level in MF recognition for IHC-guided annotation. The expert was able to visually overlay both slides and thus identify MFs in the H&E image by visual correlation to signals in the PHH3-stain. We expect the created ground truth labels to be of considerably higher quality than using H&E alone, especially with regard to the sensitivity, since active signals are much easier to recognize in the PHH3 stain. These labels served as a ground truth definition for our experiment.

We used the set of ground truth annotations $\mathcal{A}_{GT}$ and the annotations by the expert i which we denote as $\mathcal{A}_i$ to create a the set of all object annotations

$$\mathcal{A} = \mathcal{A}_{GT} \cup \bigcup_{i=1}^{23} \mathcal{A}_i \tag{1}$$

We then created a dataset of potential MF center coordinates $\mathcal{D} = \{(\mathbf{x}_i, y_i)\}_{i=1}^m$ which allowed us to frame the object detection task as a classification task of all recognized objects by any expert. For this, we started with an empty set $\mathcal{D}$ and then iteratively took elements from $\mathcal{A}$ and matched them against the objects of the dataset $\mathcal{D}$ using a distance metric of 25 px (approximately the size of a nucleus) between the centers of the objects. In case of a match, we used the newly found object to refine the center of the object in the dataset using averaging of all annotations attributed to the same object. If no match was found, a new entry in $\mathcal{D}$ was created. The cardinality of $\mathcal{D}$ was 7151 samples.

Finally, with $\mathcal{D}$ being fully constructed, we matched all individual $\mathcal{A}_i$ as well as the ground truth annotations $\mathcal{A}_{GT}$ against $\mathcal{D}$ using a ball tree with the same distance threshold as before to indicate objects that were classified as MF (cl_1) or non-MF (cl_0). Using this methodology, our dataset $\mathcal{D}$ was classified ($y_i \in \mathcal{Y} = \{cl_1, cl_0\}$) into 2,631 MFs ($cl_1$) and 4,520 non-MF ($cl_0$) corresponding to a baseline accuracy of $63.2\%(= 4520/7151)$.

2.2 Base classifiers C and majority vote ensembles $\mathcal{M}(C)$

By the construction of $\mathcal{D}$, we translated an object detection problem into a classification task, in which the experts or (base-) classifiers C are asked to predict the class $y \in \mathcal{Y}$ of the samples $\mathbf{x} \in \mathcal{X}$

$$c : \mathcal{X} \to \mathcal{Y} \qquad (2)$$

Here $c \in C$ denotes an individual classifier and $C = \{c_i\}_{i=1}^k$, $k = 23$. The performance of a classifier c is assessed by its accuracy, sensitivity (cl_1) and specificity (cl_0) on $\mathcal{D}$.

Naturally the question arises if the predictions of the base classifiers C can be combined to achieve a better performance in predicting the class labels of $\mathcal{D}$. Various fusion architectures have been designed for the aggregation of label predictions [7]. We focus on the majority vote ensembles $\mathcal{M}(C)$ that predict the class label of an object according to the following consensus of a subset of base classifiers C

$$c_{\mathcal{E}}(\mathbf{x}) = \begin{cases} cl_1 & \text{if} \quad \sum_{c \in \mathcal{E}} \mathbb{I}_{[c(\mathbf{x})=cl_1]} > \frac{|\mathcal{E}|}{2} \\ cl_0 & \text{else} \end{cases} \qquad (3)$$

where $\mathcal{E} \subseteq C$, $\mathcal{E} \neq \emptyset$ denotes the ensemble of base classifiers that were selected for the majority vote. For a fixed set of base classifiers $2^{|C|} - 1$ majority vote ensembles exist. Note that if $|\mathcal{E}| = 1$ the ensemble is equivalent to a single base classifier ($C \subseteq \mathcal{M}(C)$).

3 Experiments

The aim of this study was to derive upper bounds on the performance of majority vote ensembles $\mathcal{E}$ of the classifiers C in predicting the class labels of dataset $\mathcal{D}$ correctly. This was achieved by an exhaustive evaluation all possible non-empty ensembles of the available base classifiers $\mathcal{E} \subseteq C$, $\mathcal{E} \neq \emptyset$. That is, the exact landscape of all $2^{|C|} - 1$ majority vote ensembles was analyzed [8]. No other majority vote exist. We report the achieved accuracies, sensitivities (cl_1) and specificities (cl_0).

As we did not try to learn an optimal ensemble $\mathcal{E}^*$, the reported numbers don't take into account effects of the training process on the ensembles' generalisation performance (e.g. suboptimal choices due to overfitting). The reported numbers are therefore overoptimistic when compared to the results of learning experiments. More precisely, the result of learning experiments can only be as good as those reported in our screening. The optimal results of our screening can therefore be reported as exact upper bounds on the performance of majority votes $\mathcal{M}(C)$ designed for classifying $\mathcal{D}$.

4 Results

The results of the experiments with majority vote ensembles are given in Figure 1. Accuracies between 88% (16 ensembles) and 69% (1 ensemble) were achieved (Panel 1A). All results pass the baseline. The mode of accuracies lies at 85% ($\sim 3.4 \cdot 10^6$ ensembles). For increasing ensemble sizes k the ranges of accuracies decline ($k = 1$: 69% – 85%; $k = 20$: 84% – 86%). At the same time the modes of the accuracy distributions increase ($k = 1$: 80%; $k = 20$: 85%) suggesting that for larger k accuracies are getting better and more stable. However, the best accuracy was also achieved earlier ($k = 7$). An excerpt of 100 most accurate ensembles is provided in Figure 2. The sensitivity-specificity pairs of the screening are given in Panel 1B. Over all experiments sensitivities between 82% - 25% (1/1 ensembles) and specificities between 100% - 66% (42/1 ensembles) were achieved. The mode lies at 65% ($\sim 8.7 \cdot 10^5$ ensembles) for sensitivity and 97% ($\sim 3.8 \cdot 10^6$ ensembles) for specificity. Again larger ranges can be observed for smaller k. Here, especially higher sensitivities were gained. Larger ensembles seem to be suboptimal in this regard.

After this observation, we reanalyzed the performance of the pathologists $c \in C$ in classifying the samples in $\mathcal{D}$. The number of correct predictions k per sample were recorded. The corresponding overview is given in Figure 3. We observed that many samples of class cl_1 received a correct classification rather seldom: For example, 34.1% of all samples received the correct class label cl_1 by less than 50% of all pathologists ($k \leq 11$). 7.0% were not detected at all (Panel 3B). A post-hoc analysis of these

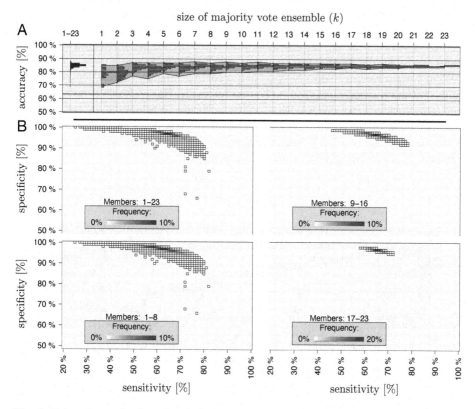

Fig. 1. Exhaustive evaluation of majority vote ensembles. The figure provides the exhaustive evaluations of all $2^{|C|} - 1$ majority vote ensembels constructed from base classifiers in C. Panel A provides an overview on the achieved accuracies. They are organized according to the size $k = |\mathcal{E}|$ of the of the majority vote ensembles $\mathcal{E} \subseteq C$. For each $k \in \{1, \ldots, 23\}$ a histogramm on the frequencies of the achieved accuracies is shown. They are normalized to the mode of the histogram. The leftmost histogram provides an overview over all sizes. The baseline accuracy is indicated in red. Panel B provides two-dimensional histograms of the frequencies of sensitivity-specificity pairs. They are again grouped according to the sizes k.

unrecognized cells revealed MF in prophase in 46% of cases, and visual ambiguities created by either the cut-angle or high similarity with pyknosis in 48% of cases. Only 27.2% of all samples received the correct class label by 90% of all pathologists ($k \geq 21$). This distribution severely differs from the corresponding distribution of class cl_0: Here, only 3.1% of all samples were classified correctly by less than 12 pathologists. Only one sample was totally misclassified. Over 75.5% of all samples were classified correctly by more than 90% of all pathologists (Panel 3C).

5   Discussion

Labeling MF in images is a difficult task and challenging even for experienced experts. Our exhaustive analysis of majority votes revealed ensembles that outperform the individual classifiers. However, the performance of a majority votes clearly depends on size of its ensemble and the performance of its members. Optimal majority votes are rather rare but also occur for smaller ensemble sizes. Robust criteria are required to identify those ensembles during an initial design or training phase. As our current analysis was designed as a screening, it does not take into account potentially (decreasing) influences of this selection process and tends to be overoptimistic. However, due to its exhaustive nature it provides exact upper bounds on the performance achievable by any majority vote ensemble of our (fixed) set of base classifiers (max Acc.: 88%, max Sens.(cl_1): 82%, max Spec.(cl_0): 100%). Note, that these bounds do not hold for other consensus strategies [7], which might be favourable for rating MF.

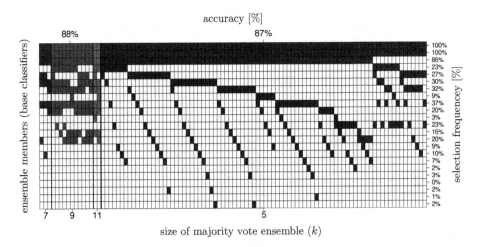

Fig. 2. Top-100 majority vote ensembles. The figure provides an excerpt of the 100 best majority vote ensembles according to accuracy. The ensembles are given column-wise and the non-white patches indicate their members. The ensembles are grouped according to accuracy and size indicated by the different colors.

Fig. 3. Distribution of the number of correct predictions of the pathologists (per class). A: Overview on the percentages of samples that have been correclty classified by a certain number of pathologists in C ($k \in \{0, \dots, 23\}$ correct predictions). Note that each majority vote ensemble $\mathcal{E} \subseteq C$ is guaranteed to fail in predicting the class label of a sample $\mathbf{x}$ if the corresponding $k < |\mathcal{E}|/2$ (class y_1) or $k \leq |\mathcal{E}|/2$ (class y_0). B: Random selection of mitotic figures that were not detected at all. C: Random selection of mitotic figures that were detected by > 20 pathologists.

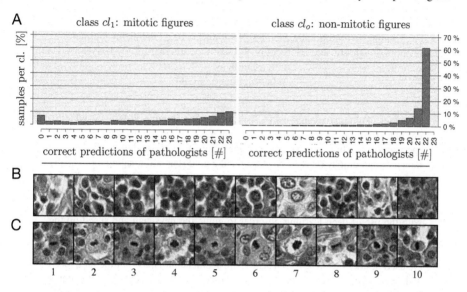

References

1. Meyer JS, Alvarez C, Milikowski C, Olson N, Russo I, Russo J et al. Breast carcinoma malignancy grading by Bloom-Richardson system vs proliferation index: reproducibility of grade and advantages of proliferation index. Mod Pathol. 2005;18(8):1067–78.
2. Veta M, Van Diest PJ, Jiwa M, Al-Janabi S, Pluim JP. Mitosis counting in breast cancer: object-level interobserver agreement and comparison to an automatic method. PLoS One. 2016;11(8):e0161286.
3. Cardoso JR, Pereira LM, Iversen MD, Ramos AL. What is gold standard and what is ground truth? Dental Press J Orthod. 2014;19:27–30.
4. Anonymous. Removed for peer review. 2022.
5. Tapia C, Kutzner H, Mentzel T, Savic S, Baumhoer D, Glatz K. Two mitosis-specific antibodies, MPM-2 and phospho-histone H3 (Ser28), allow rapid and precise determination of mitotic activity. Am J Surg Pathol. 2006;30(1):83–9.
6. Jiang J, Larson NB, Prodduturi N, Flotte TJ, Hart SN. Robust hierarchical density estimation and regression for re-stained histological whole slide image co-registration. PLoS One. 2019;14(7):e0220074.
7. Kuncheva L. Combining Pattern Classifiers: Methods and Algorithms. Wiley-Interscience, 2004.
8. Lausser L, Szekely R, Schmid F, Maucher M, Kestler HA. Efficient cross-validation traversals in feature subset selection. Sci Rep. 2022;12(1):21485.

Detection of Pulmonary Embolisms in NCCT Data Using nnDetection

Linda Vorberg[1,2], Florian Thamm[1,2], Hendrik Ditt[2], Marius Horger[3], Florian Hagen[3], Andreas Maier[1]

[1]Pattern Recognition Lab, Friedrich-Alexander-Universität, Erlangen-Nürnberg, Germany
[2]Computed Tomography, Siemens Healthineers AG, Forchheim, Germany
[3]Department of Diagnostic and Interventional Radiology, Eberhard Karls-University Tübingen, Germany
linda.vorberg@fau.de

Abstract. Pulmonary embolism (PE) is a life-threatening disease for which a prompt diagnosis is important and challenging as its symptoms are mostly non-specific. In the clinical workflow of diagnosing PE, computed tomographic pulmonary angiography (CTPA) has become the gold standard imaging tool. As the performance of a CT scan with contrast agent sometimes can be contraindicated and is associated with high costs, identifying the embolism with a non-contrast CT (NCCT) scan is desirable. We automated the detection of PE in NCCT scans with the use of deep learning, in order to guide the physician and speed up the clinical workflow. We used nnDetection, designed for medical object detection, to accomplish this task. nnDetection gets informed by additional channels which are used besides the NCCT scan. These are segmentation masks of the lung lobes and vessels which are also used for post-processing. In a study with 99 patients that all presented with PE, nnDetection was shown to detect a PE in 71% of the cases when considering the first 10 boxes with the highest probability containing a PE.

1 Introduction

Pulmonary embolism (PE) is the blockage of an artery in the lungs that most commonly originates from a deep venous thrombosis in the legs [1]. It is the third most common cause of death from cardiovascular disease, where the majority of cases of preventable death occur due to a missed diagnosis but not due to failure of therapy [2]. Therefore, a rapid and correct diagnosis can reduce the fatality rate and is crucial for the patient's prognosis [3]. In the context of diagnostic tools for PE, computed tomographic pulmonary angiography (CTPA) has become the gold standard imaging test, as the pulmonary filling defect can be visualized with the help of contrast agent [3].

Current research has proven the success of computer-aided diagnosis of PE in CTPA images using machine learning methods, which is an important step considering the high amount of daily performed CT scans and the demand for a prompt diagnosis [4, 5]. Weikert et al. evaluated the performance of an AI-powered algorithm for PE detection using CTPA scans [4]. This algorithm includes two stages, a region proposal stage, a 3D CNN, and a false positive reduction stage. Evaluation of the algorithm with the institution's test data set (n = 1499) yielded 92.7% sensitivity and 95.5% specificity.

However, the performance of a CT scan with contrast agent can be contraindicated and is a cumbersome procedure. In comparison, a non-contrast CT scan (NCCT) is less difficult to acquire and can also reduce the high costs associated with contrast agents. Up to now, research has only reported on the manual detection of PE in NCCT images by radiologists. The clots, depending on their age, mostly presenting as hyperdense structures could be identified in unenhanced scans, but in most studies, only acute central PE could be detected. For example, Mohamed et al. reported a sensitivity of 64.7% and a specificity of 98.6% for the detection of central PE [6].

As shown, human performance is limited in the task of PE detection in NCCT data as it is not accurate enough for a reliable detection. This work presents a tool to detect PE automatically and in this way, can even excel human capabilities. Other work has already proven the success of AI-based detection of PE in CTPA data [5], whereas we are, to the best of our knowledge, the first ones to propose a tool for the automated PE detection in unenhanced scans.

2   Materials and methods

2.1   Data

The data set used in this study comprises NCCT and CTPA images of 99 patients (60 male/39 female) that all presented with PE. 58 out of 99 patients (58.6%) were examined with a Somatom Definition Flash scanner (Siemens Healthineers), and the remaining 41 patients (41.4%) with a Naeotom Alpha scanner (Siemens Healthineers). The latter, a photon-counting scanner, delivers images with a higher resolution (1024×1024) reconstructed with a smaller slice thickness of 1 mm than the conventional scanner (512×512) which allowed thicknesses of 1.5 mm. To provide the data in a standardized spacing and resolution, the photon-counting data was down-sampled to 512×512 pixels and 1.5 mm slice thickness. Each patient's CTPA images were used to identify the PE and annotate the NCCT image with a segmentation of the embolism drawn by hand which serves as ground truth label for the model.

2.2   Methodology

The proposed method is based on nnDetection, but includes prior knowledge about the anatomy of the lung. nnDetection is a self-configuring method that involves the automated pre-processing, set up of the network architecture and training [7]. It allows the input of several channels into the network. We use the multi-channel feature by additionally feeding segmentation masks of the lung lobes and vessels into the model. Fig. 1 shows the model pipeline. The NCCT image is used as input, from which the segmentation of the lung lobes is generated using an algorithm based on thresholding, as described in [8]. The second part of the segmentation algorithm is based on fuzzy connectedness as also described in [8] and performs the segmentation of the lung vessels with the help of the before computed lobe mask, the original NCCT volume and seed points that are placed inside the vessels by hand. In an ablation study, nnDetection is fed with only the NCCT image, the NCCT image and both masks or the NCCT image with only the lung lobe or the lung vessel mask as additional channel. These experiments are performed to analyze the influence of the image segmentations on the model's performance. Independent of the input into nnDetection, the segmentation masks are used again in the post-processing step, which is applied to the candidate boxes predicted by the detection model. To eliminate predictions mistakenly made at locations outside the lung or in the air, the lung lobe mask is used to evaluate whether the predicted candidate box intersects ("Inter ") or, alternatively, fully overlaps with the mask ("Over"). Another approach is to use the vessel mask and determine whether the center of the predicted box is located inside a vessel ("Vessel").

2.3   Evaluation

To estimate the model's performance on unseen data, we used cross-validation with five folds, which splits the data into five different tasks. One fold (20% of the data) always serves as the test set. In this way, every patient is part of the test set once. To ensure that every fold is representative of the data, the "photon-counting"and the "conventional"data are split into five equal parts separately and taken together in the test set, such that every fold contains data of both image acquisition types.

The primary metric used for evaluating the model's performance in this work is the Top N Rank. It is based on the rank of the first correct prediction that the model makes, averaged over the whole test data set. The top N rank is more suitable for the underlying task than classical detection metrics as it allows to estimate the number of candidate proposal that are necessary for a use in clinical practice. This metric is defined on patient-level and denotes in how many cases (in %) at least one embolism per patient can be successfully detected when considering the first N predictions made

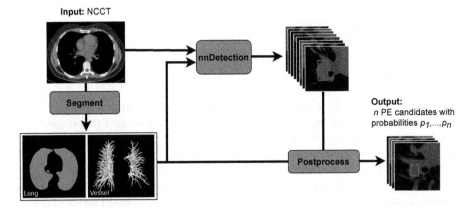

Fig. 1. Proposed model pipeline. In the first step, segmentation masks of the lung lobes and vessels are generated from the NCCT image. The input image is fed into the nnDetection model together with the segmentation masks as additional channels. Bounding boxes around the potential embolisms paired with a confidence score form the output of the model. They are postprocessed using the lung lobe or vessel mask in the last step.

by the model. For example, a top 10 rank of 71% means that for 71% of the cases, at least one embolism is detected among the first 10 candidates predicted for the patient. An example of a top N curve is shown in Fig. 2, where the maximum value of 0.81 is reached at rank 20.

The output of nnDetection is a bounding box around the suspected PE, specified by its coordinates. The boxes are first post-processed with the segmentation masks, as described above, and then sorted in descending order by their confidence score. Finally, the first correctly detected embolism is identified by comparison with the ground truth. The PE is denoted as correctly identified if the Intersection over Union (IoU) of the ground truth box and predicted box is above 0.1.

Additionally, the COCO metric mean average precision (mAP) over several IoU thresholds, in this case, 0.1 to 0.5 in steps of 0.05, at a maximum of 100 detections per image is evaluated, denoted as mAP@[.1:.5;.05]. AP@0.1 is reported as the average precision for an IoU of 0.1 and a maximum of 100 predictions.

3 Results

nnDetection was trained with different inputs to investigate the influence of additional channels, in the form of segmentation masks of the lung lobes ("L") and lung vessels ("V"). Furthermore, the resulting boxes of each experiment were post-processed using the same segmentation masks. The results of the top 20 rank of these different experiments are shown in Tab. 1. To obtain a better generalizability of the results, bootstrapping

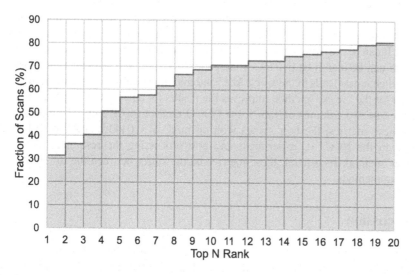

Fig. 2. Top 20 Rank for the best performing model: NCCT and lobe mask as input and post-processing by determining the intersections with the lobe mask. The AUC is 0.623 and the maximum value is 0.81 at rank 20.

Tab. 1. Results of the channel ablation experiments and different post-processing methods. Mean and std top 20 rank AUC and Max with corresponding 95% confidence interval (determined by bootstrapping) and object detection metrics evaluated on the complete data set. "L"stands for "Lobe"and "V"for "Vessel".

Experiment	Postprocessing	Top 20 AUC ± Std CI	Max ± Std CI	mAP@ [.1:.5;.05]	AP@0.1
NCCT	None	.57 ± .039[.49, .65]	.75 ± .042[.67, .83]	.03526	.08859
NCCT	Inter	**.62 ± .036[.55, .70]**	**.81 ± .038[.74, .88]**	.04208	.10368
NCCT	Over	.57 ± .042[.48, .65]	.69 ± .045[.60, .77]	.03612	.08575
NCCT	Vessel	.61 ± .039[.53, .68]	.74 ± .042[.65, .82]	.03780	.09096
NCCT+L+V	None	.54 ± .039[.47, .61]	.71 ± .046[.62, .80]	.03358	.08452
NCCT+L+V	Inter	.54 ± .039[.46, .61]	.70 ± .045[.61, .78]	.03388	.08486
NCCT+L+V	Over	.53 ± .040[.45, .60]	.68 ± .047[.59, .76]	.03220	.07371
NCCT+L+V	Vessel	.52 ± .040[.45, .60]	.67 ± .047[.57, .75]	.03384	.07908
NCCT+V	None	.57 ± .038[.50, .65]	.72 ± .043[.64, .80]	.03658	.08668
NCCT+V	Inter	.58 ± .038[.51, .65]	.75 ± .043[.66, .83]	.03744	.08833
NCCT+V	Over	.57 ± .041[.48, .64]	.70 ± .047[.60, .79]	.03677	.08078
NCCT+V	Vessel	.57 ± .040[.49, .64]	.71 ± .046[.61, .79]	.03726	.08413
NCCT+L	None	.58 ± .038[.50, .65]	.75 ± .041[.67, .83]	.04312	.11344
NCCT+L	Inter	.59 ± .038[.52, .66]	.76 ± .041[.68, .84]	**.04430**	**.11608**
NCCT+L	Over	.57 ± .041[.48, .64]	.73 ± .044[.64, .81]	.04020	.10020
NCCT+L	Vessel	.58 ± .040[.49, .65]	.74 ± .043[.66, .82]	.04172	.10435

was performed and yields the top 20 AUC and maximum values with mean, standard deviation and 95% confidence interval. Considering the top 20 AUC and the maximum value of the top 20 curve, the model with only the NCCT image as input and post-processing with the "inter"method delivers the best results. A maximum value of 0.81 is scored at rank 19, with an AUC of 0.62. The top 20 curve of this experiment is also shown in Fig. 2. It can be seen that when considering the first 10 output candidates, at least one embolism can be identified in 71% of the patients. Using both segmentation masks as additional channels leads to the worst AUC and maximum values. Post-processing with the "inter"or the "vessel"method improves the results for nearly every experiment.

In the last two columns of Tab. 1, the COCO metrics, mAP and AP are presented. Across these metrics, the best values with an mAP of 0.0443 and AP of 0.116 are achieved in the NCCT+L experiment and post-processing the resulting boxes with the "inter"method. In general, these metrics hardly differ between the different post-processing methods.

4   Discussion

In this work we presented, to the best of our knowledge, the first work that could support physicians in the clinical workflow of diagnosing PE using NCCT images. We used nnDetection, guided by lung lobes and vessel masks followed by post-processing. Classical object detection metrics exhibited very poor scores, which is plausible due to the difficulty of the problem at hand. The results showed that for the entirety of predictions, the additional lobe channel is beneficial for the network. But, in clinical practice it is important to have a limited number of reliable PE candidates that predict the true embolism. This is represented by the top N rank. Considering the top 20 rank, feeding the model with only the NCCT image as input and post-processing the predictions with the lobe mask achieves the best results. Hereby, at least one PE could be detected in 71% of the patients considering the best 10 candidates. When regarding 19 boxes with the highest confidence score, a maximum of 81% could be achieved. In this case, additional channels might be misleading for the network, which seems counter intuitive. This behavior might result from the sparsity of the binary lobe or vessel masks which are concatenated to the NCCT image. But, post-processing the predictions with the segmentation masks to exclude unrealistic PE candidates improves the model's performance.

Future work should extend this research by including also PE-negative cases into the data set. This study is limited in its application in clinical practice as it only incorporated patients that presented with at least one embolism.

References

1. Lapner ST, Kearon C. Diagnosis and management of pulmonary embolism. Bmj. 2013;346.
2. Fedullo PF, Tapson VF. The evaluation of suspected pulmonary embolism. N Engl J Med. 2003;349(13):1247–56.
3. Abdellatif W, Ebada MA, Alkanj S, Negida A, Murray N, Khosa F et al. Diagnostic accuracy of dual-energy CT in detection of acute pulmonary embolism: a systematic review and meta-analysis. Can Assoc Radiol J. 2021;72(2):285–92.
4. Weikert T, Winkel DJ, Bremerich J, Stieltjes B, Parmar V, Sauter AW et al. Automated detection of pulmonary embolism in CT pulmonary angiograms using an AI-powered algorithm. Eur Radiol. 2020;30(12):6545–53.
5. Soffer S, Klang E, Shimon O, Barash Y, Cahan N, Greenspana H et al. Deep learning for pulmonary embolism detection on computed tomography pulmonary angiogram: a systematic review and meta-analysis. Sci Rep. 2021;11(1):1–8.
6. Mohamed ND, Othman MH, Hassan LS, Yousef HA et al. The accuracy of non-contrast chest computed tomographic scan in the detection of pulmonary thromboembolism. Journal of Current Medical Research and Practice. 2019;4(1):61.
7. Baumgartner M, Jäger PF, Isensee F, Maier-Hein KH. nndetection: A self-configuring method for medical object detection. Med Image Comput Comput Assist Interv. Springer. 2021:530–9.
8. Kaftan JN, Kiraly AP, Bakai A, Das M, Novak CL, Aach T. Fuzzy pulmonary vessel segmentation in contrast enhanced CT data. Medical Imaging 2008: Image Processing. Vol. 6914. SPIE. 2008:585–96.

Exploring the Effects of Contrastive Learning on Homogeneous Medical Image Data

Robert Mendel, David Rauber, Christoph Palm

Regensburg Medical Image Computing (ReMIC), OTH Regensburg
christoph.palm@oth-regensburg.de

Abstract. We investigate contrastive learning in a multi-task learning setting classifying and segmenting early Barrett's cancer. How can contrastive learning be applied in a domain with few classes and low inter-class and inter-sample variance, potentially enabling image retrieval or image attribution? We introduce a data sampling strategy that mines per-lesion data for positive samples and keeps a queue of the recent projections as negative samples. We propose a masking strategy for the NT-Xent loss that keeps the negative set pure and removes samples from the same lesion. We show cohesion and uniqueness improvements of the proposed method in feature space. The introduction of the auxiliary objective does not affect the performance but adds the ability to indicate similarity between lesions. Therefore, the approach could enable downstream auto-documentation tasks on homogeneous medical image data.

1 Introduction

Unsupervised representation learning with algorithms like SimCLR [1] and momentum contrast (MoCo) [2] have been effective tools to pretrain large neural networks on large datasets and learn transferable representations. However, applying contrastive approaches directly to medical datasets can pose domain-specific complications. The ImageNet dataset contains 1000 approximately equally distributed classes. Consequently, batches with a size of less than 1000 are unlikely to have repeated classes. Contrastive approaches can use this property to their advantage by maximizing the similarity of one sample's augmentations and the difference to all other samples in the batch. The composition of each batch on datasets with large amounts of classes of similar frequency can lead to an approximation of supervised learning, although labels are never used [1].

However, on a dataset with fewer classes and less pronounced inter-class differences, the positive and negative samples present in each batch are likely to contain many repeated classes that are visually less distinct. This work focuses on images of the upper gastrointestinal tract containing Barrett's esophagus (BE) and Barrett's esophagus-related neoplasia (BERN), a domain that exhibits this characteristic. We investigate an approach to avoid the limitations inherent in the standard contrastive loss by not focusing on class differences. Instead, we encourage the model to learn and retain visual features that can be used to find similar lesions. We devise a data sampling strategy to select positive samples from a single patient or lesion data pool and combine it with a masked contrastive objective that ensures negative samples are exclusively from different patients or lesions. Supervised models can learn to ignore input details that are unnecessary to achieve a minimal loss. Our strategy, on the other hand, causes the model to preserve details identifying a lesion. Recognizing and differentiating between seen and unseen lesions could enable downstream retrieval tasks or automatic documentation built around this training procedure.

We integrate the contrastive objective into a multi-task training procedure with a four-class segmentation objective and three auxiliary classification tasks. The learned representations are analyzed with respect to the contrastive objective of improving attribution performance while preserving segmentation and classification performance.

2 Materials and methods

2.1 Dataset

Still images and videos of upper gastrointestinal procedures were used evaluating the presence of BE and collected over several years at the University Hospital in Augsburg, Germany. They can be divided into:

- a *multimodal subset (MMS)*: near-focus view of a single lesion shown in up to four modalities: white light and narrow-band imaging with and without vinegar applied, respectively. Images are fully annotated, i.e., with a label for diagnosis, modality, and a manual segmentation with up to four classes: background, BE, BERN, and risk region. The subset consists of 1007 images with an average of four images per lesion.
- a *general subset (GES)*: less structured than MMS; can show multiple regions per patient, contains near-focus and overview images of the esophagus (see Fig. 1). GES is partially labeled. Most of the images are annotated with the diagnosis and a manual segmentation. It consists of 2073 with an average of 12 images per patient.
- a *video subset (VIS)*: screenshots extracted from videos with a duration between five seconds to several minutes. The bitrate of the video files is between 5 mbit/s to 35 mbit/s. The VIS is weakly labeled, with the diagnosis being known for 20% of the images. It consists of 140k images with an average of 1160 frames per video.

2.2 Partitioning and sampling strategy

In unsupervised contrastive learning, a single image is augmented into two views that act as positive samples. Our approach extends the pool of possible positive samples to

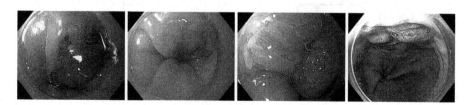

Fig. 1. Examples from a single patient in the GES subset.

the lesion level. The sampling strategy differs for each subset and takes on its respective characteristic.

In MMS, we sample randomly with replacement from each lesion. Thus, on average, the positive set contains images from the same lesion, but from different modalities.

For subsets like VIS where a large amount of data is available per lesion, the data is further subdivided into smaller anchor pools. The larger the pool size, the more underrepresented the lesion is in an epoch compared to its actual sample size. With a pool size of one, so each video frame being directly part of the epoch, the balance between the fully labeled MMS and the only in part weakly labeled VIS would be lost. The strategy is depicted in Figure 2. In VIS, we utilize frames that are uniformly selected in a five-frame range around an anchor frame. The range depends on the number of frames extracted per second. This range can be extended in a high frame rate video where every frame is used. If the capture rate is substantially lower than the frame rate, this should be reflected in a smaller range to preserve visual similarities between anchor and related samples. In GES, anchor and associated samples are selected from the same image, because it is far less structured than MMS and VIS. Hence, visual similarities cannot be guaranteed when both are chosen randomly.

The sampling strategy encourages the model to recognize defining characteristics of the input independent of the geometry. We support this behavior by further applying a local-global cropping strategy. For both the anchor and associated samples, each input is randomly resized to a local size with a larger scaling factor and a global size with a smaller non-overlapping scaling factor. Even if the anchor and related sample originate from the same image, the different scaling ensures a level of variance between the inputs. During training, the positive sets consist of a local anchor to the global related sample and the global anchor to the local associated sample.

2.3   Masked contrastive loss

Contrastive learning requires a large number of negative samples to be effective and thus is a limiting factor to model choice and input resolution. MoCo introduced a momentum encoder that predicts the projected representations for the positive and negative samples

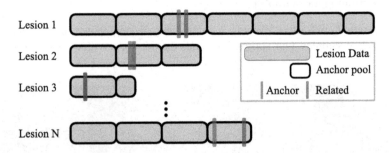

Fig. 2. For selection of anchors and associated samples, the lesion data are subdivided into smaller anchor pools. During training, the ordering of the groups is shuffled; each batch contains one anchor and one associated image sampled with replacement from the selected group.

and maintains a fixed-sized queue of past projections to increase the collection of available negative samples. The increased pool of negative samples enables successful training at the level of SimCLR with a much smaller batch size [2].

We adopt the momentum model and queue for our experiments and introduce the masked contrastive loss $L(q)$ by adding a second queue. Apart from the momentum projections, the method enqueues the lesion IDs during training. Queued samples that stem from the same lesion as the current positive samples can then be masked to keep a clean separation between positive and negative samples.

Given a temperature parameter τ, a query projection q encoded from an anchor image x, a related positive projection k_+ from a related image y, and a set of negative projections K^-, where K^- is a subset of the queued projections excluding samples from the same lesion or patient, then $L(q)$ is calculated as

$$L(q) = -\log \frac{\exp(q \cdot k_+/\tau)}{\exp(q \cdot k_+/\tau) + \sum_{k \in K^-} \exp(q \cdot k/\tau)} \tag{1}$$

The distinction between the regular NT-Xent [3] and our masked loss is the restriction of the negative set to sample from K^-.

2.4 Clustering representations

In order to show the effects of the contrastive objective, we cluster the image features of each validation set into N clusters with KMeans, where N is the number of lesions present in the validation set. We calculate the lesion cohesion and cluster uniqueness rate for each validation set. The cohesion rate is defined as

$$C := \frac{1}{N} \sum_i 1/|L_i| \tag{2}$$

where L_i is the set of cluster centers assigned to the data from lesion i and $|\cdot|$ is the cardinality of the set. Similarly, uniqueness is defined as

$$\mathcal{U} := \frac{1}{N} \sum_i 1/|C_i| \tag{3}$$

with C_i being the set of lesion sources applied to each cluster. Both metrics are bounded between 0 and 1. They are at an optimum if, for C, only a single cluster is assigned to all images per lesion, and in the case of $\mathcal{U}$ if only data from one lesion is allocated to each cluster. Since the calculation is performed only for data used to fit KMeans, division by zero is not an issue in this case.

C calculates the intra-lesion distances but does not take into account when several lesions are close to each other in feature space. $\mathcal{U}$ measures these inter-lesion distances.

In combination, the metrics help to understand individual groupings as well as the larger geometry of the feature space. Suppose the data can be separated both cohesively and uniquely. In that case, the learned representations preserve details and can be used to align closely related samples while being distinct enough to draw boundaries around these samples.

Tab. 1. Classification AUC and segmentation dice for the baseline and contrastive models.

Model	AUC		Dice	
Baseline	80.14	±1.62	63.97	±1.34
Contrastive	79.42	±2.49	63.75	±0.93
Contrastive + sampling	80.32	±2.49	63.76	±1.32

2.5 Architecture

We perform the experiments with a DeepLabv3+-based model [4] pretrained on ImageNet. The auxiliary classification tasks: differentiating between the four modalities,
detecting the near-focus perspective and predicting the presence of BERN, source their
inputs from second and third residual blocks in the backbone [5] and the pooled global
features in the ASPP module. We mirror MoCo for the representations q and k. For the
classification and segmentation objectives the model is trained to minimize the cross
entropy loss with label smoothing of 0.1. During training, classification and contrastive
losses are down-weighted with a factor of 0.4 compared to the segmentation objective.
We train the models with 16 anchor- and 16 related samples per batch for 25 000 iterations with SGD and initial learning of 0.01 polynomially decayed over the iterations.
Apart from the local-global cropping strategy outlined in Section 2.2, we randomly
rotate and flip the input and apply color jittering and random blurring.

3 Results

3.1 Validation method

In order to show the statistical significance, we conduct the 5×2 cv test [6]. All available
labeled patient data is split into two folds, each used once for training and validation.
This step is repeated five times with random assignments for each run. The shown results
are the average per-fold performance of the momentum model without early stopping.

3.2 Measuring performance, cohesion and uniqueness

Comparing the AUC score for the image-level BERN classification and the mean dice
score for the pixel-level predictions (Tab. 1) shows that with or without the proposed

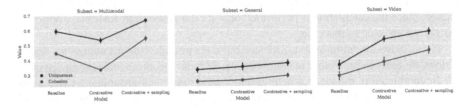

Fig. 3. Comparison of $\mathcal{U}$ and C on the validation sets separated by model and data subset. On
every dataset, the sampling strategy leads to the most expressive representations.

sampling strategy, adding an auxiliary contrastive objective does not result in a statistically significant difference ($p > 0,05$) over the baseline. Although the contrastive approaches had access to a larger data set, this inclusion did not increase detection or delineation performance. Evaluating the performance on the main training objectives suggests that contrastive learning did not affect the learned representations.

Looking at the ability to cluster the validation data offers a different view of the state of the models and opens the view to the results beyond simple performance criteria. By measuring the proposed cohesion and uniqueness scores for individually clustered subsets (Fig. 3), learning with the proposed sampling strategy produces statistically significant improvement ($p < 0.05$) in the information of the representations compared to the vanilla model.

4 Discussion

In this work, we proposed a sampling strategy for contrastive learning and evaluated its influence on the learned representations on an endoscopic dataset. Although the proposed method did not improve the target classification and segmentation metrics, the feature space analysis shows the representations benefitting from the method. This is especially important, as this analysis also highlighted that contrastive learning without the sampling strategy can deteriorate the quality of the learned representations, exemplified by reduced cohesion and uniqueness. On inspection of lesions with low cohesion, there appear to be visually distinct perspective shifts, so lower values do represent the properties of the subset. The four samples in Figure 1 highlight such an example. Especially on the MMS, the anchor-related sampling significantly differs from the vanilla approach. A high cohesion between different views of one lesion could benefit downstream applications. The learned representations could improve image retrieval and documentation tasks or enable the model to be more robust towards domain shifts through the detail preserved in the feature space.

References

1. Chen T, Kornblith S, Norouzi M, Hinton G. A simple framework for contrastive learning of visual representations. Proceedings of the 37th International Conference on Machine Learning. Vol. 119. PMLR, 2020.
2. He K, Fan H, Wu Y, Xie S, Girshick R. Momentum contrast for unsupervised visual representation learning. Proceedings of the IEEE/CVF Conference on Computer Vision and Pattern Recognition (CVPR). 2020.
3. Sohn K. Improved deep metric learning with multi-class N-pair loss objective. Advances in Neural Information Processing Systems. Vol. 29. 2016.
4. Chen LC, Zhu Y, Papandreou G, Schroff F, Adam H. Encoder-decoder with atrous separable convolution for semantic image segmentation. Proceedings of the European Conference on Computer Vision (ECCV). 2018.
5. He K, Zhang X, Ren S, Sun J. Deep residual learning for image recognition. Proceedings of the IEEE Conference on Computer Vision and Pattern Recognition (CVPR). 2016.
6. Dietterich TG. Approximate statistical tests for comparing supervised classification learning algorithms. Neural Comput. 1998;10.

Dataset Pruning using Evolutionary Optimization

Luisa Neubig, Andreas M. Kist

Department Artificial Intelligence in Biomedical Engineering, Friedrich-Alexander-Universität
Erlangen-Nürnberg
andreas.kist@fau.de

Abstract. Data is key to training deep neural networks. A common demand for individual data units is their abundance and diversity. However, it is barely investigated what is actually an informative data unit and how the amount of data relates to the neural network performance. In this study, we utilize evolutionary algorithms to optimize data usage during deep neural network training. We test multiple medical classification and segmentation datasets as being key tasks in medical imaging and found that this so-called dataset pruning removes rather unimportant data elements. Depending on how much we punished the incorporation of data, we found that across tasks and datasets, a critical amount of data is incorporated by the algorithm itself. This shows that future research not only needs to incorporate abundant data but rather relevant data.

1 Introduction

One of the key components in training deep neural networks is the used data. In general, it is assumed and common knowledge that the larger the dataset, the better. Or in other words, if the dataset is too small, the approximation will be poor. Especially in a medical context, it is essential to increase diversity in the dataset to acknowledge the considerable variation across individuals, such as images in medical imaging problems.

However, it is barely investigated what the role or the contribution of a single data point in a given dataset actually is, as well as how large a dataset needs to be to successfully allow generalization. If we were able to estimate each data point's contribution to the generalizability of a dataset, we could not only make assumptions regarding the complexity of the task itself but also on the relevant vs. perceived variance, as well as of the minimal size of a given dataset/task pair. This would allow further insights into the task and the dataset, how we need to arrange datasets accordingly, and provide guidelines for assembling new datasets.

To test each data point's contribution, one may consider a naïve leave-one-out approach. This may be feasible in very small datasets, however, contemporary datasets for medical imaging, such as the medical segmentation decathlon consists of thousands of images for each subset. In this case, this approach would one barely ever get an estimate of the contribution of a single image.

In this study, we utilize evolutionary optimization that allows us to sample randomly from the whole dataset and optimizes the subset through generations. Using an appropriate fitness function incorporating not only the model's accuracy but also relative dataset size, we select appropriate dataset subsets and provide insights into given task complexities.

© Der/die Autor(en), exklusiv lizenziert an
Springer Fachmedien Wiesbaden GmbH, ein Teil von Springer Nature 2023
T. M. Deserno et al. (Hrsg.), *Bildverarbeitung für die Medizin 2023*,
Informatik aktuell, https://doi.org/10.1007/978-3-658-41657-7_30

Tab. 1. Overview of analyzed datasets used for the two tasks classification (C) and semantic segmentation (S).

Task	Dataset	Modality	ROI	Total patients	Total images
C	Chest X-Ray Images [1]	X-Ray	Lung	N/A	5,856
C	Brain Tumor MRI Dataset [2]	MRI	Brain	N/A	7,023
C	Medical MNIST [3]	Multiple	Multiple	N/A	58,954
S	BAGLS [4]	Endoscope	Glottal area	640	55,750
S	Medical Decathlon - Task04 [5]	MRI	Hippocampus	394	13,769
S	Medical Decathlon - Task09 [5]	CT	Spleen	61	5,277

2 Materials and methods

2.1 Datasets

We selected three different medical image datasets for each task, also considering different modalities. Table 1 shows the task and corresponding dataset. We analyzed the Chest X-Ray Image dataset [1], the Brain Tumor MRI Dataset [2], and the Medical MNIST dataset [3] for image classification. The Medical MNIST dataset contains medical images of the abdomen, breast, chest, head, hand from different modalities, namely X-Ray, CT, and MRI. The segmentation task was performed on the BAGLS [4] dataset, which contains frames from high-speed endoscopy with the segmentation of the glottal area. The segmentation was performed by three experts. Additionally, we evaluated the datapruning for the segmentation on two different tasks of the Medical Segmentation Decathlon (MSD) [5], namely segmenting the hippocampus and the spleen. The MSD combines data from retrospective datasets, which includes only the rating of one human expert [5].

We used the images in grayscale, which were resized to a uniform size of 224×224 px, and a normalized pixel intensity to the range from 0 to 1. The datasets were split into train, validation, and test subsets. The split of the dataset relied on the structure of the dataset, whether a validation and test set was explicitly given or not. If train and test samples were given, 20% of the training subset was used for validation. The dataset was divided into 70% for train, 10% for validation, and 20% for test samples if no prior structure of the dataset was defined.

2.2 Evolutionary optimization

Each dataset is represented as a one-dimensional vector with the same length as the dataset size (Fig. 1). For a given individual, we create a copy of this one-dimensional vector, which resembles the individual's DNA. We decide to include each data point in the training procedure or skip it. This is represented as Boolean values: True (included) and False (not included, skipped). For each run, we create a population of 24 individuals with a random DNA, meaning that included data points are random. We set a hyperparameter θ that defines the percentage of total data points included. For example, $\theta = 0.1$ means that 10% of the total data points are included. For each individual, a neural network is trained using the specified data for that individual (training procedure see later paragraphs). After training, the fitness F_i is evaluated for each individual i

$$F_i = \Psi_i + \alpha \cdot (1 - \theta_i) \tag{1}$$

where Ψ_i is the maximum validation accuracy or Intersection over Union (IoU) score, θ_i is the amount of data included for that given individual and α is a hyperparameter that balances accuracy and dataset size. After each generation, the top ten individuals with the highest fitness F are bread. To bread a new individual, we select two random top ten individuals and choose one of the two following procedures: (i) we ensure that the newborn individual's θ is the same as its parent's θ (constrained mode) or (ii) we cross-over randomly the two parental DNAs and may change θ. Next, we apply mutations (randomly inserting and removing data points) using the same condition: (i) for each added datapoint we remove a datapoint to keep θ constant, or (ii) we add and remove data randomly. In general, the breeding and mutation strategy is either constrained (i) or unconstrained (ii). We breed again 24 new individuals in order to gain a new population using the top 8 individuals ranked according to their fitness. This process is repeated for 15 generations.

2.3 Deep neural networks

We mined two computer vision tasks: classification and semantic segmentation. For each task, we followed the same protocol.

For classification, we chose EfficientNetB0 [6] as the classification network. We removed the top layer and added after a GlobalAveragePool2D layer, a fully connected layer with 256 units and ReLU activation, a Dropout layer with probability 0.2, and another fully connected layer with linear activation and a total of N units, where N is the number of available classes. We trained each network for 20-30 epochs depending on the baseline convergence using a constant learning rate of 0.5×10^{-3} and chose Adam as the optimizer.

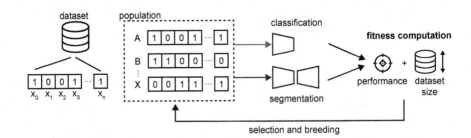

Fig. 1. Evolutionary optimization. Each individual of the total population is represented as a one-dimensional vector of dataset size N with a binary value for each data unit (1 included, 0 excluded). For each generation, the respective neural network (classification or semantic segmentation) is trained using the data provided by the individuals. After computing the fitness of each individual, the fittest individuals are selected and bred to gain a new population in the next generation.

Tab. 2. Baseline performance across tasks (C for classification, S for segmentation) and datasets.

Task	Dataset	Accuracy (train)	Accuracy (validation)	IoU (train)	IoU (validation)
C	MedicalMNIST	1.000	1.000		
C	Chest X-Ray	1.000	0.973		
C	Brain Tumor MRI	1.000	0.941		
S	BAGLS			0.870	0.871
S	Hippocampus			0.651	0.614
S	Spleen			0.942	0.932

For semantic segmentation, we relied on a custom U-Net architecture [7] where we replaced Transpose Convolutions with a combination of nearest neighbor two-dimensional upsampling operations and ordinary two-dimensional convolutional layers. Each bottleneck block consists of a Conv2D operation, followed by Instance Normalization and Leaky ReLU activation. We follow the convolutional filter distribution approach of [7] but start with an initial filter of 16 instead of 64, therefore optimizing a total of 1,373,473 parameters. The final layer consists of a point-wise convolution with a single convolutional filter and a sigmoid function.

3 Results

We first evaluated the baseline fitness of all datasets by analyzing the classification accuracy or the IoU score for semantic segmentation tasks. When incorporating 100% of the available data, our baseline deep neural networks (EfficientNetB0 for classification and U-Net for semantic segmentation) yielded acceptable performance across tasks and datasets (Tab. 2), similar to previous reports [2–4].

Next, we hypothesized that we could use the evolutionary metaheuristic shown in Fig. 1 to determine the data units with the most informative content to train successfully

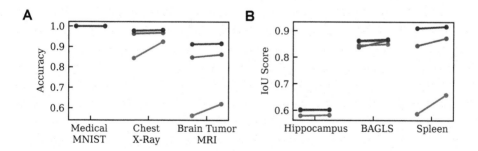

Fig. 2. Evolutionary optimization in constrained mode. (A) Accuracy on validation dataset across datasets on evolutionary optimization start and peak during optimization. Color code according to fixed data percentage (20% red, 40% green, 80% blue). (B) IoU score on validation dataset across datasets on evolutionary optimization start and peak during optimization. Color code as in panel A.

a neural network on a given task by scaling the dataset accordingly. In other words, constraining the training data to a given percentage of the total data, we asked what is the best potential performance. We tested three different percentages, namely 20%, 40% and 80%. As shown in Fig. 2, our data confirms that the more data you feed during training, the better the performance. In some task/datset settings, such as MedicalMNIST for classification and BAGLS for semantic segmentation, even a low percentage can yield very good performance, suggesting that the total amount of data is abundant. In the case of Brain Tumor MRI and the Spleen dataset, incorporating more data drastically enhances the performance. We can further confirm that the evolutionary algorithm is capable to find data units resulting in improved performance (Fig. 2). Taken together, our data suggest the evolutionary algorithm has some effect on the performance, especially when data abundance is low, however, the main contribution to the performance is due to the total data amount.

The results in the previous experiment suggest that the data amount is key for performance. We, therefore, tasked the evolutionary optimization algorithm to select as

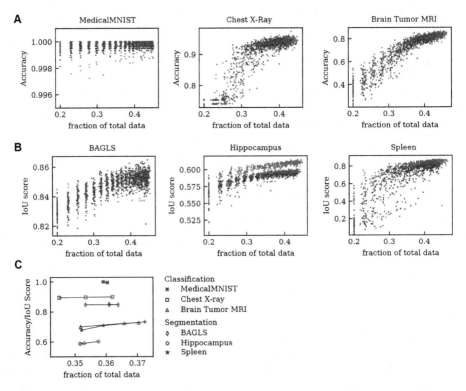

Fig. 3. Evolutionary optimization in unconstrained mode. (A) Accuracy on validation dataset vs. fraction of total data used for training. Color code according to alpha value in Eq. 1 (1 red, 2 green, 10 blue). (B) IoU score on validation dataset vs. fraction of total data used for training. Color code as in panel A. (C) Overview of mean fraction of data and mean performance across tasks and datasets. Color code as in panel A.

much of the available data to perform well on the given task and dataset. Starting with 20% of the full dataset, we allowed the evolutionary algorithm to incorporate as much data as it needed using cross-overs and mutations, however, punishing the incorporation of more data in the fitness function (Eq. 1). Overall, our results confirm our previous observation that the incorporation of more data results in better performance (Fig. 3a,b). In some cases, a drastic change in performance is observed by crossing a critical threshold of 30% (Chest X-Ray, Fig. 3a). Interestingly, the performance across datasets seems to converge around 40% of total data used for training (Fig. 3a,b). When changing the penalty term for incorporating new data by scaling the α in Eq. 1, we are able to lower the average data amount while keeping a constant performance (Fig. 3c). This shows that our proposed method would allow us to select a subset of a given dataset to maximize informative content.

4 Discussion

In this study, we show that we can utilize evolutionary algorithms to gain the best prediction accuracy given (i) the constrained data amount (Fig. 2) or (ii) an unconstrained fitness function allowing us to maximize performance while self-constraining the amount of data used (Fig. 3) for training. Our approach differs from other previous attempts as we are not eliminating data units or instances [8], but rather selecting the most informative.

In future studies, we will evaluate how these images that were selected as training pairs relate to each other and if one can delineate a common representation of what makes an image a worthy data unit.

Disclaimer. The authors declare no competing interests.

References

1. Kermany D. Labeled optical coherence tomography (OCT) and Chest X-Ray images for classification. Mendeley. 2018.
2. Nickparvar M. brain tumor MRI dataset. Kaggle. 2021.
3. Lozano AP. Medical MNIST Classification. GitHub. 2017.
4. Gómez P, Kist AM, Schlegel P, Berry DA, Chhetri DK, Dürr S et al. BAGLS, a multihospital benchmark for automatic glottis segmentation. Sci Data. 2020;7(1):186.
5. Antonelli M, Reinke A, Bakas S, Farahani K, Kopp-Schneider A, Landman BA et al. The medical segmentation decathlon. Nat Commun. 2022;13(1):4128.
6. Tan M, Le Q. Efficientnet: rethinking model scaling for convolutional neural networks. International conference on machine learning. PMLR. 2019:6105–14.
7. Ronneberger O, Fischer P, Brox T. U-net: convolutional networks for biomedical image segmentation. International Conference on Medical image computing and computer-assisted intervention. Springer. 2015:234–41.
8. Wilson DR, Martinez TR. Instance pruning techniques. ICML. Vol. 97. (1997). 1997:400–11.

Abstract: Towards Real-world Federated Learning in Medical Image Analysis using Kaapana

Klaus Kades[1,2], Jonas Scherer[1,3], Maximilian Zenk[1], Marius Kempf[4], Klaus Maier-Hein[1,5]

[1]Division of Medical Image Computing, German Cancer Research Center (DKFZ), Heidelberg, Germany
[2]Faculty of Mathematics and Computer Science, Heidelberg University, Heidelberg, Germany
[3]Medical Faculty, Heidelberg University, Heidelberg, Germany
[4]Karlsruhe Service Research Institute (KSRI), Karlsruhe, Germany
[5]Pattern Analysis and Learning Group, Heidelberg University Hospital, Heidelberg, Germany
k.kades@dkfz.de

The radiological cooperative network (RACOON) is dedicated to strengthening Covid-19 research by establishing a standardized digital infrastructure across all university hospitals in Germany. Using a combination of structured reporting together with advanced image analysis methods, it is possible to train new models for a standardized and automated biomarker extraction that can be easily rolled out across the consortium. A major challenge consists in providing generic and robust tools that work well on relevant data from all hospitals, not just on those where the model was originally trained. Potential solutions are federated approaches that incorporate data from all sites for model generation. In this work, we therefore extend the Kaapana framework used in RACOON to enable real-world federated learning in clinical environments. In addition, we create a benchmark of the nnU-Net when applied in multi-site settings by conducting intra- and cross-site experiments on a multi-site prostate segmentation dataset [1].

References

1. Kades K, Scherer J, Zenk M, Kempf M, Maier-Hein K. Towards real-world federated learning in medical image analysis using kaapana. Distributed, Collaborative, and Federated Learning, and Affordable AI and Healthcare for Resource Diverse Global Health. Ed. by Albarqouni S, Bakas S, Bano S, Cardoso MJ, Khanal B, Landman B et al. Cham: Springer Nature Switzerland, 2022:130–40.

© Der/die Autor(en), exklusiv lizenziert an
Springer Fachmedien Wiesbaden GmbH, ein Teil von Springer Nature 2023
T. M. Deserno et al. (Hrsg.), *Bildverarbeitung für die Medizin 2023*,
Informatik aktuell, https://doi.org/10.1007/978-3-658-41657-7_31

Compact Convolutional Transformers on Edge TPUs

Yipeng Sun, Andreas M. Kist

Department Artificial Intelligence in Biomedical Engineering, Friedrich-Alexander-Universität
Erlangen-Nürnberg
andreas.kist@fau.de

Abstract. Medical image processing on edge devices is the key to local and efficient data processing. In the last decade, convolutional neural networks (CNNs) have dominated and achieved top performance in various medical imaging applications. However, CNNs are limited in their performance due to their inability to understand long-distance spatial relationships. The recently proposed vision transformer (ViT) learns long-distance spatial relationships of images based on self-attention, but these require large datasets for training. Hence, ViT-based architectures can be combined with CNNs to solve this problem. Yet, their use of edge devices has been barely explored. In this work, we investigate compact convolutional transformers (CCTs) and their ability to be deployed to edge devices. Using strategic design decisions, we were able to deploy CCT to Google Edge TPUs. In comparison to a reference CNN (ResNet50) that was also deployed to the Edge TPU, we reduce the model parameters by a factor of 35 and obtain a 7× inference time speed-up while obtaining competitive accuracy.

1 Introduction

Edge computing is an extension of cloud computing that computes data closer to where it is generated.

One major advantage is real-time data processing. As both, data storage and computation tasks, are performed at the edge computing nodes, it reduces the intermediate data transmission process ensuring faster processing and reduced latency [1]. As the data to be processed does not need to be uploaded to the cloud computing center, the load on network bandwidth and the energy consumption of devices is reduced [2]. Since edge computing is only responsible for tasks within its own range, the processing of data is local, so the security of the data can be guaranteed. These features are essential to enable real-time medical data processing and to handle latency and information-sensitive medical data.

Edge computations can be sped up using special hardware accelerators. In the case of AI applications, the Coral Edge TPU provides an inexpensive and powerful (2 TOPS/W) ecosystem, that further has a small size of 5×5 mm allowing fast TensorFlow Lite model inference [3].

Vision Transformer (ViT) is the first model to handle computer vision tasks with transformers [4]. ViT generalization is not satisfactory when trained on insufficient data, because transformers lack some generalization bias inherent to CNNs. However, in the medical field, rarely do ImageNet-sized datasets exist. To improve the dependence of the transformer-based structure of neural networks on large amounts of data, a recent

© Der/die Autor(en), exklusiv lizenziert an
Springer Fachmedien Wiesbaden GmbH, ein Teil von Springer Nature 2023
T. M. Deserno et al. (Hrsg.), *Bildverarbeitung für die Medizin 2023*,
Informatik aktuell, https://doi.org/10.1007/978-3-658-41657-7_32

study proposed Compact Convolutional Transformer (CCT), a transformer architecture combined with convolutional operations [5] (Fig. 1).

In this work, we further optimized the architecture of CCT using strategic design decisions to deploy CCT on Edge TPU. This should allow fast and efficient edge computing to realize real-time image classification tasks. We described the detailed deployment strategy and the optimizations made for CCT to accommodate the Edge TPU environment and verified the multidimensional advantages of CCT over our baseline ResNet50 and for edge computing on multiple medical image classification datasets.

2   Materials and methods

2.1   Compact convolutional transformers

Our design still follows the architecture of CCT with a small CNN called Convolutional Tokenizer, the transformer encoder, and the sequence pool, but changes the layout of each component. In order to introduce an inductive bias into the model, patch and embedding in ViT are replaced with Convolutional Tokenizer which consists of several simple convolutional blocks. In our implementation, these blocks follow conventional MobileNetV1 design [6], introducing the Depthwise Separable Convolution aiming for parameter reduction (Tab. 1). For an input of size $h \times w$ with k input channels, the block outputs a tensor of size $\frac{h}{2} \times \frac{w}{2}$ with k' output channels. Since the use of ReLU in low-dimensional space has a tendency to lead to information loss, which causes the convolution kernel of the depthwise convolution to be more easily trained to be wasted, meaning that after training many of the convolution kernels are empty. To alleviate this problem, we use PReLU to preserve more information. In addition, since Depthwise

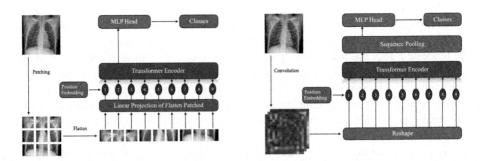

Fig. 1. *Left:* The structure of ViT. The image is segmented into fixed patches, each patch is then linearly embedded and positional embedding is added. The resulting vector sequence is fed into a standard transformer encoder. To perform the classification, a learnable MLP is added after the transformer encoder. *Right:* The images are first fed into a small CNN to preserve the local information and then undergo a reshaping operation to obtain the desired vector sequence. The obtained vector sequence is fed into a standard transformer encoder. For classification, a Sequence Pool method (SeqPool) pools the entire sequence of tokens generated by the transformer encoder, and a learnable MLP is added to the SeqPool afterward. Position embedding here is optional.

Tab. 1. Convolutional block transforming from k to k' channels, with strides=2, realizing the downsampling at the mean time.

Input	Operator	Output
$h \times w \times k$	3×3 Conv2D	$h \times w \times k'$
$h \times w \times k'$	BatchNormalization + PReLU	$h \times w \times k'$
$h \times w \times k'$	7×7 DepthwiseConv2D, s=2	$\frac{h}{2} \times \frac{w}{2} \times k$
$\frac{h}{2} \times \frac{w}{2} \times k'$	BatchNormalization + PReLU	$\frac{h}{2} \times \frac{w}{2} \times k'$

Separable Convolution cannot expand the dimension, we use a 7×7 convolution kernel for downsampling to retain more information.

The convolutional layer in the Convolutional Tokenizer performs better than standard methods for encoding location information. Since the resolution of traditional position embedding techniques is fixed, when the test and training resolutions are not the same, position embedding techniques like in ViT require interpolation, which often leads to performance degradation [7]. Therefore, in our implementation, the Convolutional Tokenizer already implements the feature of location encoding, so the traditional position embedding is removed.

Output tensor of Convolutional Tokenzier is then rearranged in order to be fed into the transformer encoder, using the reshape operation: $\mathbb{R}^{h' \times w' \times d} \rightarrow \mathbb{R}^{n \times d}$, h' is feature height, w' is feature width, n is sequence length which equals to $h' \times w'$ and d is the total embedding dimension. Since Edge TPU does not support fully connected layers with multidimensional outputs, we removed the multilayer perceptron from the transformer encoder. In our experiments, we did not see significant performance deterioration.

To further reduce the computational effort, Hassani, Ali, et al. proposed SeqPool, an attention-based method for pooling output sequences [5]. They argue that the output sequence contains relevant information about different parts of the input image. Therefore, retaining this information can improve performance without additional parameters compared to learnable tokens used in ViT. In light of the limitations previously noted for Google Edge TPU, we incorporated convolution into SeqPool. This operation consists of mapping the output sequence using the transformation $T : \mathbb{R}^{n \times d} \rightarrow \mathbb{R}^d$

$$x_L = f(x_C) \in \mathbb{R}^{n \times d} \tag{1}$$

where x_L is the output of an L layer transformer encoder f and x_C is the output from the convolutional tokenizer. x_L is reshaped and fed to a single filter convolutional layer with a kernel size of 1×1 and then reshape back to the same dimension as the tensor in the transformer encoder. The reason for this complex process is that only 2D convolution can be fully mapped to the Edge TPU. Softmax activation is applied to the output to get the attention weight w_A

$$w_A = \text{Softmax}\left(\text{Reshape}\left(\text{Conv}\left(\text{Reshape}\left(x_L\right)\right)\right)^{\text{T}}\right) \in \mathbb{R}^{1 \times n} \tag{2}$$

This generates a critical weight for each input token, which is applied as follows

$$z = w_A \times x_L \in \mathbb{R}^{1 \times d} \tag{3}$$

By flattening, the output $z \in \mathbb{R}^d$ is produced. This output can then be fed to the classifier head to achieve classification.

2.2 Edge TPU deployment

CCTs are deployed to the Edge TPU in several steps. First, TensorFlow models are converted to the TFLITE format. As the model needs to be quantized (int8 or uint8) for Edge TPU processing, the model was either trained in quantize-aware mode or post-trained quantized. With post-training quantization, we use a representative dataset of 100 samples to optimize the quantization conversion. We used the Edge TPU compiler for TFLITE conversion in version 16.0.384591198 [3]. This compiler specifies which operations are performed on the Edge TPU.

2.3 Activation-based attention map

We utilize activation-based attention maps to indicate the image's local importance [8]. In this work, considering tensor $A \in \mathbb{R}^{H^A \times W^A \times C}$ is the activation of the convolution layer in Seqpool, H^A is the feature map height, W^A is the feature map width and C is the feature channel. Attention map MAP_A is calculated accordingly

$$\text{MAP}_A = \text{Resize}\left(\sum_{i=1}^{C} \text{abs}(A_i)\right) \in \mathbb{R}^{H \times W} \tag{4}$$

where $A_i = A(:, :, i)$ (using NumPy notation), H and W are the sizes of the input image of the CCT model. Thus, the heatmap can be easily plotted on the input image to visualize the attention map.

2.4 Datasets and training

We validated our CCT on three different scales of datasets: Medical MNIST [9], Chest X-Ray Images (Pneumonia) [10] and Breast Ultrasound Images [11]. The Medical MNIST dataset contains 58954 medical images belonging to 6 classes with 64×64 resolution, while the Pneumonia dataset includes 5863 X-Ray images and 2 categories (resized to 128×128 px). The Breast Ultrasound Images dataset consists of 780 images belonging to 3 classes (resized to 224×224 px). The models in our experiments were trained using TensorFlow 2.10. We used the AdaBelief optimizer with the learning rate set to 4×10^{-4} and applied RAdam's learning rate rectification. Learning rate decay was set to 4×10^{-6}. The training was performed on an RTX3090 GPU as a worker with a batch size of 128.

3 Results

For descriptive purposes, we make the following definition: For CCT variants, CCT is combined with the subscript denoting the number of convolution and transformer encoders: for original CCT, CCT-2/2 has 2 transformer encoders, where the number of heads of the multi-head attention mechanism is 4, and its convolutional tokenizer

Tab. 2. Comparison of model accuracy, FPS, and several parameters based on three datasets. The structure chosen for the Original CCT is CCT-2/3 and for our CCT is CCT-2/3 as well. The original CCT was tested on an Intel Xeon CPU with a frequency of 2.20 GHz.

Model	Edge TPU	Top-1 Accuracy Medical MNIST	Pneu-monia	Breast Ultrasound	FPS Medical MNIST	Pneu-monia	Breast Ultrasound	Parameters
ResNet50	Yes	100%	93.42%	87.76%	24.97	23.04	22.72	23.8M
Original CCT	No	99.57%	88.14%	82.06%	87.71	18.9	5.81	0.68M
Our CCT	Yes	99.97%	90.06%	82.06%	196.07	181.81	81.30	0.64M

contains *2 convolutional layers* with 3 × 3 kernel size. For our modified CCT, CCT-2/2 denotes that the model has *2 transformer encoders*, where the number of heads of the multi-head attention mechanism is 4 and *2 convolutional blocks* in its tokenizer.

Our experiments indicate that both the original CCT and our CCT have a competitive accuracy compared to the baseline ResNet50 with only about 1/35 of the number of parameters of ResNet50 (Tab. 2). Also, owing to our strategic redesign, our CCT is marginally ahead of the original CCT in terms of accuracy, with a slight reduction in the number of parameters. Compared to the original CCT, our CCT deployed on Edge TPU gains up to more than 13× improvement in FPS. Our CCT demonstrates an improvement of more than 7 times the FPS when compared to ResNet50 deployed on Edge TPU (Tab. 2).

Our analysis of the model's training process revealed that the convergence of our CCT was slightly slower compared to the original CCT, due to the alteration in the transformer encoder. ResNet50 had the fastest convergence among the three models. We also visualized the pattern that our CCT learned on the three datasets, the attention map and Grad-CAM [12] showed that our model was trained correctly. In addition, we plotted the confusion matrix to provide a visual representation of the performance of our CCT (Fig. 2).

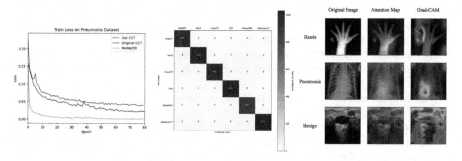

Fig. 2. *Left:* Training loss comparison for three models on pneumonia dataset. *Center:* Confusion matrix for our CCT on Medical MNIST. *Right:* Attention map and Grad-CAM of our CCT on three datasets.

4   Discussion

In this work, we successfully deployed Compact Convolutional Transformer to Edge TPU for the task of medical image classification with competitive accuracy and FPS that has surpassed the baseline by an order of magnitude, while providing a detailed deployment procedure. This demonstrates the possibilities of the transformer architecture for edge computing and provides a complete guide for future deployments of various advanced transformer architectures to Edge TPU. Potential applications include image segmentation and object detection in medical scenarios.

Disclaimer. The authors declare no competing interests.

References

1. Cao K, Liu Y, Meng G, Sun Q. An overview on edge computing research. IEEE access. 2020;8:85714–28.
2. Dong P, Ning Z, Obaidat MS, Jiang X, Guo Y, Hu X et al. Edge computing based healthcare systems: enabling decentralized health monitoring in internet of medical things. IEEE Network. 2020;34(5):254–61.
3. Sun Y, Kist AM. Deep learning on edge TPUs. 2021.
4. Dosovitskiy A, Beyer L, Kolesnikov A, Weissenborn D, Zhai X, Unterthiner T et al. An image is worth 16x16 words: transformers for image recognition at scale. arXiv preprint arXiv:2010.11929. 2020.
5. Hassani A, Walton S, Shah N, Abuduweili A, Li J, Shi H. Escaping the big data paradigm with compact transformers. arXiv preprint arXiv:2104.05704. 2021.
6. Howard AG, Zhu M, Chen B, Kalenichenko D, Wang W, Weyand T et al. Mobilenets: efficient convolutional neural networks for mobile vision applications. arXiv preprint arXiv:1704.04861. 2017.
7. Valanarasu JMJ, Patel VM. UNeXt: MLP-based rapid medical image segmentation network. arXiv preprint arXiv:2203.04967. 2022.
8. Zagoruyko S, Komodakis N. Paying more attention to attention: improving the performance of convolutional neural networks via attention transfer. arXiv preprint arXiv:1612.03928. 2016.
9. apolanco3225. Medical MNIST classification. https://github.com/apolanco3225/Medical-MNIST-Classification. 2017.
10. Kermany DS, Goldbaum M, Cai W, Valentim CC, Liang H, Baxter SL et al. Identifying medical diagnoses and treatable diseases by image-based deep learning. Cell. 2018;172(5):1122–31.
11. Al-Dhabyani W, Gomaa M, Khaled H, Fahmy A. Dataset of breast ultrasound images. Data Brief. 2020;28:104863.
12. Selvaraju RR, Cogswell M, Das A, Vedantam R, Parikh D, Batra D. Grad-cam: visual explanations from deep networks via gradient-based localization. Proceedings of the IEEE international conference on computer vision. 2017:618–26.

Automated Thrombus Segmentation in Stroke NCCT Incorporating Clinical Data

Alexandra Ertl[1], Philipp Maas[2], Wiebke Rudolph[3], Johanna Rümenapp[2], Eren B. Yilmaz[4], Claus-C. Glüer[4], Olav Jansen[2], Michael Müller[1]

[1]mbits imaging GmbH, Heidelberg
[2]Department of Radiology and Neuroradiology, University Medical Center Schleswig-Holstein, Kiel
[3]Faculty of Medicine, Christian-Albrechts-University of Kiel, Kiel
[4]Section Biomedical Imaging, Department of Radiology and Neuroradiology, University Medical Center Schleswig-Holstein, Kiel
ertl@mbits.info

Abstract. The hyperdense artery sign (HAS) in cranial non-contrast computed tomography (NCCT) is one of the earliest indicators of an ischemic stroke. We present a deep-learning-based method which incorporates symptomatic information to segment these findings. Our dataset consists of 114 NCCT scans. We include the entire cerebrovascular system, with most occlusions appearing in the M1 or M2 segment of the middle cerebral artery (MCA). Our method is based on the nnUNet framework. We evaluated the inclusion of the information regarding the side of the body on which the stroke symptoms occurred by encoding it in the second input channel. Doing so enhanced nnUNet's Dice score on the 34 test cases from 0.44 to 0.52. A Dice score of > 0.1, indicating that the thrombus was located correctly, was found in 76 % of the cases. Thereby strong differences in the performance depending on the type of occlusion were observed: for M1 and M2 occlusions a Dice score of > 0.1 was present in 89 % and 73 % of the test cases, whereas the value for the other occlusions was only 25 %. Our study not only confirms the general suitability of the nnUNet for HAS segmentation but also proposes an effective method for incorporating symptom information to enhance the network's performance. To the best of our knowledge, we are the first to incorporate individual clinical information to enhance HAS segmentation.

1 Introduction

In Europe each year about 1.1 million people suffer from stroke, resulting in death in about 20 % of the cases while survivors are often left disabled. This makes stroke the second leading cause of death and one of the main reasons for disability. The most common type of stroke is the ischaemic stroke, which is caused by an occlusion of a brain-supplying artery. Time-efficient thrombus localization is crucial for successful treatment and a precondition of advanced therapies like intravenous thrombolysis or mechanical thrombectomy. An early and specific indicator of an arterial blockage is the hyperdense artery sign (HAS). It is visible in the non-contrast computed tomography (NCCT) of about half of all stroke patients [1]. The HAS most commonly occurs in the middle cerebral artery (MCA), one of the three main paired cerebral arteries. An

T. M. Deserno et al. (Hrsg.), *Bildverarbeitung für die Medizin 2023*,
Informatik aktuell, https://doi.org/10.1007/978-3-658-41657-7_33

advantage of detecting HAS for stroke diagnosis is the non-necessity of contrast-agent. This can accelerate treatment decisions and increase availability, as NCCT is the most common modality and contrast-agent is contraindicated in cases of an allergy. Most research efforts on automatic detection of HAS focus on large vessel occlusions (LVO), generally limited to proximal thrombi in the internal carotid artery (ICA) up to the M1 segment of the MCA. However, studies often do not provide precise information on the location of the occlusions involved. Distal medium vessel occlusions (DMVOs) in the M2 MCA segment or more distal vessels are often disregarded and also commercial software solutions show a lower accuracy for detecting these thrombi [2–6]. In contrast, it is exactly these occlusions where neuroradiologists most urgently need support, as they are easily overlooked [7].

Many research groups have addressed the detection of HAS on NCCT. Popp et al. [8] trained a 2D U-Net to segment thrombus candidates in the entire cerebrovascular system. An additional graph neural network (GNN) classified whether a candidate was a thrombus. Using 634 scans, a ROC AUC of 0.85 was reported. To segment MCA and ICA occlusions, Lucas et al. [4] first created a bounding box around the respective area before applying a 2D U-Net. They used 216 CTs and achieved a Dice score of 0.5. To further enhance their results they trained a 2D convolutional neural network (CNN) which subsequently classifies the segmentations as thrombus or not. Thereby an AUROC of 0.99 was achieved. Tolhuisen et al. [5] detected LVOs by a CNN, which simultaneously processed mirrored patches of both hemispheres to capture asymmetries. They also restricted the input image to the region of the M1 segment of the MCA. Using 187 scans, thrombi were located correctly with a sensitivity of 0.86 and precision of 0.75. You et al. [6] detected LVOs in a binary classification by combining image information with structured patient data. The image features were extracted from the latent space of a 2D U-Net trained for segmenting HAS. Based on 300 studies, an XGBoost algorithm classified LVO cases with an AUC of 0.95.

While thrombus detection is often approached as a classification problem [5, 6], we aim to segment the HAS to provide clinicians with the exact localization. Segmentation further yields more insight into the model's decisions, enhancing usability and explainability. Addressing limitations of earlier studies we include LVOs as well as DMVOs and evaluate our approach individually for the different types of occlusions [4–6]. For reasons of simplicity and performance we want to achieve segmentation by a single-stage model, unlike other efforts [4, 8]. Furthermore, to improve the accuracy of our approach, we investigate the incorporation of clinical data into our model. Information like the body side on which stroke symptoms occurred can be crucial, as it indicates the brain hemisphere suffering from ischemia. Neuroradiologists accordingly consider this side information as well when assessing the images. Contrarily, combining clinical and image data is a rarely explored subject in the context of stroke. While You et al. [6] combined clinical and image features for classification, we are not aware of any efforts on incorporating clinical data to enhance segmentation.

The goal of our study is to develop a deep-learning-based method for segmenting the HAS in the entire cerebrovascular system on NCCT. We thereby explore whether including information about the symptomatic body side can help to improve the model.

2   Materials and methods

The dataset consists of 114 NCCTs showing HAS and was provided by a single clinical site. The scans were created by 5 different scanner types, using 3 different reconstruction protocols. Each CT has about 60 slices with a slice thickness of 3 mm. The inclusion criteria for a case was the term "hyperdense artery sign" to be found in the report. To create the labels, the HAS was segmented in each scan by a trained medical expert under the supervision of an experienced neuroradiologist. The dataset consists mainly of HAS in the M1 and M2 MCA segments but also includes other thrombi in the M3 MCA segment, the anterior and posterior cerebral arteries, the basilar artery, the vertebral artery, and the ICA. The randomly split training/test dataset consists of 80/34 scans including 39/19 M1, 29/11 M2, and 12/4 other HAS. Fig. 1 shows axial NCCT slices of two patients with an M1 and M2 MCA occlusion, respectively.

In addition, for each case, we have the information on which side of the body stroke symptoms occurred. Our dataset contains 46 left-sided, 53 right-sided, and 15 cases with no assignment to a side. To incorporate this information into our model, we created a second input for each CT scan. It consists of a volume filled with ones on the respective half corresponding to the hemisphere, which according to the symptoms might suffer from ischemia, and with zeros on the other half. Fig. 1 (right) shows a slice of the volume as an overlay over the corresponding scan. The overlay thereby covers the side of the scan where the occlusion is likely to be. To account for differences in the position of the patients, the overlay covers not 50 % but 60 % of the volume. If the symptoms could not be attributed to one side, the entire volume was filled with ones. This symptomatic volume is used as a second input channel to the network.

As a basis for our method, we chose the nnUNet, a self-configuring segmentation framework which already proved itself in various medical image segmentation tasks. It was developed by Isensee et al. [9] and is based on the U-Net architecture by Ronneberger et al. [10]. We used the default TrainerV2 class, 3D full resolution configuration, and trained using five-fold cross-validation for 1000 epochs without early stopping. We

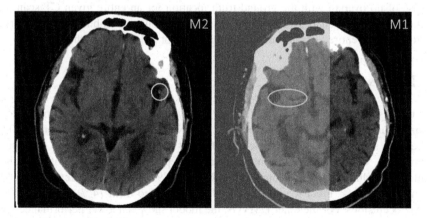

Fig. 1. NCCT showing HAS (circled in blue) in the M2 (left) and M1 (right) segment of the MCA. The second symptom-related input is shown as a grey overlay (right).

Tab. 1. Results on the test dataset. Dice score, Recall and Precision are calculated voxel-wise, while the Dice > 0.1 column gives the proportion of CT scans with a Dice score > 0.1 (n=34).

	Dice	Recall	Precision	Dice > 0.1
nnUNet	0.44	0.45	0.66	0.68
nnUNet+	0.52	0.53	0.68	0.76

Tab. 2. Results on the test dataset for nnUNet+, evaluated on a thrombus level and calculated individually for M1, M2 and other occlusions.

	M1	M2	Others	Total Testset
N	19	11	4	34
Recall	0.89	0.73	0.25	0.76
Precision	0.74	0.80	0.25	0.70

also experimented with the TrainerV2_focalLoss trainer class and the 2D and ensemble configurations but didn't achieve better cross-validation results. We trained the nnUNet once with only the NCCTs to obtain a baseline for comparison. We then trained with the NCCTs and the symptomatic volume as a second input which is further referred to as nnUNet+.

On the test data, the Dice score, Recall, and Precision were calculated on a voxel-based level. We further show the proportion of test samples with a Dice score > 0.1 to give an impression on how many HAS were located correctly by the network and treat the task as a detection problem. Segmentations with a Dice score > 0.1 arguably hold enough correctly labeled voxels to provide useful localization information for the user to detect the thrombi. Since HAS structures are small and variations in the predicted and labelled segmentations strongly affect the Dice score, we further evaluated the model on a per thrombus level. Here each connected component of the predicted segmentation was either assigned as true positive, in case it overlapped with the ground truth or as false positive in case of no overlap. Per test case only one true positive finding was possible. In case of no overlap with the ground truth location for an entire given CT scan, the prediction was counted as a false negative. The evaluation at thrombus level was carried out for both the entire test data set and individually for M1, M2 and other thrombi.

3 Results

The test results in Tab. 1 show that adding the symptomatic information in a second channel numerically improved all metrics. nnUNet+ achieved a Dice score of 0.52 and a Dice score of > 0.1 was present in 76 % of the cases. Tab. 2 shows the results of nnUNet+, evaluated on a thrombus level and depending on the type of occlusion. While M1 occlusions were detected with a Recall of 89 %, the metric decreased for M2 occlusions to 73 %. Precision on the other hand increased from 74 % for M1 to 80 % for M2 occlusions. For the other DMVOs, the model showed a lower performance with a Recall and Precision of 25 %. Fig. 2 presents examples of the predicted segmentation (yellow) compared to the ground truth (blue) to qualitatively evaluate the performance.

4 Discussion

Our study demonstrates the general suitability of the nnUNet for the task of thrombus segmentation in NCCT. Tab. 1 confirms that integrating the symptomatic side information enhances the segmentation model. This is attributed to the increasing probability of an occlusion being present in the corresponding hemisphere. Encoding this increased probability as a second input is effective for this kind of information, as it has direct spatial relevance. The voxels in the second symptomatic input carry the information for the corresponding voxels in the NCCT input. Our method allows the model to directly incorporate this probability at an early stage of processing. We chose to use a second input channel instead of cropping the scans to the respective hemisphere to not restrict the model too strongly and to be more robust in cases of wrong or missing information. Also, our proposed method is simple to implement, as no change in architecture is necessary. While other approaches combine clinical and image features for classification or use anatomical information to crop the images [5, 6], we are the first to incorporate individual symptom information to enhance segmentation, to the best of our knowledge.

While most work on thrombus detection is limited to LVOs [4–6], we included a broader variety of occlusions. The strong variability of the model's performance shown in tab. 2 indicates the importance of taking this data heterogeneity into account and giving transparency regarding the kind of occlusion to be detected. Compared to M1 thrombi, the sensitivity of the model is noticeably lower for M2 and especially for the other occlusions. These results are not surprising, as distal thrombi are smaller and less prominent visible in NCCT. Also, the Others group is comparably small in our dataset, which might lead to a reduced performance of the model for insufficiently represented occlusion types.

Compared to the literature we reached a competitive accuracy [4] while training on a smaller dataset, indicating the efficiency of our method. On the other hand, our small dataset is a strong limitation of our work. To improve the model performance and increase the significance of the results, further evaluation of our method on a larger dataset is necessary. Particularly, more distal occlusions should be included to improve the segmentations of the model for these. Further, we'd strive to obtain ground truth segmentations from multiple readers to enhance the label quality. Since the segmentation

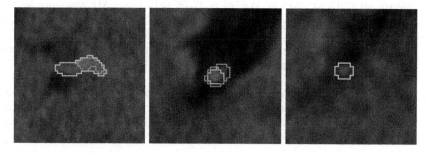

Fig. 2. Qualitative comparison of the ground truth (blue) and predicted segmentation (yellow) showing over-segmented (left), under-segmented (middle), and false positive predictions (right) in axial NCCT slices of stroke patients.

of the tiny HAS structures is difficult, the ground truth is prone to be uncertain and some inter-reader variability is to be expected. In future work, we plan to adjust the segmentation threshold between the background and foreground classes to optimally balance Recall and Precision against each other. This will be particularly beneficial for detecting M2 occlusions, where the model shows a comparably low Recall but a high Precision. As for medical applications missing a pathology generally comes with much greater harm than showing false positives, a higher Recall at the cost of a lower Precision is usually preferable.

To conclude, we successfully evaluated the performance of the nnUNet for segmenting HAS in NCCT. Further, we demonstrated a simple yet effective way to incorporate individual symptom information, hoping to inspire further research on combining medical images and clinical data.

References

1. Mair G, Boyd EV, Chappell FM, Kummer R von, Lindley RI, Sandercock P et al. Sensitivity and specificity of the hyperdense artery sign for arterial obstruction in acute ischemic stroke. Stroke. 2015;46(1):102–7.
2. Yahav-Dovrat A, Saban M, Merhav G, Lankri I, Abergel E, Eran A et al. Evaluation of artificial intelligence powered identification of large-vessel occlusions in a comprehensive stroke center. AJNR Am J Neuroradiol. 2021;42(2):247–54.
3. Olive-Gadea M, Crespo C, Granes C, Hernandez-Perez M, Ossa NP de la, Laredo C et al. Deep learning based software to identify large vessel occlusion on noncontrast computed tomography. Stroke. 2020;51(10):3133–7.
4. Lucas C, Schöttler JJ, Kemmling A, Aulmann LF, Heinrich MP. Automatic detection and segmentation of the acute vessel thrombus in cerebral CT. 2019. Ed. by Handels H, Deserno TM, Maier A, Maier-Hein KH, Palm C, Tolxdorff T:74–9.
5. Tolhuisen ML, Ponomareva E, Boers AMM, Jansen IGH, Koopman MS, Sales Barros R et al. A convolutional neural network for anterior intra-arterial thrombus detection and segmentation on non-contrast computed tomography of patients with acute ischemic stroke. Appl Sci (Basel). 2020;10(14).
6. You J, Tsang ACO, Yu PLH, Tsui ELH, Woo PPS, Lui CSM et al. Automated hierarchy evaluation system of large vessel occlusion in acute ischemia stroke. Front Neuroinform. 2020;14.
7. Duvekot MHC, Es ACGM van, Venema E, Wolff L, Rozeman AD, Moudrous W et al. Accuracy of CTA evaluations in daily clinical practice for large and medium vessel occlusion detection in suspected stroke patients. Eur Stroke Jl. 2021;6,4:357–66.
8. Popp A, Taubmann O, Thamm F, Ditt H, Maier A, Breininger K. Thrombus detection in non-contrast head CT using graph deep learning. 2022. Ed. by Maier-Hein K, Deserno TM, Handels H, Maier A, Palm C, Tolxdorff T:153–8.
9. Isensee F, Jaeger PF, Kohl SAA, et al. nnU-Net: a self-configuring method for deep learning-based biomedical image segmentation. Nat Methods. 2021;18:203–11.
10. Ronneberger O, Fischer P, Brox T. U-Net: convolutional networks for biomedical image segmentation. 2015. Ed. by Navab N, Hornegger J, Wells WM, Frangi AF:234–41.

Geometric Deep Learning Vascular Domain Segmentation

Robert Kreher[1,2], Annika Niemann[1,2], Libin Kutty[1], Viju Sudhi[1], Bernhard Preim[1], Daniel Behme[3], Sylvia Saalfeld[1,2]

[1]Research Campus STIMULATE, Otto-von-Guericke University, Magdeburg, Germany
[2]Department of Simulation and Graphics, Otto-von-Guericke University, Magdeburg, Germany
[3]Clinic for Neuroradiology, University Hospital Magdeburg, Germany
robert.kreher@ovgu.de

Abstract. For rupture risk assessment of intracranial aneurysms, 3D surface model extraction might be time-consuming but supports calculation of morphological and hemodynamical parameters. We present a geometric deep learning approach to segment the intracranial vascular domain of interest in 3D surface meshes comprising only the aneurysm and surrounding vessels to speed up this process. This fast and automatic segmentation supports mesh cutting needed for further mesh processing and subsequent rupture risk assessment. With deep learning on patient-specific 3D geometries, the vascular domain could be segmented with an accuracy of 88 percent.

1 Introduction

Intracranial aneurysms (IAs) are balloon-shaped pathologic deformations of vessel walls in the brain with the risk of rupture, occurring in around 3% of the population [1]. Although their rupture might cause fatal consequences, treatment can be challenging especially for complex IAs shapes or bad accessibility. As imaging techniques are more commonly used in clinical routine, the number of incidentally found aneurysms is rising. To avoid unnecessary treatments of IAs which are associated with very low rupture risk, IA rupture risk assessment is an active research area.

Rupture risk assessment often involves analysis of morphological attributes, e.g., maximum IA diameter, and blood flow characteristics, e.g., analysis of wall shear stresses [2]. While complex morphological parameter calculation based on surface meshes of the aneurysms and the inclusion of hemodynamic simulations show promising results in assessing the rupture risk, the necessary effort hinders the integration of the findings in clinical routines [3].

Aiming at an simplification of labor- and time-intensive mesh processing for the subsequent morphological and hemodynamical parameter extraction, we analyzed a data base of IA patient data. This data base was curated over several years and includes the medical image datasets, as well as further analyses and intermediate results for an interdisciplinary aneurysm research. In the database, the medical image data is segmented to obtain a large 3D model of the intracranial vessel tree. Afterwards, the mesh was cropped to obtain only the aneurysm, its parent vessel and outlet vessels in the vicinity of the aneurysm.

Deep learning has been applied to the detection of aneurysms in medical images [4]. In contrast, geometric deep learning for 3D surface models of medical organs or pathologies has great potential which has not been sufficiently used yet.

Hanocka et al. [5] presented MeshCNN for deep learning classification and segmentation of triangle meshes. They introduced pooling and unpooling layers for meshes based on an edge-collapse operation. The neural net architecture for the segmentation resembles a U-Net [6] working on the edges of the mesh. Yang et al. [7] extracted small vessel segments and segmented them into aneurysm and vessel. They compared several deep learning segmentations on point clouds and meshes. They reduced the meshes to 2,250 edges and the point clouds to 2,048 points. A higher number of points/edges tends to yield better results. This problem was addressed by Schneider et al. [8] by introducing MedMeshCNN, an extension of MeshCNN. Compared to MeshCNN, MedMeshCNN is more memory-efficient and uses a weighted loss function to address class imbalance problems. It was applied to segment aneurysms meshes into vessels, inlet vessel, bifurcations and aneurysm. The area around the aneurysm represented in the mesh was larger than the segments used by Yang et al. [7].

A second approach would be to use a variational graph autoencoder (VGAE) [9], which is an extension of a variational auto-encoder (VAE) and uses various latent variables to learn an interpretable representation for the graph.

In contrast, we want to use geometric deep learning for identification of the region of interest, i.e., the aneurysm and its surrounding, of the surface model. This should accelerate the cropping of the mesh.

2 Materials and methods

To create a data set for the segmentation task, 50 meshes were randomly selected from an internal database representing the vascular area around an aneurysm. To create the ground truth, each mesh was divided into two areas (Fig. 1). Here, the important vascular structure includes inflow and outflow vessels to the aneurysm, which are important for later evaluations. The unimportant vascular region includes all vessels that have no, or very little, effect on the aneurysm. The segmentation of the ground truth was performed manually by experts and requires a high level of expertise, as both knowledge and experience are necessary, since no fixed rules for the segmentation are given.

Subsequently, the data set was divided into 5 folds (40 training, 10 evaluation) to work out a suitable static evaluation of the following approaches. To obtain the best possible segmentation, the two approaches MedMeshCNN and variational graph autoencoder (VGAE) were compared.

MedMeshCNN is used to segment surface meshes. To prepare the dataset for the network, all meshes were remeshed to an equal number of 19,200 faces. The number of faces was chosen such that the smallest possible number would still sufficiently reflect the shape of the mesh as well as possible. The edges in the region of interest were labeled as 1 and all other edges, which should be removed from the mesh, as 0. To determine the hyperparameters of the network, a combination of parameters was used as the starting point, which has given good results in previous studies. First, the number of pooling layers and the size of the kernels in the convolutional layers

Tab. 1. Hyperparameter selection for best performing MedMeshCNN Network.

Parameters		Parameters	
Batch size	2	Residual blocks	1
Maximum input edges	30,000	Number of augmented meshes	20
Convolution filters	16; 32; 64; 128; 256	Learning rate policy	lambda
Pooling layers	25,000; 20,000; 10,000; 5,000	Learning rate	0.001

were adjusted. After a suitable segmentation accuracy was achieved, fine tuning was performed by replacing the crossentropy loss with a weighted crossentropy loss to counteract the uneven distribution. Finally, the variance in the size of the input meshes was analyzed. Parameters such as batch size, learning rate, learning rate optimizer and number of augmentations were not further adjusted from the starting point, as they were determined by the given computational resources and time to train. The hyperparameters are summarized in Table 1.

In the second part, a VGAE was evaluated as an viable option to the edge-based segmentation method. To prepare the dataset for the network, the input meshes are not remeshed, but transformed to an undirected graph. Each vertex becomes a node. The connection between the nodes are determined by the edges defined by the faces of the mesh. To add spatial information to the graph representation, several node features are assigned to each node. Features like spacial coordinates, vertex normal, edge length, vertex angle and face angles describe the position of a vertex in relation to the surrounding vertices. The division into two classes is modeled as a node classification problem. Each node represents a vertex of the mesh and is labeled 1 or 0.

While spacial coordinates and vertex features have a fixed length, the length of the number of face angles depends on the number of faces which include the vertex. To address this problem, two ideas were evaluated. Taking the mean of all face angels and zero padding, where the features vector is padded with 0 to the maximum number of face angels. This results in a feature vector of size 15 or 41 for each node. To test whether

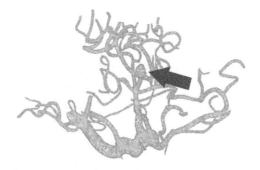

Fig. 1. Example of initial 3D model containing an aneurysm (arrow) with surrounding vessels. The vascular domain that is important is color-coded in red. The vascular domain that is unimportant is color-coded in cyan.

Tab. 2. Results of MedMeshCNN with different label weights.

Weights	[0.4, 0.6]	[0.125, 0.125]
Accuracy	86	88
IoU vessel	84	85
IoU vascular domain	59	61
IoU mean	72	73

edges are a factor in the segmentation task, two options were explored. A constant edge weight of one or the edge length. A dedicated network was constructed for this task. As in the first section, the general structure of the network was first determined by determining the number of graph layers that form the feature vector for the classifier. Due to resource limitations, only one fully connected layer was used for the classifier and a batch size of 1 was selected. Learning rate, learning rate optimizer and number of training epochs were kept the same as in the MedMeshCNN experiments.

3   Results

The analysis of the experiments shows that in a 5 fold test the MedMeshCNN could achieve an accuracy of 88 percent when both labels were weighted by 0.125. With a weighting of 0.4 for label 0 and 0.6 for label 1, the accuracy is only slightly worse, as shown in Table 2, where IoU denotes the intersection over union.

A larger impact could be observed based on the variance in the dataset. With a reduced dataset, where the number of vertices ranged from 24k to 36k compared to the whole dataset up to 159k vertices before remeshing, an IoU of 0.81 percent was reached. The neural network segmented a connected region surrounding the aneurysm for most of the records. However, in some cases, fine vessels in the vicinity of the aneurysms were not detected, as shown in Figure 2.

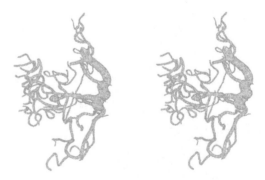

Fig. 2. Prediction of MedMeshCNN (left) of the vascular domain compared to the labeled test data set (right). Some smaller branches are not segmented. The vascular domain is color-coded in red.

Tab. 3. Influence of coordinates as feature and edge length as edge weight inclusion of coordinates.

	No coordinates	Coordinates	Edge weight	Edge length
Accuracy	76	76	76	76
IoU vessels	76	76	76	76
IoU vascular domain	0.03	5	0.03	5
IoU mean	38	38	38	38

The analysis of the experiments shows that in a 5 fold test the graph neural net could achieve an accuracy of 76 percent, but only an IoU of 76 percent for the vessel area and only 0.03 percent for the vascular domain, as shown in Table 3. Visual inspections also confirmed that while a high accuracy was reached, the segmentation was insufficient (Fig. 3).

Further experiments showed that both methods of representing the face angle did not change the accuracy, although the available information of some nodes was reduced. Adding the coordinates as node features improved the IoU from 0.03 to 5 percent (Table 3). The introduction of the edge length as connection weights in the graph representation of the network, on the other hand, did not improve the metrics, compared to a connection weights of 1, as shown in Table 3.

In summary, the MedMeshCNN method was able to achieve higher accuracy of 88 percent and mean IoU of 73 percent, than the variational graph autoencoder method, which had an accuracy of 76 percent and mean IoU of 38 percent.

4 Discussion

Segmentation of the vascular domain is a complex and, as automatic solutions are unavailable, time-consuming task. The main difference between the mesh segmentation presented in this work and previously described aneurysm mesh segmentation [7, 8] is the arbitrary character of the segmentation. While bifurcations and aneurysms are distinctive geometric properties of the mesh, the vascular domain is more complex to

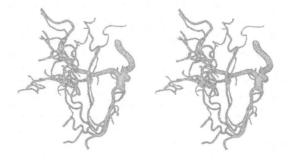

Fig. 3. Prediction of mesh GNN (left) for the region of interest of the vascular domain compared to the labeled test data set (right). The vascular domain that is important is color-coded in red. The vascular domain that is unimportant is color-coded in cyan.

define. Vessels included in the vascular domain and vessels outside of the domain mainly differ in their position relative to the aneurysm but not in shape. The vascular domain normally includes part of the vessel the aneurysm occurs at. The length of the included vessel area is not well defined and there is no change in the mesh itself marking the end of the vascular domain. It can be influenced by the distribution of other vessels along the parent vessel and near the aneurysm and the study goal. Especially for hemodynamic simulations for parameter extraction, where extrusion of the outlets is desired, cutting the vessel in a way to leave space for extrusion of the outlet can be challenging. Due to the limited amount of data, the mesh segmentation process cannot be reliably extended to all aneurysms yet.

However, first experiments show promising results and suggest that automation might be possible once sufficient data is collected. Especially with MedMeshCNN the prediction of the vascular domain is possible. While a variational auto-encoder did not yield as good results as MedMeshCNN, there are various design choices which are not tested yet. The experiments showed that a lower number of features did not change the accuracy and a constant edge weight decreased the segmentation quality. Adding coordinates as node features did slightly improve the results. In the future, other node features might further improve the segmentation with a variational auto-encoder.

References

1. Toth G, Cerejo R. Intracranial aneurysms: review of current science and management. Vascular Medicine. 2018;23(3):276–88.
2. Xiang J, Tutino VM, Snyder KV, Meng H. CFD: computational fluid dynamics or confounding factor dissemination? The role of hemodynamics in intracranial aneurysm rupture risk assessment. AJNR Am J Neuroradiol. 2014;35(10):1849–57.
3. Neyazi B, Swiatek V, Skalej M, Beuing O, Stein KP, Hattingen J et al. Rupture risk assessment for multiple intracranial aneurysms: why there is no need for dozens of clinical, morphological and hemodynamic parameters. Ther Adv Neurol Disord. 2020;13.
4. Yang J, Xie M, Hu C, Alwalid O, Xu Y, Liu J et al. Deep learning for detecting cerebral aneurysms with CT angiography. Radiology. 2021;298(1):155–63.
5. Hanocka R, Hertz A, Fish N, Giryes R, Fleishman S, Cohen-Or D. MeshCNN: a Network with an edge. ACM Transactions on Graphics (TOG). 2019;38(4):90:1–90:12.
6. Ronneberger O, Fischer P, Brox T. U-Net: convolutional networks for biomedical image segmentation. Springer International Publishing, 2015:234–41.
7. Yang X, Xia D, Kin T, Igarashi T. IntrA: 3D intracranial aneurysm dataset for deep learning. Proceedings of the IEEE/CVF Conference on Computer Vision and Pattern Recognition (CVPR). 2020.
8. Schneider L, Niemann A, Beuing O, Preim B, Saalfeld S. MedmeshCNN - Enabling meshcnn for medical surface models. Comput Methods Programs Biomed. 2021;210:106372.
9. Kipf TN, Welling M. Variational graph auto-encoders. 2016.

CNN-based Whole Breast Segmentation in Longitudinal High-risk MRI Study

Initial Findings on Quality vs. Quantity of Training Annotations

Ani Ambroladze[1,2], Horst K. Hahn[1,2], Heba Amer[3,4], Michael Ingrisch[5], Annika Gerken[2], Markus Wenzel[2], Michael Püsken[6], Andreas Mittermeier[5], Christoph Engel[7], Rita Schmutzler[6], Eva M. Fallenberg[3]

[1]Dept. of Comp. Science, University of Bremen, Germany
[2]Fraunhofer MEVIS, Institute for Digital Medicine, Bremen, Germany
[3]Technical University of Munich, Germany
[4]Zagazig University, Egypt
[5]University Hospital, LMU Munich, Germany
[6]University Hospital Cologne, Germany
[7]University of Leipzig, Germany

Abstract. Segmentation of breast MRI in a longitudinal high-risk cohort is challenging due to considerable variability in image quality and artefacts, imaging protocols, scanner types and field strengths, and not least anatomy. Automated segmentation of the whole breast is a prerequisite for quantitative tissue characterization in early detection as well as image-based risk modeling and predictive machine learning. We investigated the behavior of a 2D U-net architecture when being faced with a large set of error-prone training input and compared the results to the training on a smaller but human-corrected high-quality annotation set, both when being used for fine-tuning and training from scratch. Our dataset consists of a total of 876 pre-contrast axial T1 weighted MRI volumes from 166 subjects acquired between 2006 and 2021 in a longitudinal high-risk breast cancer screening cohort study. All images were previously segmented using a fully automated heuristic algorithm, resulting in error-prone segmentation masks, which were used in an initial 'human-free' experiment. We randomly separated on a per-subject level 102 volumes from 23 subjects, for which an expert radiologist manually corrected these segmentation masks, providing the basis for the additional two experiments. Our results indicate a subclass of input errors can be compensated for by the regularization capacity of standard deep convolutional neural networks while other errors are learnt or even newly introduced. In particular, tissue boundaries in axial directions were missed in our experiment. In the inner region, the median Dice coefficient of our fine-tuning U-net exceeded 98% at a reasonable robustness and consistency, which is promising given the simplicity of our approach. Future work will address efficient learning schemes, aiming at boosting the segmentation quality with minimal human input, and the boundary issue.

1 Introduction

Breast MRI is an essential tool for breast cancer care and prevention due to its superior sensitivity. Automated and quantitative assessment of breast MRI strongly benefits from an accurate automatic breast tissue segmentation, serving as prerequisite for more detailed analysis steps. Relevant quantitative breast tissue parameters consist of, e.g., the amount and structure of dense fibroglandular tissue [1, 2] or background parenchymal enhancement [3]. However, breast MRI sequences and image quality are variable both across and within sites. Often, different scanners are in use and MRI methodology continues to evolve over time. As a consequence, in particular in longitudinal studies, the development of a robust automated breast MRI tissue analysis method is challenging.

We base our work on a previously published algorithm by Wang et al. [4], which was designed in a rather simple, heuristic fashion to segment the breast tissue for axial non-fat-saturated (non-FS) T1 weighted (T1w) breast MRI. We follow the hypothesis that a suitable U-net can improve the robustness especially in anatomical variable situations and in studies with varying image quality (cf. Fig. 2). Anatomically, the frontal pectoral muscle interface in case of dense breast represents one of the main segmentation challenges, besides significant inter-subject variability.

Existing methods often comprise heuristic approaches [2–8], model- or atlas-based [9–11], but also machine-learning and deep learning-based methods [1, 8, 12, 13].

2   Materials and methods

Our dataset includes a total of 876 axial, non-FS T1w breast MRI volumes from 166 subjects (average: 5.3 acquisitions per subject) obtained in a high-risk program from 2006 to 2021. During that time, different MR scanners were used for breast imaging comprising several 1.5T closed systems and one 1.0T open MRI. Sequences used in our dataset are, e.g., dynamic TFE, FFE, HR SENSE, and dynamic Dixon.

The image resolution ranged from 0.47x0.47 to 0.70x0.70 mm^2, and the slice thickness was 1.5 mm in most cases, plus some with 2.5 mm. We applied a slice-wise resampling to the average pixel size of 0.64x0.64 mm^2 using a Lanczos-3 filter, and linear (2;98) percentile gray-value normalization to an 8-bit target range of (0;255) for all volumes. The number of slices was unchanged from the original DICOM series.

Data was randomized following a strict per-subject scheme. Subjects were randomly allocated to three groups, each holding a predefined number of subjects: training set (128 subjects with 694 volumes), validation set (15 subjects with 80 volumes), and test set (23 subjects with 102 volumes).

For all training, validation, and test cases, we had initial breast masks available, generated using a previously published heuristic, fully-automated segmentation algorithm [4]. The resulting automated breast masks for the training and validation sets, despite being error-prone in many cases, were used as input for training a level-5 2D U-net (symbol 'A' in Fig. 1) with 32 3x3 base filters and random-weight initialization. Training parameters were 92x92 padding, 228x228 patch size, batch normalization, 500 validation batch size, 25% dropout, Dice loss, 10^{-4} learning rate, plus data augmentation including random transformations (shifting, rotations, scaling, x-flipping).

Then, for the 102 volumes of our 23 test subjects, an expert radiologist manually corrected all initially generated automated breast masks using brush drawing and interpolation tools of a web-based annotation toolkit until an acceptable reference mask was achieved on all slices. The test set with these corrected annotations were used in a strict per-subject 5-fold cross-validation mode for unbiased training of further U-nets (symbols 'B' and 'C') using the same architecture and training parameters as above. Consequently, for each fold, we used data from 16 or 17 subjects for training, from 2 subjects for validation, and tested the resulting network on the data from the 4 or 5 remaining subjects, respectively. We performed this cross-validation twice with different weight initialization: Once starting from the pre-trained weights of the network 'A' (cf. above). This fine-tuning approach is registered with symbol 'B'. And once with random weight initialization ('C').

3 Results

Our first experiment ('A'), which was fully based on automated training and validation masks of 774 MR volumes from 143 subjects, followed the hypothesis that a U-net would be able to correct for occasional errors in the training material, if trained on a sufficiently large dataset. The third experiment ('C') provides the counterpart, with training and testing being performed on subsets of the test set of experiment 'A'. Due to the relatively small size of this high-quality data set, we performed 5-fold cross-validation, as described above. The procedure for 'B' is identical to 'C', but conducted as fine-tuning with weights initialized from the best network configuration resulting from experiment 'A'.

In order to discriminate errors made in particular in the challenging pectoral muscle region from those in the outer boundary regions in lateral and axial direction, we defined in a pragmatic ad-hoc manner a so-called 'inner region', where we removed for all test cases the cranial (upper), caudal (lower), and lateral (left and right) 20% from the 3D bounding box around all voxels annotated by our expert radiologist. We label the

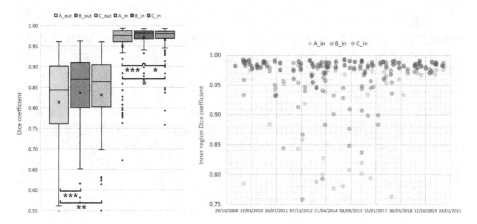

Fig. 1. Left: Box plots for three different U-net configurations 'A', 'B', and 'C' (cf. text body) of Dice coefficients measured on test set vs. corrected reference masks, both for outer region (first three bars, 'out') and inner region (second three bars, 'in'). The two-tailed Wilcoxon signed-rank test showed significance at $p<10^{-5}$ (***), $p<0.001$ (**), and $p<0.01$ (*), respectively. Right: Scatter plot of Dice coefficients (inner region) over acquisition date for all 102 test cases.

remainder of the volumes 'outer region', where it is even for humans challenging to agree on reproducible cutoff lines in lateral and axial directions (cf. Fig. 2 c–e).

We measured Dice coefficients versus the expert reference masks for all 102 test volumes in the three experiments. Fig. 1 (left) summarizes these results as box and whisker plots with indicated first and third quartiles, median, and average values, plus outliers. A largely varying quality with a median Dice in the range of 0.84–0.88 can be observed for the outer region evaluation. The similarity in the inner region, which was the main focus of our work due to the importance of the pectoral muscle interface, is much higher with median Dice scores around 0.98. Significance levels between the three experiments are provided in the chart. Fig. 1 (right) shows how the inner region Dice scores on the test cases are distributed over acquisition date for all three experiments.

4 Discussion

One motivation for our work was to compare the training on a large but error-prone dataset ('A') to a smaller but high-quality dataset ('C'). The image number ratio between these two was roughly 9:1. But still, the smaller dataset outperformed the larger due to

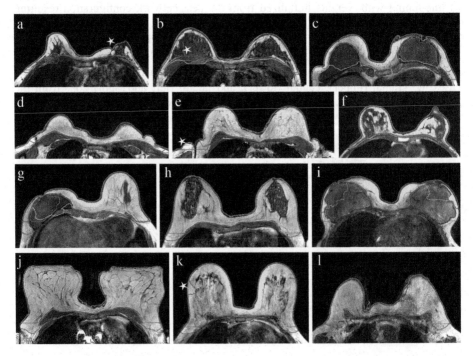

Fig. 2. Segmentations for 12 example test images, four contours each: Expert reference contour (green region), automated contours [4] (cf. input to experiment 'A', pale blue), U-net outputs from 'A' (auto-training, yellow) and 'B' (fine-tuning, pink). (Contours 'C' omitted due to close proximity to 'B'.) These examples highlight the variability of our dataset with anatomic anomalies (a), dense breast tissue (a, b, f), large size (h, j, k), small size (a, f), and implants (c, g, i).

the higher quality of the expert-corrected training masks. This difference was significant at p<0.001 for the outer and p<0.01 for the inner region, respectively (cf. Fig. 1 left). Having a closer look at some of the datasets in Fig. 2, larger errors of the automated mask generator (blue lines) occurred in unusual situations such as implants (Subfig. c, g, and i) and in lateral directions around the axilla (d and e). It is therefore not surprising that such problems are also not well solved by the network 'A' solely trained on these error-prone masks. The hypothesized error-correction ability was observed only to a limited extent in our experiment 'A'.

In order to combine the two experiments, we designed a simple fine-tuning approach, where the cross-validation networks trained on expert annotations were initialized with the best weight configuration from 'A'. While in the outer region, only a slight (non-significant at p<0.1) improvement was found, this fine-tuning was able to outperform the networks trained on the corrected data alone significantly in the inner region (p<0.01). In addition, the number of outliers could be greatly reduced (cf. Fig. 1 left and right).

Given the vanilla neural network design and the difficulty of the task, the anatomical consistency in experiments 'B' and 'C' on the unseen test data was rather impressive. The posterior breast tissue boundary was matched well in many cases, even in case of implants. However, a number of occasional segmentation errors need to be carefully examined (cf. asterisk symbols in Fig. 2 b and k). We found that these tend to occur in large breasts (j and k) and very dense breast tissue (b), which could be due to a too small effective receptive field, which could be solved by increasing the target voxel size or adapting the network architecture.

Our preliminary findings indicate some classes of anatomical errors contained in the input masks can be compensated based on the consistency principle within deep neural network learning. For the particular problem of the outer boundaries in axial directions, no solution was found here. If no breast tissue was seen anymore on the given slice, the 2D U-nets probably suffered from a lack of information. We hypothesize that the axial boundaries would be segmented in a similarly robust fashion as the lateral boundaries with the use of 3D U-nets or orthogonal 2D ensembles instead of axial 2D alone.

5   Conclusion and future work

We conducted experiments on a longitudinal clinical-grade breast MRI dataset with 876 volumes from 166 subjects in three different learning paradigms: auto-trained on a large dataset, expert-supervised on a small dataset, and fine-tuning combining the two. Despite its simplicity, we found in particular the fine-tuning approach to perform well in the important pectoral muscle delineation. Even with implants, a good segmentation quality was achieved. The robustness of the method is also notable given the longitudinal nature of our dataset, containing data from different scanners and protocols, with significant anatomical variability, acquired over more than 12 years. Compared to most existing papers, our work comprised a higher number of cases, both for training and for testing, and probably a higher level of difficulty due to the longitudinal nature of the dataset. The median Dice of over 98% in the inner region is promising for addressing the extraction of breast tissue related predictive imaging biomarkers. We also need to investigate how accurate a segmentation needs to be for different clinical applications [2].

In our future research, we will continue to evaluate the error sub-classes and their relation to the error-correction ability of segmentation networks, also depending on the chosen network architecture and learning strategy. Moreover, we will investigate to what extent a few manual corrections on difficult cases could further improve the segmentation performance and compare different weakly-supervised training and hybrid learning approaches with mixed input quality, including inter-reader variability. Not least, the segmentation of fat-suppressed scans, which becomes increasingly important in multicenter real-world data evaluations, can be achieved through deformable image registration against a non-FS scan, if both were acquired, or transfer learning, similar to the work by Zhang et al. [13].

Acknowledgement. Partially funded by DFG SPP 2177.

References

1. Ma X, Wang J, Zheng X, et al. Automated fibroglandular tissue segmentation in breast MRI using generative adversarial networks. Phys Med Biol. 2020;65(10):105006.
2. Doran SJ, Hipwell JH, Denholm R, et al. Breast MRI segmentation for density estimation: do different methods give the same results and how much do differences matter? Med Phys. 2017;44(9):4573–92.
3. Niell BL, Abdalah M, Stringfield O, et al. Quantitative measures of background parenchymal enhancement predict breast cancer risk. Am J Radiol. 2021;217(1):64–75.
4. Wang L, Platel B, Ivanovskaya T, et al. Fully automatic breast segmentation in 3D breast MRI. Proc. IEEE Int Symposium Biomed Imaging (ISBI). 2012:1024–27.
5. Pandey D, Yin X, Wang H, et al. Automatic and fast segmentation of breast region-of-interest (ROI) and density in MRIs. Heliyon. 2018;4(12):e01042.
6. Thakran S, Chatterjee S, Singhal M, et al. Automatic outer and inner breast tissue segmentation using multi-parametric MRI images of breast tumor patients. PLoS One. 2018;13(1):e0190348.
7. Giannini V, Vignati A, Morra L, et al. A fully automatic algorithm for segmentation of the breasts in DCE-MR images. Annu Int Conf IEEE Eng Med Biol Soc. 2010:3146–49.
8. Verburg E, Wolterink JM, Waard SN de, et al. Knowledge-based and deep learning-based automated chest wall segmentation in magnetic resonance images of extremely dense breasts. Med Phys. 2019;46(10):4405–16.
9. Fooladivanda A, Shokouhi SB, Ahmadinejad N. Localized-atlas-based segmentation of breast MRI in a decision-making framework. Australas Phys Eng Sci Med. 2017;40(1):69–84.
10. Lin M, Chen JH, Wang X, et al. Template-based automatic breast segmentation on MRI by excluding the chest region. Med Phys. 2013;40(12):122301.
11. Gubern-Mérida A, Kallenberg M, Martí R, Karssemeijer N. Segmentation of the pectoral muscle in breast MRI using atlas-based approaches. Proc. Med Image Comput Comput Assist Interv (MICCAI). Vol. 15. (Pt 2). Springer, 2012:371–78.
12. Wang Y, Morrell G, Heibrun ME, et al. 3D multi-parametric breast MRI segmentation using hierarchical support vector machine with coil sensitivity correction. Acad Radiol. 2013;20(2):137–47.
13. Zhang Y, Chan S, Chen JH, et al. Development of U-Net breast density segmentation method for Fat-Sat MR images using transfer learning based on Non-fat-sat model. J Digit Imaging. 2021;34(4):877–87.

Automatic Lung Nodule Segmentation in CT Imaging using an Improved 3D-Res2Unet

Pavan Tummala, Georg Hille, Sylvia Saalfeld

Department of Simulation and Graphics, Faculty of Computer Science, University of Magdeburg, Germany
`georg.hille@ovgu.de`

Abstract. Lung cancer represents one of the most common and lethal types of cancerous pathologies and lung nodules are an early indicator for pulmonary cancer. Hence, a precise and reliable segmentation of lung nodules could enhance early diagnosis and therapy and thus, increase patients' survival rates. This work proposes a modified 3D-Res2Unet, combining an Unet-style neural network architecture with residual blocks and attention mechanisms. This network was tested on the publicly available LUNA16 CT dataset and achieved on average 91.27 ± 6.49 %. Therefore, the proposed method indicates state-of-the-art performance and could represent an important tool for early diagnosis of lung cancer.

1 Introduction

Among cancer related deaths per year, lung cancer represents by far the most common cause for the death of cancer patients [1]. One reason for the high morbidity lies in the mostly non-symptomatic early stages of the disease resulting in unnoticed growth, that leads to delayed diagnosis in later stages and thus, valuable treatment time has passed. Lung cancer is commonly found in the form of malignant lung nodules, which are among the leading radiological indicators. Since the malignancy depends on their size, accurate and early identification is of utmost importance. Therefore, a computed tomography (CT)-aided lung nodule segmentation has the great potential too improve early diagnosis and treatment of lung cancer [2]. However, the identification and segmentation are highly challenging due to the vast shape and size variability, as well as the heterogeneous image signals of adjacent tissue. Traditionally, lung nodule segmentation has been performed manually by trained clinical experts, who must carefully review and annotate each scan. However, this is a time-consuming and subjective process and may lead to inconsistencies in the annotations. In addition, manual annotations represent a significant workload for medical professionals, and may not be feasible for large datasets. To address these challenges, image processing methods were applied with varying degree of automation and user interaction. Besides more traditional model-based approaches [3], fully automatic deep learning-based methods have become increasingly popular in recent years. These methods exclusively or largely use convolutional neural networks (CNNs) to automatically learn and extract features from 2D or 3D lung images, e.g., from publicly available databases, achieving an increasingly better accuracy [4–8]. This work proposes a deep learning-based approach for lung nodule segmentation in CT imaging. For this

© Der/die Autor(en), exklusiv lizenziert an
Springer Fachmedien Wiesbaden GmbH, ein Teil von Springer Nature 2023
T. M. Deserno et al. (Hrsg.), *Bildverarbeitung für die Medizin 2023*,
Informatik aktuell, https://doi.org/10.1007/978-3-658-41657-7_36

purpose, a Unet-style architecture was combined with residual blocks and attention mechanisms in order to accurately segment lung nodules of various sizes and shapes. The presented method was trained and tested, along with three additionally implemented networks on the LUNA16 CT dataset [9]. Approaches with a reasonable segmentation accuracy have the potential to reduce the workload of clinicians, save valuable time in clinical practise and objectify the outcome of such radiological annotations. But most importantly, it could support early detection of lung nodules, which lead to early treatment with benefits for patients' life expectancy.

2   Material and methods

2.1   Image data

For this work, data of the LUng Nodule Analysis 2016 (LUNA16) challenge [9] established by the NIH and NCI of the United States was primarily used. This challenge provided a dataset comprised of 888 3D chest scans in DICOM format screened from the much larger Lung Image Database consortium (LIDC) and Image Database Resource Initiative (IDRI) [10] database of 1018 low-dose lung CT scans from 1010 lung cancer patients. LUNA16 thereby is a sub-set of this database where slices with a thickness greater than 2.5 mm are excluded, which leaves a dataset of 888 CT scans. Radiologists made in total 36,378 annotations and overall, 1186 nodules were marked as $\geq 3mm$ in diameter. The typical image volume size ranged between $432 \times 306 \times 214$ and $512 \times 512 \times 652$. Samples from the LUNA16 dataset can be seen in Fig. 1.

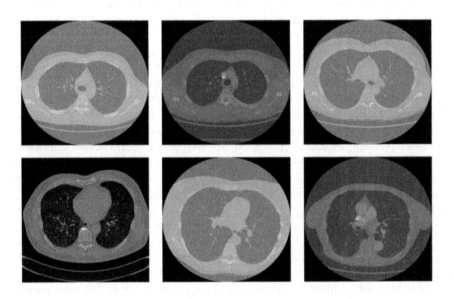

Fig. 1. Exemplary patient cases from the LUNA16 CT dataset.

2.2 Preprocessing

Since three dimensional thoracic scans contain, in terms of lung nodule segmentation, a high proportion of irrelevant image information around the lungs, the first step was to minimize the search space for the presented method by extracting a region of interest (ROI). The LUNA16 dataset already provides such lung ROIs, which were used as the image input for the task of lung nodule segmentation in this work (see Fig. 3). However, a common Unet was additionally trained and tested to self-produce such masked lung ROIs, in order to provide the whole image processing pipeline. With use of the LIDC/IDRI database and their 'pylidc' tool, in total 950 patient cases were available. The accuracy for whole lung segmentation was on average 98 ± 4 %. Any further processing, i.e., training and validation of the proposed model was applied to these lung ROI images (see Fig. 3), which were of the same image size as the original CT volumes. In order to improve training performance and resulting segmentation accuracies a few augmentation techniques were applied to the imaging data. This included flipping, rotations by a random angle between -15 and 15 degrees, the addition of Gaussian noise, as well as affine transformations, which involved scaling and shearing.

2.3 Methods

In order to address the challenges of lung nodule segmentation, i.e., their highly variable size, shape and morphology as well as complex semantic information surrounding them, the proposed approach combined architectural elements of different state-of-the-art networks. The principal structure resembled the commonly known Unet as proposed by [11], extended it to 3D image input and combined it with residual connections derived from the Res2Net as proposed by [12]. The latter used a multi-scale residual block that contained multiple branches with different scales, which allowed the network to learn complex, hierarchical features at multiple scales simultaneously and could therefore, improve the network's performance on segmenting small image objects, e.g., lung nodules. The resulting network is the 3D-Res2UNet as proposed by [5]. To further improve the performance of the 3D-Res2UNet architecture for lung nodule segmentation, this work presents several modifications that were made to the network architecture. Most importantly, attention blocks were added to the up-sampling path of the network and in conjunction with skip connections to combine features at different scales. Such attention gates guide the network's focus on targeted regions while suppressing feature activation in merely irrelevant image regions. Furthermore, batch normalization was introduced to the 3D-Res2UNet to normalize the activation of the network. Finally, Glorot initialization [13] was used, which initializes the weights to be drawn from a uniform distribution with a range determined by the number of input and output units, which helps preventing vanishing or exploding gradients. The modified 3D-Res2UNet network is shown in Fig. 2. The model was trained using Adam optimization with a learning rate of 3e-4, ReLu activation and batch size of 32. For evaluation purposes, 5-fold cross-validation was used.

3   Results

In order to assess the networks' capability to accurately segment lung nodules in CT images, the Dice similarity coefficient and intersection over union (IoU) between ground truth and network prediction of each patient case were determined. The stated results represent the average over all patient cases in the validation set per fold and subsequently averaged over all five folds (see Table 1).

Compared with the additionally implemented Unet [11], 3D-Unet [14] and original 3D-Res2UNet [5], the proposed network achieved superior results with on average 91.27 ± 6.49 % Dice score on the CT images of the LUNA16 dataset. Since this dataset additionally provide information about the nodule size, it was possible to assess the network's performance on nodules with a diameter of < 3 *mm*. Although, such small nodules were regarded as not relevant by the radiologists, which annotated the LUNA16 datasets, they could play a decisive role for early lung cancer diagnosis prospective monitoring cases. As expected, the average Dice score drops to 79.32 ± 11.39 %, due to the increasing challenge of locating and contouring smaller nodules. Fig. 3 displays exemplary patient cases.

4   Discussion

This work presented an approach to automatically segment lung nodules in CT imaging. For this purpose, the 3D-Res2Unet proposed by [5], which showed promising segmentation accuracy, was modified by the incorporation of attention blocks in the up-sampling path and the skip connections, as well as by an advanced initialization method and batch normalization. Furthermore, to ensure direct comparability, a traditional 2D- [11] and 3D-Unet [14] was implemented along with the approach of Xiao et al. [5]. Although, there are related works targeting lung nodule segmentation using other datasets, this discussion will, for the sake of comparability, focus on those works, which tested their approaches on the LUNA16 dataset.

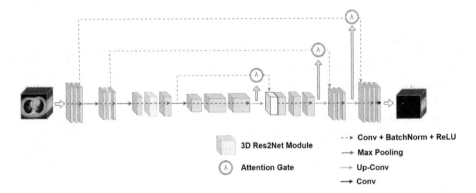

Fig. 2. The proposed modified 3D-Res2UNet network with attention gates and batch normalization.

Tab. 1. Results comparison on the LUNA16 CT data. While methods marked with an asterisk indicate, that they were re-implemented for this work, the other results were taken from the respective publication.

Method/Work	DSC [%]	IOU [%]
UNet* [11]	81.39 ± 8.67	82.17 ± 10.01
3D-UNet* [14]	86.73 ± 6.99	86.99 ± 8.06
3D-Res2UNet* [5]	89.32 ± 7.01	90.19 ± 7.03
Khosravan et al., 2018 [8]	91	
Huang et al., 2019 [7]	79.3	
Keetha et al., 2020 [6]	82.82 ± 11.71	
Ours	91.27 ± 6.49	91.01 ± 7.77

The proposed approach achieved state-of-the-art results, whereas the modifications made to the 3D-Res2Unet proposed by [5] led to a slight improvement of its performance. In comparison to other works, which trained and tested their networks on the LUNA16 dataset, the proposed approach yielded mostly superior results or is on par, e.g., with the work of Khosravan et al. [8], who also achieved on average Dice scores of 91 %. In contrast to the approach of this work, Khosravan et al. utilized already cropped image ROIs of candidate nodule regions with a size of 40×40×6 as an image input for network training and validation. Those ROIs were generated by the annotating radiologists of the LUNA16 dataset and provided with the original CT scans. The usage of such ROIs simplifies the segmentation task due to significantly reducing the search space, but it would require an highly accurate nodule detection procedure as a preprocessing step in

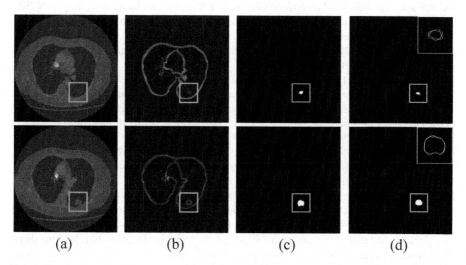

(a)　　　　　(b)　　　　　(c)　　　　　(d)

Fig. 3. Results for two exemplary patient cases of the LUNA CT dataset. Shown are the original CT image (a), the lungs ROI after preprocessing (b), the ground truth nodule annotation (c) and the network's segmentation (d).

clinical practice. The proposed approach avoids such a detection task as a prerequisite and locates and segments nodules in the whole lung parenchyma. In conclusion, the proposed deep learning-based approach, combined a Unet-style architecture with residual and attention blocks and achieved state-of-the-art results on lung nodule segmentation in CT imaging. Accurate segmentations have the potential to reduce workload of clinicians and time needed for diagnostic procedures in clinical practise, as well as support early stage diagnosis and treatment of lung cancer.

References

1. Siegel RL, Miller KD, Jemal A. Cancer statistics, 2019. CA Cancer J Clin. 2019;69(1):7–34.
2. Kamble B, Sahu SP, Doriya R. A review on lung and nodule segmentation techniques. Advances in Data and Information Sciences: Proceedings of ICDIS 2019. 2020:555–65.
3. Carvalho Filho AO de, Sampaio WB de, Silva AC, Paiva AC de, Nunes RA, Gattass M. Automatic detection of solitary lung nodules using quality threshold clustering, genetic algorithm and diversity index. Artif Intell Med. 2014;60(3):165–77.
4. Pezzano G, Ripoll VR, Radeva P. CoLe-CNN: context-learning convolutional neural network with adaptive loss function for lung nodule segmentation. Comput Methods Programs Biomed. 2021;198:105792.
5. Xiao Z, Liu B, Geng L, Zhang F, Liu Y. Segmentation of lung nodules using improved 3D-UNet neural network. Symmetry (Basel). 2020;12(11):1787.
6. Keetha NV, Annavarapu CSR et al. U-Det: a modified U-Net architecture with bidirectional feature network for lung nodule segmentation. arXiv preprint arXiv:2003.09293. 2020.
7. Huang X, Sun W, Tseng TLB, Li C, Qian W. Fast and fully-automated detection and segmentation of pulmonary nodules in thoracic CT scans using deep convolutional neural networks. Computerized Medical Imaging and Graphics. 2019;74:25–36.
8. Khosravan N, Bagci U. Semi-supervised multi-task learning for lung cancer diagnosis. 2018 40th Annual international conference of the IEEE engineering in medicine and biology society (EMBC). IEEE. 2018:710–3.
9. LUng Nodule Analysis 2016 (LUNA16). https://luna16.grand-challenge.org/Home/. Accessed: 2010-09-30.
10. Armato III SG, McLennan G, Bidaut L, McNitt-Gray MF, Meyer CR, Reeves AP et al. The lung image database consortium (LIDC) and image database resource initiative (IDRI): a completed reference database of lung nodules on CT scans. Med Phys. 2011;38(2):915–31.
11. Ronneberger O, Fischer P, Brox T. U-Net: convolutional networks for biomedical image segmentation. CoRR. 2015;abs/1505.04597.
12. Gao SH, Cheng MM, Zhao K, Zhang XY, Yang MH, Torr P. Res2Net: a new multi-scale backbone architecture. IEEE Transactions on Pattern Analysis and Machine Intelligence. 2021;43(2):652–62.
13. Glorot X, Bengio Y. Understanding the difficulty of training deep feedforward neural networks. Proceedings of the thirteenth international conference on artificial intelligence and statistics. JMLR Workshop and Conference Proceedings. 2010:249–56.
14. Çiçek Ö, Abdulkadir A, Lienkamp SS, Brox T, Ronneberger O. 3D U-Net: learning dense volumetric segmentation from sparse annotation. 2016.

Automated Deep-learning-based Vertebral Body Localization and Instance Segmentation for Osteoporosis Assessment using CT

Nicolai R. Krekiehn[1], Eren B. Yilmaz[1,2], Hannes C. Kruse[2], Carsten Meyer[2,3], Claus C. Glüer[1]

[1]Section Biomedical Imaging, Dept. of Radiology and Neuroradiology, University Medical Center Schleswig-Holstein (UKSH), Campus Kiel
[2]Dept. of Computer Science, Ostfalia University of Applied Sciences, Wolfenbüttel, Germany
[3]Dept. of Computer Science, Faculty of Engineering, Kiel University, Germany
nicolai.krekiehn@rad.uni-kiel.de

Abstract. Osteoporosis is an important disorder that is underdiagnosed. We aim to develop a robust automated CT-based vertebral label-independent approach for localization and instance segmentation of the vertebral bodies (VB) which permits assessment of bone mineral density (BMD) and generates VB center data for subsequent fracture assessment tools. We utilize an nnU-Net adapted for segmentation of the surface vs interior of the VBs vs background. This allows delineation of individual VBs, segmentation of the cortical surface encompassing the cancellous bone for BMD assessment, and localization of VB centers. After training the performance was evaluated on an external test data set. Our approach detected 97.5% of the vertebral bodies showing robustness to spinal degenerations like osteophytes. VB centers were determined with residual errors of 3.5 ± 0.9 mm, sufficiently accurate as input for our fracture detection tool. BMD evaluated in Hounsfield Units (HU) correlated with ground truth values with $r^2 = 0.96$, RMS error $= 11.3$ HU, sufficiently accurate for automated diagnosis and CT-based opportunistic screening for osteoporosis.

1 Introduction

Osteoporosis (OPO) is a highly prevalent disease, leading to pain and disability, and huge financial costs – and prevalence will grow due to increasing life expectancy [1]. 3-D imaging methods such as computed tomography (CT) and magnetic resonance imaging (MRI) provide essential diagnostic information. However, indicators for disease are often overlooked in the daily clinical routine (e.g. less than 50% of vertebral fractures are recognized by radiologists [2]). Automated image analysis procedures as proposed for opportunistic screening [3] could help closing this resulting diagnostic gap. Deep learning (DL) based methods have proven to be particularly promising, also for tackling musculoskeletal disorders [4]. Several approaches have been developed for automatic vertebra localization, segmentation and labeling; For a review and comparison of methods for CT images, see [5]. Most approaches either directly localize the center of the vertebra or vertebral body (VB) by regressing a pseudo-probability map [6, 7] or use encoder-decoder convolutional neuronal networks (CNN) like the U-Net [8]. However, current approaches have some limitations specifically in the context of osteoporosis

© Der/die Autor(en), exklusiv lizenziert an
Springer Fachmedien Wiesbaden GmbH, ein Teil von Springer Nature 2023
T. M. Deserno et al. (Hrsg.), *Bildverarbeitung für die Medizin 2023*,
Informatik aktuell, https://doi.org/10.1007/978-3-658-41657-7_37

assessment. (i) Most segmentation approaches target the entire vertebra including the vertebral arches and processi[5]. There are only few studies which explicitly focus on the VB [9]. However, osteoporotic fractures occur in the VB and evaluation of bone mineral density (BMD) as indicator of future vertebral fracture risk require automated delineation of the VB from the rest of the vertebra along with assessment of vertebral body properties (VBPs like center point, height and gray level distributions). (ii) Automatic vertebra labeling is still a serious problem especially in case of limited field-of-view, pathologies (including vertebral fractures and infrequent vertebrae like T13) and imaging artifacts [5]. VBPs are more important than a correct labeling: it is more important to know how many fractures are present in a patient, not which vertebrae are fractured; it is more important to know a vertebra's BMD and fracture status than its label. (iii) While both MRI and CT are strong for diagnosing prevalent fracture only CT offers accurate estimates of BMD and bone strength and allows assessment of cortical bone properties. These considerations have guided us in our strategy for developing an automated DL approach for assessment of osteoporosis. We aim to develop an automated CT-based vertebra label-independent approach for localization and instance segmentation of the vertebral bodies which is robust to spine degenerations like osteophytes, allows assessment of BMD, and generates accurate VBPs for subsequent fracture assessment tools (e.g. [10])

2 Materials and methods

2.1 Algorithm

Our pipeline solves the problem that only whole vertebra data is available [5], but information about the VB is needed as mentioned in the introduction. We use the nnU-Net framework [12] as a backbone for automatic segmentation of the vertebrae with

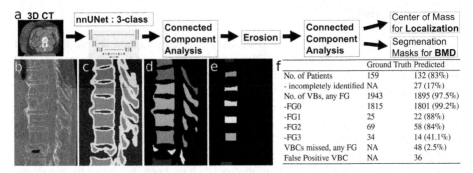

Fig. 1. *a*: Overview of our algorithm, from input to output. *b*: Sagittal slice of a test case with osteophytes and osteoporotic fracture. *c–e*: Outputs of the individual steps of our pipeline: *c*: 3-class segmentation, *d*: vertebra instances by connected component analysis, and *e*: final vertebral body segmentations after erosion. *f*: Evaluation metrics on a per-patient and per-vertebra basis. The per-vertebra results are also split into Genant [11] fracture grades FG 0 – 3.

default settings for the "3d full resolution" network[1]. The algorithm is shown in Fig. 1a. A binary segmentation of VBs vs background (BG) turned out to be insufficient to separate all VBs, specifically if bridging occurs in the presence of osteophytes (Fig. 1b), a very common spinal degeneration in the elderly. Therefore, we introduced a third class separating the vertebra surface (VS class) from the inner vertebra volume (IVV class) and BG which allows erosion steps to resolve this issue. First, the model assigns each CT-voxel to one of three classes: BG, VS and IVV (Fig. 1c), trained on publicly available annotated vertebra segmentation masks [5]. Next, ignoring VS and BG voxels a connected component analysis (CCA) using 26-connectivity is performed on the IVV voxels[2], yielding individual vertebra instances, but not all of the vertebrae separated yet (Fig. 1d, 3 cyan-colored). The generated vertebra segmentations are reduced to the VBs with an erosion procedure (any VS or IVV voxel the 26 neighbours of which do not belong to the same class is removed). Erosion is applied five times, followed by a final connected component analysis to yield separated VBs (Fig. 1e). For each VB center of mass can be computed as vertebral body center (VBC) (Fig. 2).

2.2 Data

Vertebra annotations provided in the VerSe database [5] were used to train the 3-class model. VerSe is a large scale, multi-detector, multi-site, CT spine database consisting of 374 scans from 355 patients scanned with a standard dose bone CT protocol. Using only 1 scan per patient, we evaluated 4363 annotated vertebrae. Vertebral labels are ignored and replaced by the 3 classes BG, VS and IVV. The official training (n=1520) and validation (n=1465) splits were combined and used as training database in a five-fold cross-validation for the nnU-Net. The official VerSe test split (n=1378) was used as a interim test dataset to evaluate the interim step vertebra segmentation performance. As independent test data the "Diagnostik Bilanz" (DB) of the BioAsset project dataset [13] was used. Unlike VerSe, low-dose CT images were used (159 patients, 1943 vertebrae, from 7 centers). Ground truth data was available on VBC and VB fracture grades for T4 to L4 and on trabecular BMD (in HU) of T9 to L2 (except T11) for 2 centers (n=419 VBs). Fractured VBs were excluded from BMD analysis, since BMD values are biased in these VBs.

2.3 Evaluation metrics

We assess the localization performance of our algorithm on the DB dataset on a per-vertebra and on per-patient basis using the following metrics. The (unlabeled) *localization error* [14] is defined as the distance between a predicted VBC to the closest annotated VBC. Vertebrae were considered as identified if a predicted VBC was observed within a radius of 10 mm around an annotated VBC, otherwise as missed. The level of 10mm was selected for the following reason. Predicted VBCs are to be used as anchor point for placing bounding boxes around each VB in available fracture detection model [10] and the size of those bounding boxes is large enough to still encompass the

---

[1]https://github.com/MIC-DKFZ/nnUNet/tree/aa53b3b87130ad78f0a28e6169a83215d708d659
[2]CCA is used to create bounding boxes to calculate erosion only in these sections.

entire vertebral body even if the center is misplaced by as much as 10 mm. We also have
false positive predicted VBCs (V-FP in Fig. 2a) – no true VBC was observed within
10mm radius. We also investigated whether missing a VB might be due to fractures.

3   Results

3-class nnU-Net segmentation of BG, VS and IVV voxels of the entire vertebrae assessed
on the VerSe test split based on five-fold cross-validation resulted in the following Dice
scores: IVV Class: 0.93 ± 0.02, VS Class: 0.87 ± 0.03, BG Class: 0.999 ± 0.001,
comparable to results in [15]. Our evaluation results on the DB dataset are summarized
in Fig. 1f. 1895 (97.5%) of 1943 annotated VBs were correctly localized. 48 (2.5%) VBs
were missed. For 28 VBs, the distance between ground truth and predicted VBC was
larger than 10mm and for 20 of these there was no predicted VBC within the VB volume
at all. 34 of the 48 VB missed had an osteoporotic fracture (marked as black boxes in
Fig. 3, n=128, Fig. 1f). For 83%, 10%, and 7% of the patients there were 0, 1, and 2 or
more missed vertebrae, respectively. As the Genant fracture grade increases from 1 to
3, the rate of missed VBs increases from 12% to 59% because the compressed fractured
volume may be completely dissolved during the erosion step (Fig. 1b–e, second vertebra
from bottom). On the other hand our algorithm was robust to degenerative pathologies
(marked as grey boxes in Fig. 3, n=1005) correctly localizing 99.2% of all non-fractured

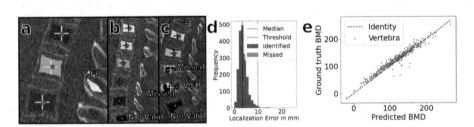

Fig. 2. *a-c*: CT slices overlayed with segmentation masks, VBC predictions (red dot) and annotations ("+"), visualizing in general good performance along with some problems. *a*: false positive
VBC on the processus of a vertebra (V-FP) due to insufficient erosion. *c*: two missed VBCs, one
without any prediction (missed) and one with a prediction >10 mm from true VBC (missed). *b,c*:
here the bottom VB displays reasonably predicted VBC in vertebral bodies near the border of
the scan without ground truth VBCs ("not valid"); such cases were excluded from the analysis
d: Histogram of localization errors in mm *e*: Correlation of ground truth and predicted (n=419
available) BMD (HU) values calculated within VB segmentation masks.

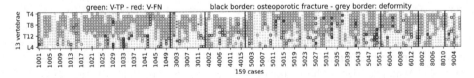

Fig. 3. Vertebra localization results on the DB dataset. Patients (ID) at horizontal, vertebrae at
vertical axis. Vertical black lines mark clinical center borders.

vertebrae (Genant fracture grade 0, n=1815). Fig. 2a-c visualized the performance of our algorithm. Fig 2d) shows a histogram of the localization errors with a median of 3.5 ± 0.9 mm. The correlations of the average BMD (HU) within the VB masks with uncalibrated ground truth HUs [16] were $r^2 = 0.97$, RMS error = 9.8 HU (n=419, Fig. 2e) at the vertebral level and $r^2 = 0.96$, RMS error = 9.8 HU (n=93). When compared to a slope=1, intercept=0 line, the RMS error increased to 12.2 HU on a per-vertebra base and to 11.3 HU on a per-patient base. The localization results across the DB dataset are visualized in Fig. 3.

4 Discussion

Osteoporosis diagnosis and fracture risk assessment require determination of two main characteristics: low BMD and presence of vertebral fractures. The DL based model presented here shows performance levels sufficient to accomplish this task. BMD results in HU can be converted to BMD using internal or external calibration methods and the residual RMS error of 11.3 HU corresponds to approximately 12.9 mg/cc in the Diagnostik Bilanz study. This error is small compared to the difference of 40 mg/cc between patients with normal (120 mg/cc) vs osteoporotic (80 mg/cc) BMD [17] and thus permit accurate diagnostic categorization. Our model was not developed to detect osteoporotic vertebral fractures but to serve as an input stage for an available published vertebral fracture detection model [10]. This model solely requires detection of each VB and specification of its center coordinate, accurate enough to place bounding boxes around each vertebra. With a VB detection rate of 97.5% and residual errors of 3.5 ± 0.9 mm for the VB centers achieved here, the performance of our model is sufficient to place those bounding boxes (of typical size of $40x50x60$ mm^3). The 2.5% missed vertebrae are mainly due to vertebral fractures; fewer erosion steps might help to delineate also those instances. A comparison to state-of-the-art approaches is not straightforward since most published segmentation methods identify the entire vertebra and not only the (inner volume of) the VB, which is crucial for our aim of measuring BMD of the VB. For the same reason it is difficult to compare the residual error of vertebra center coordinates with the errors of VB center reported elsewhere. While the errors of vertebral centers were somewhat smaller (around 1 mm [5]) for the best performers in the VerSe challenge, in the VerSe challenge training and testing were performed on data with similar CT protocols whereas our model was trained on VerSe and test on Diagnostik Bilanz with a low dose protocol and data from 7 different centers[13] and thus substantially more noisy images and a larger domain mismatch. Moreover, the difference of about 1 mm vs 3 mm has little relevance for the placement of the much larger bounding boxes and comparative assessment of studies involving different datasets have to be interpreted with caution. In conclusion, our model should allow diagnostic assessment of osteoporosis through determination of BMD and, together with the available fracture detection model [10], detection of present vertebral fractures. Since these two outcomes are well established strong predictors of future fracture risk, our model should provide a powerful basis for opportunistic screening for osteoporosis status and future fracture risk.

Acknowledgement. This work has been financially supported by the Federal Ministry of Education and Research (grants 01EC1005, 01EC1908C). We thank Stefan Bartenschlager for supporting us with MIAF BMD data.

References

1. Willers C, Norton N, Harvey NC, Jacobson T, Johansson H, Lorentzon M et al. Osteoporosis in Europe: a compendium of country-specific reports. Arch Osteoporos. 2022;17(1):23.
2. Mitchell RM, Jewell P, Javaid MK, et al. Reporting of vertebral fragility fractures: can radiologists help reduce the number of hip fractures? Arch Osteoporos. 2017;12(1):71.
3. Aggarwal V, Maslen C, Abel RL, Bhattacharya P, Bromiley PA, Clark EM et al. Opportunistic diagnosis of osteoporosis, fragile bone strength and vertebral fractures from routine CT scans; a review. Ther Adv Musculoskelet Dis. 2021;13:1–19.
4. Smets J, Shevroja E, Hügle T, Leslie WD, Hans D. Machine learning solutions for osteoporosis—a review. J Bone Miner Res. 2021;36(5):833–51.
5. Sekuboyina A, Husseini ME, Bayat A, et al. VerSe: a vertebrae labelling and segmentation benchmark for multi-detector CT images. Med Image Anal. 2021;73:102166.
6. Payer C, Štern D, Bischof H, Urschler M. Integrating spatial configuration into heatmap regression based CNNs for landmark localization. Med Image Anal. 2019;54:207–19.
7. Mader AO, Lorenz C, Bergtholdt M, et al. Detection and localization of spatially correlated point landmarks in medical images using an automatically learned conditional random field. Comput Vis Image Underst. 2018;176-177:45–53.
8. Elton D, Sandfort V, Pickhardt PJ, Summers RM. Accurately identifying vertebral levels in large datasets. Medical Imaging 2020: Computer-Aided Diagnosis. SPIE, 2020.
9. Lessmann N, Ginneken B van, Jong PA de, et al. Iterative fully convolutional neural networks for automatic vertebra segmentation and identification. Med Image Anal. 2019;53:142–55.
10. Yilmaz EB, Buerger C, Fricke T, et al. Automated deep learning-based detection of osteoporotic fractures in CT images. Mach Learn Med Imaging. Vol. 12966. 2021:376–85.
11. Genant HK, Wu CY, Kuijk C van, Nevitt MC. Vertebral fracture assessment using a semiquantitative technique. J Bone Miner Res. 1993;8(9):1137–48.
12. Isensee F, Petersen J, Klein A, Zimmerer D, Jaeger PF, Kohl S et al. nnU-Net: self-adapting framework for U-Net-based medical image segmentation. Nat Methods. 2021;18:203–11.
13. Glüer CC, Krause M, Museyko O, et al. New horizons for the in vivo assessment of major aspects of bone quality microstructure and material properties assessed by quantitative computed tomography and quantitative ultrasound methods. Osteologie. 2013;22:223–33.
14. Glocker B, Zikic D, Konukoglu E, Haynor DR, Criminisi A. Vertebrae localization in pathological spine CT via dense classification from sparse annotations. Med Image Comput Comput Assist Interv. Springer, 2013:262–70.
15. Hempe H, Yilmaz EB, Meyer C, et al. Opportunistic CT screening for degenerative deformities and osteoporotic fractures with 3D DeepLab. Med Imag: Image Proc. Vol. 12032. SPIE, 2022:8.
16. Mastmeyer A, Engelke K, Fuchs C, Kalender WA. A hierarchical 3D segmentation method and the definition of vertebral body coordinate systems for QCT of the lumbar spine. Med Image Anal. 2006;10(4):560–77.
17. Engelke K, Adams JE, Armbrecht G, Augat P, Bogado CE, Bouxsein ML et al. Clinical use of quantitative computed tomography and peripheral quantitative computed tomography in the management of osteoporosis in adults. J Clin Densitom. 2008;11(1):123–62.

Mitigating Unknown Bias in Deep Learning-based Assessment of CT Images
DeepTechnome

Simon Langer[1], Oliver Taubmann[2], Felix Denzinger[1,2], Andreas Maier[1], Alexander Mühlberg[2]

[1]Pattern Recognition Lab, Friedrich-Alexander University Erlangen-Nuremberg, Germany
[2]Siemens Healthcare GmbH, Forchheim, Germany
simon.langer@fau.de

Abstract. Reliably detecting diseases using relevant biological information is crucial for real-world applicability of deep learning techniques in medical imaging. We debias deep learning models during training against unknown bias – without preprocessing/filtering the input beforehand or assuming specific knowledge about its distribution or precise nature in the dataset. Control regions are used as surrogates that carry information regarding the bias; subsequently, the classifier model extracts features, and biased intermediate features are suppressed by our custom, modular DecorreLayer. We evaluate our method on a dataset of 952 lung computed tomography scans by introducing simulated biases w.r.t. reconstruction kernel and noise level and propose including an adversarial test set in evaluations of bias reduction techniques. In a moderately sized model architecture, applying the proposed method to learn from data exhibiting a strong bias, it near-perfectly recovers the classification performance observed when training with corresponding unbiased data.

1 Introduction

Technical variation in CT scans occurs for a variety of reasons, becoming especially problematic when it is correlated with the predictive task, for instance due to prior knowledge of the clinician and/or patient of a likely diagnosis, or site-specific differences in patient selection and acquisition protocols within multi-center data sets [1].

The range of reconstruction and scan parameters affects the amount and appearance of technical variation present [2]: choosing an appropriate reconstruction kernel forces a tradeoff between detail and noise level; tube current and voltage affect the amount of noise and radiation dose. The severity and presence of beam hardening, scatter, metal, motion and truncation artifacts are influenced by such choices as well as by patient behavior and physiology. Different reconstruction kernels and additive white Gaussian noise (AWGN) serve as our two exemplary test cases, simulating such biases.

When automating image analysis with deep/machine learning (DL/ML), bias poses a fundamental challenge – consequently, there has been substantial research and industry interest in it. When tackling known bias, normalizing the input data w.r.t. technical variation in a preprocessing step is a classical approach; e.g. Choe et al. [3] employ DL to preprocess images, converting their style using convolutional neural networks

© Der/die Autor(en), exklusiv lizenziert an
Springer Fachmedien Wiesbaden GmbH, ein Teil von Springer Nature 2023
T. M. Deserno et al. (Hrsg.), *Bildverarbeitung für die Medizin 2023*,
Informatik aktuell, https://doi.org/10.1007/978-3-658-41657-7_38

which predict the image differences of reconstruction kernels. Alternatively, adversarial debiasing can be performed, i.e. a secondary network debiases while training using gradient reversal and/or min-max based approaches [4]. In contrast, there has been relatively little work in DL tackling the more general, universal case of unknown bias. Notably, a resampling preprocessing approach accounts for less frequent permutations of image properties – acquired with a variational autoencoder – by sampling the associated images more frequently [5]. In classical ML, removal of artificial voxel effect by linear regression (RAVEL) regresses unwanted features per voxel using control regions [6] and the Technome [1] combines debiasing and training in order to avoid the risk of removing informative biological information when stabilizing during preprocessing. Our work aims to transfer such ideas to the field of DL.

2   Materials and methods

2.1   DecorreLayer

Control regions (CRs) serve as surrogates, capturing the technical variation but little to no biological variation related to the detection task. To maximize similarity e.g. in streak and noise patterns, areas of the CT scan which are outside of, but close to the regions of interest (ROIs) such as surrounding air or anatomical structures are good choices, depending on the presumed general types of biases that might be present. This introduces the assumption that the confounder manifests itself not only in the task-relevant area, yet, no other knowledge about the specific nature or distribution of the bias is required.

Our novel, modular DecorreLayer is inserted into an existing classifier model, receiving features calculated by the model architecture up to that point for both the ROI and CR (applying the same computations to ROI and CR data), and returns a filtered version of the ROI features, as illustrated in Figure 1.

2.1.1   Correlation unit. DecorreLayer consists of two modules with separate tasks. The correlation unit determines what features probably depend on technical variation, comparing each feature with its control region counterpart over the batch dimension.

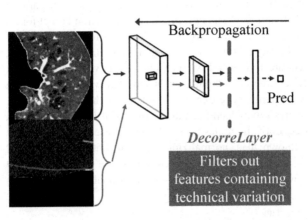

Fig. 1. Overview of a model augmented with DecorreLayer; ROI related data in dark blue (here: slice of left lung lobe), CR related data in red (here: slice of air above patient), surrounding areas are segmented out.

For the sake of simplicity, the pearson correlation coefficient (PCC) was used for this purpose in our experiments. In order to operate independently of the location of e.g. a noise pattern, a global average pooled virtual feature vector (one scalar feature as the mean over each pixel in a channel) is used if DecorreLayer's output will still be interpreted with spatial information (e.g. by a subsequent convolutional layer). While the use of PCC may appear to limit the approach to linear co-dependencies, note that it is computed on internal feature maps that are themselves non-linear w.r.t. the input data. Nonetheless, it could also be replaced with other correlation measures, linear or non-linear, if deemed appropriate – even trainable ones. We suggest inserting DecorreLayer prior to every fully connected and convolutional layer, except the first one.

2.1.2   Filter unit. The filter unit is in direct contact with the surrounding architecture. It generates filtered versions of the ROI features as DecorreLayer's output, with stronger filtering being applied when the correlation unit's output is higher: Either by multiplying with a small constant if the PCC exceeds a threshold (factor mode), or by interpreting dependency on technical variation as a dropout probability, guaranteeing dropout at $\geq g$ (dropout mode). The latter performed best, gradually reducing the reliability of a feature the more it is probably dependent on technical variation by increasing the dropout probability appropriately. With $\text{Bern}(p)$ being the Bernoulli distribution, $\mathbf{x}$ denoting all instances of one feature over the batch dimension and $\hat{d}$ the scalar PCC, the result $\hat{\mathbf{y}}$ can be described as

$$\mathbf{z} \sim \text{Bern}\left(\max\left\{0, 1 - \max\left\{0, \hat{d}\right\} \cdot g^{-1}\right\}\right) \tag{1}$$

$$\hat{\mathbf{y}} = \mathbf{x} \cdot \mathbf{z} \tag{2}$$

2.1.3   Backward pass and inference. We intentionally relax the constraint of perfectly matching the forward pass computations during the backward pass: DecorreLayer is ignored entirely, which results in a reweighting of the error tensor such that errors caused by DecorreLayer's filtering of features containing technical variation are "blamed on" the previous layers. At inference time, DecorreLayer is inactive since the model has already learned to extract features without bias, i.e. CRs are no longer needed.

2.2   Data preparation and testing setup

Our evaluation data set contains 952 lung CT scans from a single site, acquired with a SOMATOM® Force and labeled for the presence (label CE) or absence of centrilobular emphysema. As this disease is primarily visible in the upper half of the lung [7], we extract 5 evenly spaced lung-masked axial slices from that area as ROIs, and unrelated air regions above the patient from the same slices as CRs (Fig. 1a). Since each scan was reconstructed with both a soft (Br36d3) and a sharp (Bl57d3) kernel, we can simulate realistic technical variation by more frequently sampling softer images for label CE, and otherwise sharper, but noisier images (CE $\leftrightarrow$ 90% chance of soft image). In a separate experiment with artificial technical variation we apply additive white Gaussian noise (AWGN, $\mu = 0$, $\sigma = 0.5\,\sigma_{\text{ROI}}$, where σ_{ROI} denotes the standard deviation of the ROI voxel intensities) to images labeled CE with a 90% chance.

We define adversarial test sets as an inversion of the introduced manipulations, affecting every image in the test set, and argue for their adoption in future work on debiasing DL/ML since they directly display worst-bias-case performance as well as visualize the reliance of a model on technical variation (such as extra noise) not present in the original, unbiased data (full test set).

We also propose the Histogram of Correlations – a visualization technique which plots the correlations of ROI and CR activations (i.e. the correlation unit output), optionally including a comparison with unbiased and/or debiased trainings (Fig. 2). It both facilitates visually determining a reasonable hyperparameter range for DecorreLayer, and investigating our or other debiasing techniques.

Our approach is tested on three architectures: a) a small custom model consisting of 2 sets of convolutional, ReLU, MaxPool layers (6, 16 channels) followed by 3 fully connected ones, b) a medium custom model consisting of 3 wider sets of this structure (32, 64, 128 channels), followed by 4 fully connected layers, as well as c) ResNet-18 [8] with batch normalization disabled. DecorreLayer is inserted prior to every fully connected and convolutional layer (excluding the first one), and training is performed with minimal augmentations (horizontal flip, translation) using stochastic gradient descent.

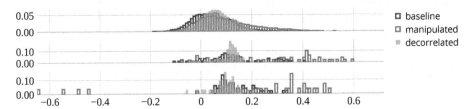

Fig. 2. Histogram of Correlations with 3 DecorreLayers inserted at depths 6, 9, 11 (their individual histograms shown top to bottom) into the small custom architecture, with the filter unit in dropout mode at $g = 0.3$. We visualize how many activations exhibit a specific (here: Pearson) correlation value (bins on x-axis), normalized by total number of activations (y-axis). Note the shift towards positive correlation when training a model on manipulated, i.e. biased data, compared to the baseline – DecorreLayer successfully reverts this effect.

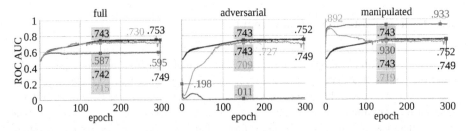

Fig. 3. DecorreLayer on the small custom architecture – Experiment S_1 in Table 1. The subplots represent the different test sets: full (unbiased), adversarial, and manipulated (same bias as training data). Color coding denotes whether training data was biased (□/■) or unbiased (□/■) and DecorreLayer was enabled (■/■) or disabled (□/□). The depicted trends in performance as training progresses are representative for the vast majority of our experiments.

Tab. 1. Mean ROC AUC model performance ± standard deviation after 150 training epochs. Each column represents a model, with which we performed 4 trainings (4 boxes □,■,□,■; solid boxes ■/■ represent DecorreLayer being active). The best results of trainings on biased and unbiased data, respectively, are highlighted in italics. S/M/R refers to small custom/medium custom/ResNet18 architecture (Sec. 2.2), ^{weak} to a weakened bias of 70% instead of 90%. When training on biased data, both the unbiased as well as adversarial ROC AUCs are almost always much higher when employing DecorreLayer (■) in contrast to not performing any debiasing (□).

Test	Training Setup		Exp. 1: Reconstruction Kernel Bias				Exp. 2: AWGN Bias		
			S_1	S_1^{weak}	M_1	M_1^{weak}	S_2	M_2	R_2
unbiased	unbiased	□	.743±.03	.743±.03	.731±.02	.731±.02	.743±.03	.731±.02	.740±.04
		■	.742±.03	.742±.03	.703±.04	.703±.04	.739±.03	.752±.03	.614±.06
	biased	□	.587±.02	.663±.02	.554±.05	.634±.08	.611±.02	.574±.08	.645±.06
		■	.715±.04	.725±.02	.713±.02	.677±.05	.686±.05	.726±.03	.699±.05
adversarial	unbiased	□	.743±.03	.743±.03	.729±.03	.729±.03	.743±.03	.729±.03	.739±.05
		■	.743±.03	.743±.03	.707±.04	.707±.04	.740±.03	.747±.04	.618±.07
	biased	□	.011±.01	.286±.06	.240±.26	.343±.20	.011±.01	.492±.15	.016±.02
		■	.709±.04	.744±.02	.749±.02	.725±.07	.622±.09	.719±.04	.652±.07

3 Results

Our results are summarized as mean ± std. dev. ROC AUC of a 5-fold cross validation in Table 1, reported after half of the (typically over-)allocated training time of 300 epochs.

Figure 3 (S_1) demonstrates the inflated score one would see when e.g. training and testing the small custom architecture on data with reconstruction kernel bias (.930 ROC AUC), compared to the dramatic impact on true (.587 ROC AUC) and especially adversarial performance (.011 ROC AUC). DecorreLayer minimizes this issue, achieving scores within .035 ROC AUC of the baseline using the recommended dropout mode.

DecorreLayer also effectively decorrelates when applied to weaker reconstruction kernel bias (S_1^{weak}) and/or incorporated into the medium custom architecture (M_1, M_1^{weak}). In further experiments (S_2, M_2) of AWGN added to most images of ill patients, the factor mode performed well. Applying DecorreLayer to the comparatively huge ResNet-18 did not work as easily (R_2) – our training decorrelated at the cost of degraded performance if no bias had been present. However, we observed promising results when performing additional testing with ResNet-18 on CIFAR-10 [9]. Also, DecorreLayer is currently incompatible with batch normalization; we argue that the mean and variance estimates of batch normalization might fluctuate significantly due to the changing number of filtered features, hence creating conflicts.

Having determined appropriate hyperparameters for DecorreLayer using the proposed Histogram of Correlations, it can even have a positive impact on training stability: for instance, we observed occasional stability issues when training an unmodified medium custom architecture on biased data, enabling DecorreLayer acted in a stabilizing/regularizing fashion, like a regular dropout layer. Finally – to determine suitable hyperparameters and gain interpretable testing results – we still consider access to a small unbiased data set vital for real-world application.

4 Discussion

To the best of our knowledge, DecorreLayer is the first method to debias DL models while exclusively training on data containing unknown biases: we teach models not to use bias present in training data as long as the confounder is also observable in image areas not directly related to the task at hand – i.e., the sources of bias do not need to be explicitly modeled. While currently working less reliably on larger architectures, as well as requiring hyperparameter values carefully adjusted using the proposed tools, in our experiments on CT lung emphysema classification, DecorreLayer was able to immensely boost generalization performance under adverse conditions of both artificially created and intentionally sampled technical variation – often near-perfectly recovering the baseline performance while training on heavily biased data.

To achieve this, instances of DecorreLayer are inserted into the model pipeline, analyzing how the model perceives control regions in addition to regions of interest, acting as smart filtering/regularization. During training, an additional forward pass is performed; in exchange, there are no additional trainable parameters as well as no added load during inference – the original architecture can perform its task without extra help.

Future work directly expanding on DecorreLayer could learn/dynamically calculate filter unit hyperparameters, or investigate new correlation units: a) applying other existing measures of dependence and, b) learning an arbitrary correlation function, which could circumvent the risk of models bypassing correlation checks by considering earlier feature maps (or even unprocessed CRs) to compare ROI features against. Future work also needs to investigate how well the approach generalizes to various modalities as well as other types of bias.

References

1. Mühlberg A, Katzmann A, Heinemann V, et al. The technome - a predictive internal calibration approach for quantitative imaging biomarker research. Sci Rep. 2020;10(1103).
2. Taubmann O, Berger M, Bögel M, et al. Computed tomography. Medical imaging systems. Ed. by Maier A, et al. Springer, 2018. Chap. 8:147–89.
3. Choe J, Lee SD, Do K, et al. Deep learning-based image conversion of CT reconstruction kernels improves radiomics reproducibility for pulmonary nodules or masses. Radiol. 2019;292 2:365–73.
4. Kim B, Kim H, Kim K, et al. Learning not to learn: training deep neural networks with biased data. Proc IEEE Comput Soc Conf Comput Vis Pattern Recognit. 2019:9004–12.
5. Amini A, Soleimany A, Schwarting W, et al. Uncovering and mitigating algorithmic bias through learned latent structure. Proc Conf AAAI/ACM AI, Ethics, and Society. 2019:289–95.
6. Fortin J, Sweeney E, Muschelli J, et al. Removing inter-subject technical variability in magnetic resonance imaging studies. Neuroimage. 2016;132:198–212.
7. Anderson AE, Foraker AG. Centrilobular emphysema and panlobular emphysema: two different diseases. Thorax. 1973;28:547–50.
8. He K, Zhang X, Ren S, et al. Deep residual learning for image recognition. Proc IEEE Comput Soc Conf Comput Vis Pattern Recognit. 2016:770–8.
9. Krizhevsky A. Learning multiple layers of features from tiny images. Tech. rep. University of Toronto, 2009.

Taming Detection Transformers for Medical Object Detection

Marc K. Ickler[1], Michael Baumgartner[1,3,4], Saikat Roy[1,3], Tassilo Wald[1,4], Klaus H. Maier-Hein[1,2]

[1]Division of Medical Image Computing, German Cancer Research Center, Heidelberg, Germany
[2]Pattern Analysis and Learning Group, Heidelberg University Hospital
[3]Faculty of Mathematics and Computer Science, Heidelberg University, Germany
[4]Helmholtz Imaging
m.baumgartner@dkfz.de

Abstract. The accurate detection of suspicious regions in medical images is an error-prone and time-consuming process required by many routinely performed diagnostic procedures. To support clinicians during this difficult task, several automated solutions were proposed relying on complex methods with many hyperparameters. In this study, we investigate the feasibility of detection transformer (DETR) models for volumetric medical object detection. In contrast to previous works, these models directly predict a set of objects without relying on the design of anchors or manual heuristics such as non-maximum-suppression to detect objects. We show by conducting extensive experiments with three models, namely DETR, Conditional DETR, and DINO DETR on four data sets (CADA, RibFrac, KiTS19, and LIDC) that these set prediction models can perform on par with or even better than currently existing methods. DINO DETR, the best-performing model in our experiments demonstrates this by outperforming a strong anchor-based one-stage detector, Retina U-Net, on three out of four data sets.

1 Introduction

Clinical decision-making is often based on the correct localization and classification of multiple pathologies throughout the entire human body. Because this task is frequently associated with an error-prone and time-sensitive diagnostic process, multiple computer-aided diagnostic (CAD) systems have been published in the past to automate this process. Most of the previous works relied on methods with anchors [1, 2] or center points suffering from complex design and manual heuristics, such as the anchor matching strategy or non-maximum suppression. Recently, a new detection paradigm was proposed [3] for natural images by reformulating the detection task as a set prediction problem. In contrast to previous methods, these models directly predict a set of objects without relying on manual heuristics such as anchors and post-processing procedures. While the first introduction of the detection transformer (DETR) [3] already demonstrated impressive performance, it suffered from reduced performance on small objects and long training times. Follow-up work [4, 5] tackled these shortcomings and is now achieving state-of-the-art (SOTA) results on the commonly used COCO benchmark.

Despite their advantages, detection transformers remain poorly studied in the medical domain. Only one study [6] employed them to detect organs on three-dimensional CT images but the basic DETR models did not show promising performance compared to an anchor-based method. More research is required to assess the potential of detection transformers in the medical field because of the restricted experiments on one task conducted thus far. In this work, we aim to study the feasibility of DETR models on a diverse set of volumetric medical object detection problems. We evaluate three set prediction models, namely DETR [3], Conditional DETR [4] and DINO-DETR [5] against the strong anchor-based baseline nnDetection [1] on four data sets (CADA [7], RibFrac [8], KiTS19 [9] and LIDC [10]).

2   Materials and methods

2.1   Network architecture

The architecture of DETR, Conditional DETR, and DINO DETR is shown in Fig. 1. DETR [3] has two special properties that differentiate it from other object detectors. Firstly, it uses a transformer, which takes in a sequence of features and outputs a set of object proposals. Owing to the global attention mechanism, the transformer is expected to detect large features in the encoder as well as prevent duplicate predictions in the decoder. Secondly, DETR predicts bounding boxes with direct set prediction. This requires a loss that is invariant to permutations of the predictions. The Hungarian algorithm finds an optimal bipartite matching between the predictions and ground truth objects that is used to calculate the classification and regression losses. By using direct set prediction, no additional post-processing steps are required, but the model has to prevent duplicate predictions. DETR was the first method that does this in a non-autoregressive way by using a transformer with parallel decoding while achieving competitive performance to current anchor-based models. Because of the attention mechanism, the model can globally reason about all objects using the pair-wise relations between queries. This novelty makes the difficult and potentially performance-degrading non-maximum-suppression obsolete.

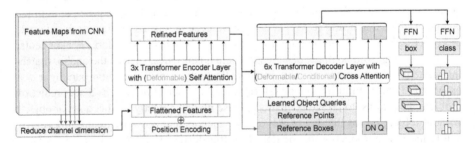

Fig. 1. A convolutional neural network (CNN) takes a patch and computes a feature map that is flattened to a sequence. After adding positional encoding, the sequence is fed through a transformer encoder and decoder. The output sequence is processed by two feed-forward networks (FFN), one predicting bounding boxes and the other class labels. Conditional DETR (green) separates content and spatial queries and uses conditional cross-attention to attend to important regions. The DINO DETR module's multi-scale features, anchors, and denoising queries (DN Q) are shown in red.

However, the vanilla DETR architecture converges slowly and struggles to detect small objects. Conditional DETR [4] introduces conditional attention and reference points to improve upon both weaknesses. In the decoder, each query predicts one reference point around which it will attend to encoder features and predict the output bounding box. Additionally, the architecture increases the number of queries and uses the focal loss instead of the cross-entropy loss to improve the classification. DINO DETR [5] utilizes a sparse attention called deformable attention, which reduces memory consumption and enables the use of multi-scale features in the transformer. In addition, it takes features from the encoder to initialize the reference boxes. These boxes are not predefined unlike anchors in other methods and are used throughout the decoder to attend to encoder features and predict bounding boxes close to them. Additional denoising queries and denoising losses are implemented to improve the training signal for faster convergence. Finally, DINO DETR also uses focal loss and even more queries than Conditional DETR.

2.2 Data sets

To cover a diverse set of problems we performed experiments on four medical object detection data sets. The CADA data set [7] has 127 objects in 109 scans and covers the low data regime. The target structures are brain aneurysms which are typically small. In the RibFrac data set [8] the task is to detect rib fractures. It represents a large medical data set with 4422 objects in 500 thin-slice CT scans. For multi-class detection, we use the LIDC data set [10] and follow the previous design of [2] to divide lesions into two categories of lung nodules that are difficult to distinguish. It comprises of 1035 CT scans where the annotated lung nodules are very small making the task even more challenging. Finally, DETRs performance on large objects is studied on the KiTS19 data set [9] that has 225 objects in 204 cases. The target structures are kidney tumors.

2.3 Experimental setup

We use a patch-wise prediction-based approach and employ nnDetection [1] as our development framework for training, inference and evaluation. Within the nnDetection augmentation pipeline, we decrease the maximum rotation to 20 degrees and increase the minimum downscaling to 0.8 to increase training speeds. For a fair comparison to Retina U-Net, all models are configured to require less than 11 GB of GPU memory. We utilize the standard nnDetection backbone (a plain convolutional encoder) and use the configured, data set-dependent patch size. For DINO DETR, the three feature maps with the lowest resolutions are fed into the transformer. We change the hidden dimension to 120 or 128 for DINO DETR and the transformer feed-forward network dimension to 1024 to adapt the model to medical data. We use a different number of queries depending on the data set and architecture (Tab. 1).

The training schedule is PolyLR with an exponent of 0.9 and a learning rate of 0.0001. The AdamW optimizer with a weight decay of 0.0001 is used. We train for 2500 batches per epoch with a batch size of 4 and adapt the number of epochs for all models to converge (Tab. 1). Other parameters were left to their default values since we found them to translate well to the medical domain.

Tab. 1. Data set specific settings for all data sets. Abbreviations: DE=DETR, CD=Conditional DETR, DI=DINO DETR. Only DINO DETR uses denoising queries.

	CADA			RibFrac			KiTS19			LIDC		
	DE	CD	DI	DE	CD	DI	DE	CD	DI	DE	CD	DI
architecture												
# queries (denoising)	6	12	20 (8)	20	50	90 (20)	6	12	20 (8)	12	24	40 (8)
# epochs	50	50	25	125	100	75	100	100	35	200	100	75

3   Results

The mean average precision (mAP) metric at an intersection-over-union (IoU) value of 0.1 is used for evaluation to reflect the clinical need for coarse localizations. Reported results were obtained by performing a five-fold cross-validation on each data set. The results are shown in Fig. 2.

All models show similar performance with a maximum discrepancy smaller than ten percent per data set. Especially on the largest data set RibFrac, the model scores are close with DETR being the worst and DINO DETR being the best model. We observe a trend clearly showing that DINO DETR performs best, followed by Conditional DETR and DETR, in agreement with our initial architectural analysis. DINO DETR and Retina U-Net achieve remarkably similar scores, with DINO DETR performing slightly better on three out of four data sets.

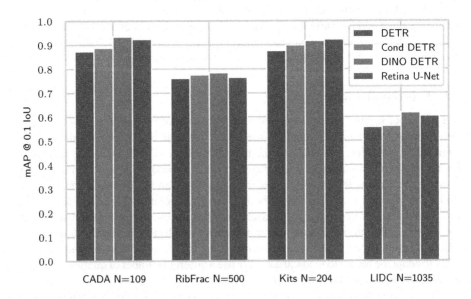

Fig. 2. Performance comparison between Retina U-Net (red), DETR (blue), Conditional DETR (orange), DINO DETR (green) on CADA, RibFrac, KiTS19, and LIDC. N denotes the number of scans in the data set.

4 Discussion

Our results in Fig. 2 illustrate that detection transformers are a viable option for medical object detection. While not on par with Retina U-Net, even the vanilla DETR model with a few modifications for volumetric input shows promising performance. Further optimized models like Conditional DETR and DINO DETR close the gap and show that competitive scores can be achieved using set prediction models.

By omitting the need for anchors and non-maximum suppression, set prediction models depend on fewer hyperparameters and therefore reduce the search space during the hyperparameter tuning process. The number of predictions is controlled by the number of queries in the transformer decoder and is one of our only data set-dependent parameters. This simplicity makes detection transformers easy to adapt to different detection problems and great candidates for self-configuring models.

Furthermore, the detection transformers only need bounding box inputs for training. Retina U-Net uses semantic segmentation as an auxiliary task to improve detection performance, making it dependent on segmentation labels which take more effort to annotate. Our experiments show that DINO DETR can achieve similar results without using an auxiliary segmentation loss.

While the performance of the models is similar, their convergence speed is not. DETR takes 200 epochs to converge on LIDC, four times more than Retina U-Net. In general, DETR and Conditional DETR need more training than Retina U-Net and DINO DETR, but the detection transformer models have the advantage of being computationally less expensive. The transformer is small compared to the backbone and forward and backward passes are approximately 1.5 times faster than for Retina U-Net (measured on a system equipped with a Ryzen 9 3900X, 64GB RAM, and an NVIDIA RTX 3090 24GB).

The most significant performance difference between DINO DETR and the other DETR models occurs on the CADA and LIDC data sets, which contain the smallest objects. We assume that the drop in performance stems from a lack of high-resolution features in the single-scale DETR models. DINO DETR uses three feature maps with the highest resolution being four times higher per dimension than the resolution of the feature maps used by DETR and Conditional DETR. This higher feature resolution improves the localization of objects in the transformer and increases performance. The resolution of DETR and Conditional DETR can be improved by decreasing the stride in the backbone and reducing the score gap to DINO, only requiring more GPU memory. To provide a fair comparison, this experiment was omitted here since we restricted the available GPU memory to 11 GB while using the same patch size as the baseline model.

Additionally, the improved performance of DINO DETR comes at the cost of model complexity. While DETR is a straightforward model which can be easily implemented and understood, DINO DETR introduces more complex features and changes to most modules of DETR. Conditional DETR only introduces slight changes to the transformer decoder of DETR, keeping it more similar.

While this study establishes the competitive nature of the class of transformer-based set prediction methods (DETR) for object detection in medical images, there also exist some limitations. Firstly, the detection transformer models used are not self-configuring, and thus per data set tuning was required. Another limitation is that because of the patch-wise training and prediction, a strategy to merge predictions from overlapping patches has to be implemented. This reintroduces the need for some post-processing, but because of far fewer predictions for detection transformers, other methods could be applied.

Considering the promising results, a future study of a self-configuring detection transformer on all ten data sets proposed by nnDetection would be of high interest. The detection transformers can also efficiently be extended to instance segmentation models.

In conclusion, detection transformers are well-suited for medical object detection. They prove to have competitive performance on a wide range of data sets without the need for predefined anchors, non-maximum-suppression, or segmentation losses.

Acknowledgement. Part of this work was funded by Helmholtz Imaging, a platform of the Helmholtz Incubator on Information and Data Science.

References

1. Baumgartner M, Jäger PF, Isensee F, Maier-Hein KH. NnDetection: a self-configuring method for medical object detection. Med Image Comput Comput Assist Interv. Springer, 2021:530–9.
2. Jaeger PF, Kohl SA, Bickelhaupt S, Isensee F, Kuder TA, Schlemmer HP et al. Retina U-Net: embarrassingly simple exploitation of segmentation supervision for medical object detection. ML4H Workshop. PMLR. 2020:171–83.
3. Carion N, Massa F, Synnaeve G, Usunier N, Kirillov A, Zagoruyko S. End-to-end object detection with transformers. Comput Vis ECCV. Springer, 2020:213–29.
4. Meng D, Chen X, Fan Z, Zeng G, Li H, Yuan Y et al. Conditional DETR for fast training convergence. Proc IEEE Int Conf Comput Vis. 2021:3631–40.
5. Zhang H, Li F, Liu S, Zhang L, Su H, Zhu J et al. Dino: Detr with improved denoising anchor boxes for end-to-end object detection. 2022.
6. Wittmann B, Navarro F, Shit S, Menze B. Focused decoding enables 3D anatomical detection by transformers. 2022.
7. Ivantsits M, Goubergrits L, Kuhnigk JM, Huellebrand M, Bruening J, Kossen T et al. Detection and analysis of cerebral aneurysms based on X-ray rotational angiography-the CADA 2020 challenge. Med Image Anal. 2022;77:102333.
8. Jin L, Yang J, Kuang K, Ni B, Gao Y, Sun Y et al. Deep-learning-assisted detection and segmentation of rib fractures from CT scans: development and validation of FracNet. EBioMedicine. 2020;62.
9. Heller N, Sathianathen N, Kalapara A, Walczak E, Moore K, Kaluzniak H et al. The KiTS19 challenge data: 300 kidney tumor cases with clinical context, CT semantic segmentations, and surgical outcomes. 2019.
10. Armato III SG, McLennan G, Bidaut L, McNitt-Gray MF, Meyer CR, Reeves AP et al. The lung image database consortium (LIDC) and image database resource initiative (IDRI): a completed reference database of lung nodules on CT scans. Med Phys. 2011;38(2):915–31.

Deep Learning-based Subtyping of Atypical and Normal Mitoses using a Hierarchical Anchor-free Object Detector

Marc Aubreville[1], Jonathan Ganz[1], Jonas Ammeling[1], Taryn A. Donovan[2], Rutger HJ. Fick[3], Katharina Breininger[4], Christof A. Bertram[5]

[1]Technische Hochschule Ingolstadt, Ingolstadt, Germany
[2]Schwarzman Animal Medical Center, New York, NY, USA
[3]Tribun Health, Paris, France
[4]Department AIBE, Friedrich-Alexander-Universität Erlangen-Nürnberg, Germany
[5]Institute of Pathology, University of Veterinary Medicine Vienna, Vienna, Austria
marc.aubreville@thi.de

Abstract. Mitotic activity is key for the assessment of malignancy in many tumors. Moreover, it has been demonstrated that the proportion of abnormal mitosis to normal mitosis is of prognostic significance. Atypical mitotic figures (MF) can be identified morphologically as having segregation abnormalities of the chromatids. In this work, we perform, for the first time, automatic subtyping of mitotic figures into normal and atypical categories according to characteristic morphological appearances of the different phases of mitosis. Using the publicly available MIDOG21 and TUPAC16 breast cancer mitosis datasets, two experts blindly subtyped mitotic figures into five morphological categories. Further, we set up a state-of-the-art object detection pipeline extending the anchor-free FCOS approach with a gated hierarchical subclassification branch. Our labeling experiment indicated that subtyping of mitotic figures is a challenging task and prone to inter-rater disagreement, which we found in 24.89% of MF. Using the more diverse MIDOG21 dataset for training and TUPAC16 for testing, we reached a mean overall average precision score of 0.552, a ROC AUC score of 0.833 for atypical/normal MF and a mean class-averaged ROC-AUC score of 0.977 for discriminating the different phases of cells undergoing mitosis.

1 Introduction

The significance of identifying and counting mitotic figures in histopathology samples has been demonstrated for many tumor types [1]. Errors of chromosome segregation that occur during cell division can appear morphologically as atypical mitotic figures (AMFs) and may correlate with genetic abnormalities [2]. AMFs can be placed into two categories including mitotic/polar asymmetry and abnormal segregation of sister chromatids [1]. Moreover, it has been long suspected [3] and recently confirmed [2, 4, 5] that not only the number of mitotic figures per unit area (the mitotic count) is of prognostic significance, but that atypical morphology is also prognostically important. Ohashi et al. were the first to investigate the significance of AMFs in breast cancer, and found that the presence of chromosome lagging and spindle multipolarity had a higher prognostic value than the mitotic figure count or Ki-67 immunohistochemistry-stained cell count [4]. In a larger study by Lashen et al. the authors found that a high atypical-

Springer Fachmedien Wiesbaden GmbH, ein Teil von Springer Nature 2023
T. M. Deserno et al. (Hrsg.), *Bildverarbeitung für die Medizin 2023*,
Informatik aktuell, https://doi.org/10.1007/978-3-658-41657-7_40

to-typical mitotic figure ratio is associated with poor breast cancer-specific survival and is a predictor of poor response to chemotherapy in triple negative breast cancer [2].

The detection and counting of mitotic figures on digital histopathology images stained with standard hematoxylin and eosin is a task that can be automated using deep learning architectures [6]. These advances are possible because of the availability of large-scale, diverse datasets such as the TUPAC16 [7] and MIDOG21 challenge [6] datasets along with the availability of modern deep learning-based object detection pipelines. Yet, there are currently no automated pipelines reported in literature that have considered detection of mitotic figures and subclassification according to their morphology into normal and atypical mitotic figures or into the various phases within the mitosis. Automated approaches are therefore necessary for investigating these aspects on a larger scale. Distinct types of abnormalities may occur in the different mitosis phases and separation of the normal mitotic figure morphologies along the cell cycle may facilitate identification of AMF. Further, identification of mitosis phase might be a valuable tool for high throughput cell analysis within the development of novel cancer targets [8].

We propose an efficient and fully automatic pipeline based upon the principle of fully convolutional one-stage object detection (FCOS) [9]. Considering the different phases of mitotic figures and the morphological variations manifested as AMF, the classes of a one-dimensional classification problem does not account for the hierarchy of classes. Thus, we extend the architecture by a hierarchical class prediction and define a tailored loss function and sampling scheme.

2 Dataset

All mitotic figures contained within the TUPAC16 [7] and MIDOG21 [6] datasets were annotated by two pathologists according to five classes, spread across two hierarchical

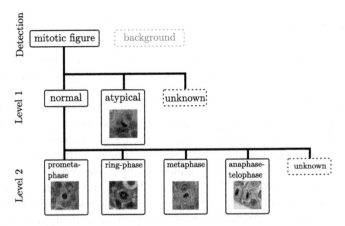

Fig. 1. Label hierarchy: We consider the detection and the subclassification of mitotic figures in two levels.

Tab. 1. Confusion matrix for subclassification of mitotic figures of expert 1 (columns) and expert 2 (rows) in our annotation experiment on the TUPAC16 and MIDOG21 datasets (total number of objects was 4,769).

| | | Atypical | | Typical | | |
			ring shape	anaphase-telophase	prometa-phase	meta-phase
Atypical		587	6	17	39	79
	ring shape (prometaphase or metaphase)	21	57	2	3	3
Typical	normal anaphase-telophase	88	0	218	3	17
	normal prometaphase	258	128	25	1200	280
	normal metaphase	176	0	12	30	1520

levels (Fig. 1 and Tab. 1): On level 1, we differentiated between atypical and normal mitotic figures. The latter was subsequently split on level 2 into prometaphase, metaphase, ring shaped mitosis, and anaphase/telophase. The category of atypical mitotic figures was not subdivided further due to the limited prevalence. For the annotation, we used the definitions used by Donovan et al. [1]. We used the alternative version of the TUPAC16 dataset [10] provided by the same authors as the MIDOG21 dataset to reduce potential label bias. For annotations, we exported all mitotic figures as image cropouts with sufficient contextual information and asked two pathologists independently to assign the respective subcategories for both hierarchy levels. We found a total agreement in 75.11% of all cells. As shown in Table 1, the agreement was the highest for normal mitotic figures, while the the lack of agreement was most significant between atypical mitotic figures and prometaphase and metaphase mitotic figures.

3 Methods

The expert disagreement in almost a quarter of cases raises the question of how to deal with the expert disagreement algorithmically. Particularly for the four-category discrimination on our secondary level (mitotic phase), incorporating the opinion of a blinded tertiary expert would not necessarily lead to a clear majority vote. Instead, our approach aimed at mitigating this disagreement: We formulate the object detection problem as a hierarchical label problem with the main object class (mitosis) being a categorical label that a majority of experts agreed upon. We introduce two subcategorical labels for each object that can be either present (in case of an unanimous vote of the experts) or absent (Fig. 1).

3.1 Deep Learning Architecture

We based our experiments on the FCOS architecture by Tian et al.[9]. Over previous approaches, FCOS does not depend on the prior definition and optimization of anchor boxes for object detection and instead predicts object classes and bounding boxes as well as the distance to the object center for each coordinate in the latent space of a feature pyramid network. As shown in Figure 2, we extended the architecture by two new heads, corresponding to the two hierarchical levels of our problem. Accounting for the significant disagreement between experts that Tab. 1 reveals, we added also an *unknown* class on each hierarchy level to account for expert disagreement. For both new subclassification heads, we added a loss-term to the FCOS loss, realized as a generalized intersection over union-dependent focal loss as in FCOS, but gated with the availability of the subclass, i.e., zeroed for object-related losses where the respective subclass is *unknown*. As a baseline, we used an unmodified, non-hierarchical FCOS approach with 6 classes: mitotic figure with unknown subclass, atypical, and the four normal classes. In both cases, we used square patches of size 1024 *px*. All prediction heads had 4 CNN layers, as in the default FCOS. We make all code available online[1].

3.2 Training

We trained and validated both models on the MIDOG21 dataset and used the less diverse (particularly regarding the scanner variability) TUPAC16 dataset as our hold-out test set. To account for variability in training, especially related to a potential domain shift between datasets, we repeated the experiments five times. We randomly assigned 20% of the MIDOG21 cases to the validation set, which we used for model selection and used the remainder of the training set for the optimization of the model weights. We

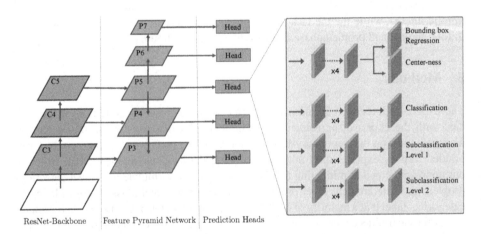

Fig. 2. Depiction of the model architecture, with two additional hierarchical label classification heads. Modified from [9].

Tab. 2. Results of the proposed hierarchical anchor-free model in comparison to a baseline non-hierarchical baseline model. Given are mean ± std values of the area under the receiver operating characteristic curve (ROC-AUC) of detected objects of five consecutive runs as well as the overall average precision (AP) and average recall (AR).

approach	ROC-AUC Level 1		ROC-AUC Level 2			Overall AP	Overall AR
	atypical/ normal	prometa-phase	ring shape	meta-phase	anaphase-telophase		
FCOS (baseline)	0.817± 0.019	0.957± 0.024	0.926± 0.011	0.924± 0.009	0.945± 0.008	0.499± 0.061	0.929± 0.012
HFCOS (proposed)	**0.833**± 0.061	**0.971**± 0.023	**0.966**± 0.023	**0.984**± 0.012	**0.987**± 0.003	**0.552**± 0.084	**0.946**± 0.013

stratified for the six classes within our sampling scheme to make sure a sufficient gradient accumulation for the classes of low occurrence. Our sampling scheme ensured that at least one mitotic figure of the selected class would be visible on the selected image patch. Additionally, we employed sampling of hard negatives examples (imposters), which are available in both datasets, in 30% of cases, which aims to make the model more robust (i.e., able to differentiate mitotic figures from mitotic figure look-alikes). The training dataset provides hard examples that can be used for this purpose. We defined an epoch as containing 2000 randomly sampled images. We then trained for up to 50 epochs, using early stopping on the validation loss with a patience of 10.

3.3 Evaluation

Average precision (AP) is commonly calculated class-specific for each of the object detection classes, based upon the score that was assigned to that object, and averaged to yield the mean average precision (mAP) score. However, having only a single class (mitosis) in our hierarchical label approach and multiple classes in the baseline, this makes the mAP metric for this case practically incomparable. Instead, we calculated for both models the overall (class-independent) AP score. For the baseline model this was achieved by ignoring the class of the object for both, the labels and the detections. Similarly, we report the overall average recall (AR). Additionally, we report the area under the receiver operating characteristic curve (ROC-AUC) of all objects that were detected by the respective approaches (using the default threshold of 0.5 for the intersection over union). For the multi-class problem in hierarchy level two, we report the ROC-AUC as one-vs-rest classification problem.

4 Results

We found that the subclassification benefits from the hierarchical approach (Tab. 2). We observed this effect both for the level 1 subclassification of atypical vs. normal mitotic figures and for the level 2 subclassification of mitotic phases. Effectively, for all observed metrics, the proposed approach outperformed the baseline. Moreover, we found a moderate variability of the results across the five runs. Further, assessing the overall cell detection, we found the AP and AR for mitotic figures overall to be increased by using the hierarchical labels model.

5 Discussion

Our results, particularly those of the annotation experiment (Tab. 1), indicate that differentiation between normal and atypical mitotic figures (AMFs) represents a difficult task. However, identification of the phases of mitosis (when clearly defined), is a more straightforward task for humans and deep learning algorithms. It is possible that a refined definition of the features of AMFs may improve agreement between experts, or that some of the subcategories of AMFs may have better agreement than others. The overall moderate AP value could be linked to a domain shift between the MIDOG21 and the TUPAC16 data set, and could be reduced by applying methods of domain generalization [6], and/or tackled by more extensive data augmentation. One limitation of the current work is that the MIDOG21 and the TUPAC16 datasets include only regions from the areas of increased mitotic activity (hotspots) within the breast cancer specimens. Thus, it is unclear how robust the trained algorithm would perform on whole slide images (WSIs), and clinical-grade solutions would need to be trained on combined data sets including fully annotated WSI. Furthermore, the MIDOG21 dataset uses data from only one hospital, and generalization might also be reduced by this. To the best of our knowledge, this approach represents the first attempt at automated mitotic figure detection and subclassification on H&E-stained tissue, both for the identification of AMFs and the mitotic phase for normal mitoses. The availability of this method enables extensive clinical research investigating the prognostic power of the ratio of AMFs to normal mitotic figures, which we will continue to expand upon in our ongoing research.

References

1. Donovan TA, Moore FM, Bertram CA, Luong R, Bolfa P, Klopfleisch R et al. Mitotic Figures—Normal, Atypical, and Imposters: A Guide to Identification. Vet Pathol. 2021;58(2):243–57.
2. Lashen A, Toss MS, Alsaleem M, Green AR, Mongan NP, Rakha E. The characteristics and clinical significance of atypical mitosis in breast cancer. Mod Pathol. 2022;35:1341–8.
3. Rubio C. Atypical mitoses in colorectal adenomas. Pathol Res Pract. 1991;187(4):508–13.
4. Ohashi R, Namimatsu S, Sakatani T, Naito Z, Takei H, Shimizu A. Prognostic utility of atypical mitoses in patients with breast cancer: a comparative study with Ki67 and phosphohistone H3. J Surg Oncol. 2018;118(3):557–67.
5. Jin Y, Stewénius Y, Lindgren D, Frigyesi A, Calcagnile O, Jonson T et al. Distinct mitotic segregation errors mediate chromosomal instability in aggressive urothelial cancers. Clin Cancer Res. 2007;13(6):1703–12.
6. Aubreville M, Stathonikos N et al. Mitosis domain generalization in histopathology images–The MIDOG challenge. Med Image Anal. 2023;84:102699.
7. Veta M, Heng YJ, Stathonikos N, Bejnordi BE, Beca F, Wollmann T et al. Predicting breast tumor proliferation from whole-slide images: the TUPAC16 challenge. Med Image Anal. 2019;54:111–21.

8. Tao CY, Hoyt J, Feng Y. A support vector machine classifier for recognizing mitotic subphases using high-content screening data. SLAS Discovery. 2007;12(4):490–6.

9. Tian Z, Shen C, Chen H, He T. Fcos: Fully convolutional one-stage object detection. Proceedings of ICCV. 2019:9627–36.

10. Bertram CA, Veta M, Marzahl C, Stathonikos N, Maier A, Klopfleisch R et al. Are pathologist-defined labels reproducible? Comparison of the TUPAC16 mitotic figure dataset with an alternative set of labels. Interpretable and Annotation-Efficient Learning for Medical Image Computing. Springer, 2020:204–13.

Abstract: Automated Detection and Quantification of Brain Metastases on Clinical MRI Data using CNNs

Irada Pflüger[1,7], Tassilo Wald[2,3,7], Fabian Isensee[2,3], Marianne Schell[1],
Hagen Meredig[1], Kai Schlamp[1], Denise Bernhardt[4], Gianluca Brugnara[1],
Claus P. Heußel[1,6], Juergen Debus[1,2], Wolfgang Wick[1,2], Martin Bendszus[1],
Klaus Maier-Hein[1,2], Philipp Vollmuth[1]

[1]Heidelberg University Hospital, Heidelberg, Germany
[2]German Cancer Research Center (DKFZ), Heidelberg, Germany
[3]Helmholtz Imaging
[4]Technical University Munich (TUM), Munich, Germany
[5]German Center for Lung Research (DZL)
[6]Translational Lung Research Center (TLRC), Heidelberg, Germany
[7]equal contribution; Full affiliations in [1]
philipp.vollmuth@med.uni-heidelberg.de

Reliable detection and precise volumetric quantification of brain metastases (BM) on MRI are essential for guiding treatment decisions. We evaluate the potential of CNNs for automated detection and quantification of BM by training models on 308 patients with BM (with a 4:1 split for training/testing) for automated volumetric assessment of contrast-enhancing tumors (CE) and non-enhancing FLAIR signal abnormality including edema (NEE). An independent test set of 30 patients was used for external testing. We assessed performance case-wise for CE and NEE and lesion-wise for CE using the case-wise/lesion-wise DICE-coefficient (C/L-DICE), positive predictive value (L-PPV) and sensitivity (C/L-Sensitivity). The performance of detecting CE lesions on the validation dataset was not significantly affected when evaluating different volumetric thresholds (0.001–0.2 cm 3 ; $P = .2028$). The median L-DICE and median C-DICE for CE lesions were 0.78 (IQR = 0.6–0.91) and 0.90 (IQR = 0.85–0.94) in the institutional as well as 0.79 (IQR = 0.67–0.82) and 0.84 (IQR = 0.76–0.89) in the external test dataset. The corresponding median L-Sensitivity and median L-PPV were 0.81 (IQR = 0.63–0.92) and 0.79 (IQR = 0.63–0.93) in the institutional test dataset, as compared to 0.85 (IQR = 0.76–0.94) and 0.76 (IQR = 0.68–0.88) in the external test dataset. The median C-DICE for NEE was 0.96 (IQR = 0.92–0.97) in the institutional test dataset as compared to 0.85 (IQR = 0.72–0.91) in the external test dataset. The developed ANN-based algorithm (publicly available at www.github.com/NeuroAI-HD/HD-BM) allows reliable detection and precise volumetric quantification of CE and NEE compartments in patients with BM. The full paper has been published at Neuro-Oncology Advances [1].

References

1. Pflüger I, Wald T, Isensee F, Schell M, Meredig H, Schlamp K et al. Automated detection and quantification of brain metastases on clinical MRI data using artificial neural networks. Neurooncol Adv. 2022;4(1). vdac138.

© Der/die Autor(en), exklusiv lizenziert an
Springer Fachmedien Wiesbaden GmbH, ein Teil von Springer Nature 2023
T. M. Deserno et al. (Hrsg.), *Bildverarbeitung für die Medizin 2023*,
Informatik aktuell, https://doi.org/10.1007/978-3-658-41657-7_41

Abstract: Determination of Unknown Biomechanical Parameters of a Screw-vertebra MBS Model

Ivanna Kramer[1], Sabine Bauer[2], Dietrich Paulus[1]

[1]Institute for Computational Visualistics, University of Koblenz, Koblenz
[2]Institute of Medical Technology and Information Processing, University of Koblenz, Koblenz
ikramer@uni-koblenz.de

In this study, we show that parameters for which values are not known a priori can be determined with sufficient accuracy using a multibody simulation (MBS) model. We propose a sensitivity analysis method that allows us to approximate these unknown parameters without the need for long simulation times. Furthermore, this method allows the MBS model to be optimized to a high degree using an iterative process. The sensitivity analysis method is applied to a simplified screw-vertebra model, consisting of an anterior anchor implant screw and vertebral body of C4. The main focus is on determining stiffness (c) and damping (d) characteristics to analyze the interaction between the implant anchor screw and the vertebral body. In the two-stage algorithm, we aim to find a tuple of the minimum stiffness and damping coefficients from the predefined values so that the maximum screw translation and the maximum screw velocity are constrained by the selected thresholds when the pullout force is applied to the cervical screw. In addition, we analyze when the static equilibrium state of the model is reached in each iteration. The proposed parameter determination is performed in two phases. In the first step, two initial sets of parameters, one set for c-values and one containing d-values, were collected. Then, for each pair of parameter values, the model simulation is executed, and the final search intervals for both parameters are determined. In the final step, a binary search is used to minimize the parameters. The optimal model parameters for the MBS model are determined to be $c = 823224 N/m$ for stiffness and $d = 488 Ns/m$ for damping. The presented method of parameter identification can be used in studies including more complex MBS spine models or to set initial parameter values that are not available as initial values for FE models [1].

References

1. Kramer I, Bauer S. Can a priori unknown values of biomechanical parameters be determined with sufficient accuracy in MBS using sensitivity analysis? Analyzing the characteristics of the Interaction between cervical vertebra and pedicle screw. Biomechanics (Basel). 2022;2(1):107–24.

Challenge Results are not Reproducible

Annika Reinke[1,2,3], Georg Grab[1,3], Lena Maier-Hein[1,2,3]

[1]Intelligent Medical Systems (IMSY), German Cancer Research Center (DKFZ), Heidelberg, Germany
[2]HI Helmholtz Imaging, DKFZ, Heidelberg, Germany
[3]University Heidelberg, Heidelberg, Germany
a.reinke@dkfz-heidelberg.de

Abstract. While clinical trials are the state-of-the-art methods to assess the effect of new medication in a comparative manner, benchmarking in the field of medical image analysis is performed by so-called challenges. Recently, comprehensive analysis of multiple biomedical image analysis challenges revealed large discrepancies between the impact of challenges and quality control of the design and reporting standard. This work aims to follow up on these results and attempts to address the specific question of the reproducibility of the participants methods. In an effort to determine whether alternative interpretations of the method description may change the challenge ranking, we reproduced the algorithms submitted to the 2019 Robust medical image segmentation challenge (ROBUST-MIS). The leaderboard differed substantially between the original challenge and reimplementation, indicating that challenge rankings may not be sufficiently reproducible[1].

1 Introduction

Robust segmentation of biomedical images is an important precursor to many new, innovative computer-assisted applications. Deep learning-based segmentation methods have proven to work successfully on a wide range of medical imaging data, including computed tomography (CT), magnetic resonance imaging (MRI), and endoscopy [1]. For benchmarking which type of model works best on a given medical domain, challenges have become an important tool, and are now commonplace in conferences such as the conference on medical image computing and computer assisted interventions (MICCAI) or the IEEE international symposium on biomedical imaging (ISBI). However, recent comprehensive analysis of challenges in the biomedical domain revealed that the current state of quality control severely limits interpretation of rankings and reproducibility, with only a fraction of the relevant information typically provided [2].

In order to concretely analyze the reproducibility of the participating methods in challenges, we aimed to reimplement the algorithms of all participating teams in a challenge only based on their submitted method descriptions. As an example, we performed our experiments for the 2019 Robust medical image segmentation challenge (ROBUST-MIS). Given the obligation to submit a detailed description of their methods together with their actual results, this challenge had a disproportionately high amount of algorithmic information available, which should in theory faciliate the reproducibility of

---

[1]Shared first authors: Annika Reinke and Georg Grab

© Der/die Autor(en), exklusiv lizenziert an
Springer Fachmedien Wiesbaden GmbH, ein Teil von Springer Nature 2023
T. M. Deserno et al. (Hrsg.), *Bildverarbeitung für die Medizin 2023*,
Informatik aktuell, https://doi.org/10.1007/978-3-658-41657-7_43

results. However, in this work, we show that even with this high amount of information available, we were not able to reproduce the challenge results.

2 Materials and methods

The ROBUST-MIS challenge [3] focused on the robustness and generalization capabilities of algorithms. A collection of surgical data with 10 040 annotated images from 30 surgical procedures across three different types of surgery served as the basis for the challenge. The challenge was validated across competing methods in three stages with a growing domain gap between the training and test data, i.e. higher stages contained more difficult images requiring a higher degree of generalization to be segmented successfully. A detailed overview of the challenge can be found in [3]. In the following experiments, we focused on the multi-instance instrument segmentation task of the challenge.

In the challenge, alongside their algorithm submission, participating teams were required to submit a document summarizing their method in detail to the point of being reproducible, such as the used network architecture, data augmentations and all hyperparameters. These method descriptions, along with the summaries included in the challenge paper [3] were used as a basis for reproducing the challenge results. In general, we aimed to stay as close to the descriptions as possible, meaning the same programming languages and libraries were used, if this information was made available.

In case of ambiguous or missing information in method descriptions, we first attempted to infer the correct meaning using literature directly cited by the method description. Only if this was not possible, secondary literature was considered. As a last resort, we filled the missing information by surveying publicly available similar implementations and taking the most popular approach that worked reasonably well on the problem domain. For example, if a team would not document the type of optimizer, and relevant citations did not explicitly mention this either, the default choice of the most popular or official implementation was used. If two interpretations were equally likely, the method was trained using both interpretations, and the one resulting in better validation performance was chosen.

In the original challenge, participants were ranked according to two different criteria, robustness and generalization capabilities, resulting in two rankings based on the multi-instance dice similarity coefficient (MI_DSC) [3, 4]. The robustness ranking was determined by calculating a metric-based ranking using the 5% quantile of MI_DSC values obtained from the testing set. The accuracy ranking was calculated as a test-based ranking using a Wilcoxon signed rank test at a 5% significance level [5]. For our calculation, we considered stage three of the test set. Additionally, we compared the rankings with Kendall's τ correlation coefficient [6], which yields a value of 1 for two perfectly agreeing rankings and -1 if rankings are reversed. Ranking variability was investigated via bootstrapping [5]. We used the *challengeR* package [5] for calculating rankings and ranking uncertainty.

3 Results

During our reimplementation, lots of ambiguities were found in the method descriptions. Fig. 1 presents a qualitative summary of the assumptions made across all descriptions. Here, the term minor deficiency was defined as an assumption that had to be taken due to missing or clearly incorrect information, but was thought to either have a minor impact on model performance or there was high confidence that the right assumption has been made from context. Major deficiencies were defined as missing design decisions either thought to have a major impact on final model performance, there was low confidence that the correct assumption had been made from context or context was unavailable. In such a case, it was highly unlikely that our choice was identical to that of the original implementation. From the figure, it can be seen that both the model selection and data augmentation showed the highest amount of major and minor deficiencies during the reimplementation, followed by the data splits and the description of inference.

When calculating the metric values of the reimplemented methods, the distribution of values substantially differed between the original challenge and the reimplementation, except for team A2. This was also visible in the rankings. Tab. 1 shows the accuracy ranking for the original challenge and the reimplementation. The original winner changed for the reimplementation and teams moved mostly up or down by one single rank with an average change of one rank. Kendall's τ was 0.59 between both rankings, indicating a high variability. The ranking variability was analyzed by applying bootstrapping. The average (median, Interquartile range (IQR) Kendall's τ over 1,000 bootstrap rankings was 1.00 (median: 1.00; IQR: (1.00, 1.00)) for the original challenge, which was thus very robust against small perturbations. The average (median, IQR) Kendall's τ for the reimplementation was slightly less with a mean (median, IQR) Kendall's τ of 0.98 (median: 0.98; IQR: (0.98, 1.00)).

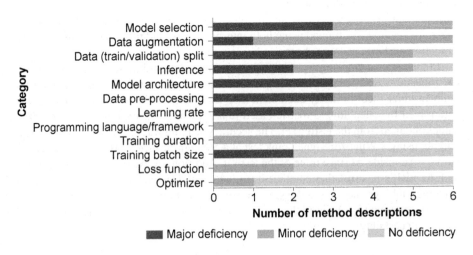

Fig. 1. Qualitative analysis of deficiency in method descriptions across several different aspects of implementation.

Tab. 1. Accuracy ranking based on the multi-instance dice similarity coefficient (MI_DSC). Accuracy is determined by the proportion of significant tests divided by the number of algorithms (Prop. Sign). The last column of (b) Δ shows the relative rank difference between the original challenge and the reimplementation of the algorithm.

Team	Prop. Sign.	Rank
A1	1.00	1
A2	0.83	2
A3	0.67	3
A4	0.33	4
A5	0.33	4
A6	0.17	6
A7	0.00	7

(a) Original

Team	Prop. Sign.	Rank	Δ
A2	1.00	1	↑ 1
A1	0.83	2	↓ 1
A4	0.67	3	↑ 1
A5	0.50	4	→ 0
A3	0.33	5	↓ 2
A7	0.17	6	↑ 1
A6	0.00	7	↓ 1

(b) Reimplementation

Tab. 2. Robustness rankings based on the 5% quantile of the multi-instance dice similarity coefficient (MI_DSC), computed for all stage 3 test cases. The last column of (b) Δ shows the relative rank difference between original challenge and reimplementation for the algorithm.

Team	MI_DSC	Rank
A5	0.31	1
A2	0.26	2
A4	0.22	3
A7	0.19	4
A1	0.17	5
A3	0.00	6
A6	0.00	6

(a) Original

Team	MI_DSC	Rank	Δ
A2	0.28	1	↑ 1
A1	0.11	2	↓ 1
A5	0.04	3	↓ 2
A3	0.00	4	↑ 2
A7	0.00	4	→ 0
A4	0.00	4	↓ 1
A6	0.00	4	↑ 2

(b) Reimplementation

Similarly, Tab. 2 shows the original and reimplemented versions for the robustness ranking. Again the winners according to this ranking changed and the average change in ranks was higher for this ranking scheme (1.3). Comparing both rankings yielded a Kendall's τ of 0.40. Notably, four algorithms failed to achieve a 5% quantile of the MI_DSC above 0 in the reimplementation, which only happened for two algorithms in the original challenge. We further found a higher ranking uncertainty for the original challenge with a mean (median, IQR) Kendall's τ of 0.85 (median: 0.98; IQR: (0.98, 1.00)). On the other hand, this ranking scheme was more stable for the reimplementation (mean: 0.97; median: 1.00; IQR: (1.00, 1.00)).

4 Discussion

In this work, we attempted to reproduce the rankings of the ROBUST-MIS challenge by means of reimplementing algorithms of participating teams given the method description they were required to submit. This attempt failed: both ranking schemes yielded results that substantially differed for the reimplementation, including changing the winners.

While training deep learning models comes with a substantial amount of non-determinism, which additionally contributes to the problem of reproducibility, we think the primary reason for failing to reproduce the results is the insufficient documentation provided by the participants. As shown in Fig. 1, the number of assumptions needed to be taken for reproducing the methods were numerous and spanned all relevant steps of model development, including data preprocessing, model architecture, and inference. For one team, we were not even able to identify the basic network architecture.

We found that complex design decisions tended to be described less accurately than design decisions that are typically simpler to document. For example, the standard choices for optimizers are limited and typically prominently visible in the source code. This may be a reason why almost all participants succeeded in unambiguously stating the utilized optimizer and associated hyperparameters.

On the other hand, model selection and data augmentation are complex processes, which were documented poorly by challenge teams. While the best-performing model is usually selected by calculating the loss on a separate validation data set, this does not necessarily have to be the case. In the ROBUST-MIS challenge, in particular, it was beneficial to select a sensitive over a specific model, since a false negative fraction of only 5% would be enough to completely fail the robustness ranking, i.e. yielding a 5% quantile of 0. Many teams either overlooked this aspect of the challenge completely in their documentation or provided incomplete information. Similarly, while the types of data augmentations were typically well reported, the respective hyperparameters were usually not documented. In addition, data augmentations can be applied individually or be combined with other data augmentation techniques. In such a case, the order and probabilities need to be specified. Finally, data augmentations complicate the exact meaning of the term 'epoch': is the original dataset extended only once with a certain percentage of augmented images, or are augmentations continually applied on the fly during training? All these choices need to be documented in detail in order to allow for faithful reimplementation.

Most design choices going into an algorithm relevant for challenge participation directly map to the source code, and thus reproducibility would be greatly improved by making the source code publicly available. However, since this is practically challenging, e.g. for teams from industry, certain aspects of the method description should be handled with great care:

- *Reasoning for complexity:* Some teams made complicated design decisions. For example, one team used a complex multi-stage approach for inference but did not elaborate on the reasoning for choosing this procedure. While a detailed explanation would have increased the understanding in general, it could also have been used to verify that an implementation was correct while reproducing the results.
- *Hyperparameters:* Although simple to document, many teams failed to properly list their chosen hyperparameters, especially for data augmentation and final threshold values for the purpose of inference.
- *Model Selection:* While most design decisions directly map to the source code, model selection is often a notable exception to this, and may involve manual analysis and comparison of several models using different performance metrics. This may be a reason why this work identified many deficiencies related to this aspect. Especially

in segmentation tasks, the considerations may go beyond minimizing the validation loss, since the final ranking methods are often not suitable for being utilized as loss functions. In any case, model selection should ideally be quantifiable and documented.

It should be noted that drawing conclusions from this work is limited since only a single challenge has been analyzed. However, for this challenge, an exceptionally high amount of information regarding the algorithms was available, strengthening our hypothesis that reproduction of challenge results is limited even if a detailed method description is required from the organizers. Furthermore, training deep learning models is inherently associated with a certain degree of non-determinism, where two identical training runs can potentially lead to severely different results [7]. Only one challenge participant addressed this limitation by employing ensembling and averaging their results during inference. Thus, ironically, this work itself may be deemed non-reproducible.

With this work, we showed that even well-documented methods are not easily reproducible. However, we think that the most effective way of reducing the issue of non-reproducibility would be publicly available source code of all participating teams of a challenge, although maybe practically challenging. Especially for the winning teams, such an action would be desirable since the winning method is typically seen as the new state-of-the-art method for a specific problem. We hope that this work will trigger further actions by stakeholders involved in policy-making for challenges.

Acknowledgement. Part of this work was funded by Helmholtz Imaging, a platform of the Helmholtz Incubator on Information and Data Science. We would like to thank Marcel Knopp and Minu D. Tizabi for proofreading the document.

References

1. Siddique N et al. U-net and its variants for medical image segmentation: a review of theory and applications. IEEE Access. 2021.
2. Maier-Hein L et al. Why rankings of biomedical image analysis competitions should be interpreted with care. Nat Commun. 2018;9(1):1–13.
3. Ross T et al. Comparative validation of multi-instance instrument segmentation in endoscopy: results of the ROBUST-MIS 2019 challenge. Med Image Anal. 2021;70:101920.
4. Dice LR. Measures of the amount of ecologic association between species. Ecology. 1945;26(3):297–302.
5. Wiesenfarth M et al. Methods and open-source toolkit for analyzing and visualizing challenge results. Sci Rep. 2021;11(1):1–15.
6. Kendall MG. A new measure of rank correlation. Biometrika. 1938;30(1/2):81–93.
7. Pham HV et al. Problems and opportunities in training deep learning software systems: an analysis of variance. Proc IEEE/ACM Int Conf Autom Softw Eng Workshops. 2020:771–83.

Abstract: Is Medical Chest X-ray Data Anonymous?

Deep Learning-based Patient Re-identification is Able to Exploit the Biometric Nature of Medical Chest X-ray Data

Kai Packhäuser, Sebastian Gündel, Nicolas Münster, Christopher Syben, Vincent Christlein, Andreas Maier

Pattern Recognition Lab, Friedrich-Alexander-Universität Erlangen-Nürnberg, Germany
kai.packhaeuser@fau.de

With the rise and ever-increasing potential of deep learning techniques in recent years, publicly available medical datasets became a key factor to enable reproducible development of diagnostic algorithms in the medical domain. Medical data contains sensitive patient-related information and is therefore usually anonymized by removing patient identifiers, e. g., patient names before publication. To the best of our knowledge, we are the first to show that a well-trained deep learning system is able to recover the patient identity from chest X-ray data. We demonstrate this using the publicly available large-scale ChestX-ray14 dataset, a collection of 112,120 frontal-view chest X-ray images from 30,805 unique patients. Our verification system is able to identify whether two frontal chest X-ray images are from the same person with an AUC of 0.9940 and a classification accuracy of 95.55 %. We further highlight that the proposed system is able to reveal the same person even ten and more years after the initial scan. When pursuing a retrieval approach, we observe an mAP@R of 0.9748 and a precision@1 of 0.9963. Furthermore, we achieve an AUC of up to 0.9870 and a precision@1 of up to 0.9444 when evaluating our trained networks on external datasets such as CheXpert and the COVID-19 Image Data Collection. Based on this high identification rate, a potential attacker may leak patient-related information and additionally cross-reference images to obtain more information. Thus, there is a great risk of sensitive content falling into unauthorized hands or being disseminated against the will of the concerned patients. Especially during the COVID-19 pandemic, numerous chest X-ray datasets have been published to advance research. Therefore, such data may be vulnerable to potential attacks by deep learning-based re-identification algorithms. This work has previously been published in Scientific Reports [1].

References

1. Packhäuser K, Gündel S, Münster N, Syben C, Christlein V, Maier A. Deep learning-based patient re-identification is able to exploit the biometric nature of medical chest X-ray data. Sci Rep. 2022;12(1):1–13.

Abstract: Pan-tumor CAnine CuTaneous Cancer Histology (CATCH) Dataset

Frauke Wilm[1,2], Marco Fragoso[3], Christian Marzahl[1], Jingna Qiu[2], Chloé Puget[3], Laura Diehl[3], Christof A. Bertram[4], Robert Klopfleisch[3], Andreas Maier[1], Katharina Breininger[2], Marc Aubreville[5]

[1]Pattern Recognition Lab, Friedrich-Alexander-Universität Erlangen-Nünberg, Germany
[2]Department AIBE, Friedrich-Alexander-Universität Erlangen-Nürnberg, Germany
[3]Institute of Veterinary Pathology, Freie Universität Berlin, Germany
[4]Institute of Pathology, University of Veterinary Medicine, Vienna, Austria
[5]Technische Hochschule Ingolstadt, Ingolstadt, Germany
frauke.wilm@fau.de

The identification of tumor regions on cutaneous tissue sections and the subsequent differentiation into individual tumor subtypes are routine tasks for veterinary pathologists. However, manual tumor delineation can be time-consuming and morphological similarities of tumor types can make the subtyping task difficult. Deep learning-based algorithms have been successfully applied for both tasks but require a large amount of annotated data to learn robust representations. Acquiring the annotations necessary to train these algorithms can be time-consuming and requires expert knowledge. Publicly available datasets reduce this annotation overhead and allow for a comparison of image analysis algorithms trained for the task at hand. We published a publicly available dataset of 350 whole slide images (WSIs) of seven different canine cutaneous tumors. These were annotated for the tumor subtypes and additionally six skin tissue classes. Overall, the database includes 12,424 polygon annotations for 13 classes, which exceeds most publicly available datasets in annotation extent and label diversity. In our dataset report, we validated the provided annotations through inter-rater experiments on a subset of the presented dataset, where three pathologists demonstrated high consistency in labeling tissue structures, especially for tumor annotations. Furthermore, we performed a technical validation by first training a deep neural network for tissue phenotyping. The model segmented the WSI into tumor and five skin tissue classes, where we achieved a class-averaged Jaccard coefficient of 0.7047 and a Jaccard coefficient of 0.9044 for tumor in particular. Afterward, we classified the segmented tumor regions into the tumor subtypes and achieved a slide-level accuracy of 0.9857. These baseline results provide a starting point for the development of more advanced algorithms. Previous works have shown that canine and human cutaneous tumors share various histologic patterns, which extends the added value of the presented dataset beyond veterinary pathology [1].

References

1. Wilm F, Fragoso M, Marzahl C, Qiu J, Puget C, Diehl L et al. Pan-tumor CAnine cuTaneous Cancer histology (CATCH) dataset. Sci Data. 2022;9:588.

T. M. Deserno et al. (Hrsg.), *Bildverarbeitung für die Medizin 2023*,
Informatik aktuell, https://doi.org/10.1007/978-3-658-41657-7_45

Multi-scanner Canine Cutaneous Squamous Cell Carcinoma Histopathology Dataset

Frauke Wilm[1,2], Marco Fragoso[3], Christof A. Bertram[4], Nikolas Stathonikos[5], Mathias Öttl[1], Jingna Qiu[2], Robert Klopfleisch[3], Andreas Maier[1], Katharina Breininger[2], Marc Aubreville[6]

[1]Pattern Recognition Lab, Friedrich-Alexander-Universität Erlangen-Nünberg, Germany
[2]Department AIBE, Friedrich-Alexander-Universität Erlangen-Nürnberg, Germany
[3]Institute of Veterinary Pathology, Freie Universität Berlin, Germany
[4]Institute of Pathology, University of Veterinary Medicine, Vienna, Austria
[5]Pathology Department, University Medical Centre Utrecht, The Netherlands
[6]Technische Hochschule Ingolstadt, Ingolstadt, Germany
frauke.wilm@fau.de

Abstract. In histopathology, scanner-induced domain shifts are known to impede the performance of trained neural networks when tested on unseen data. Multi-domain pre-training or dedicated domain-generalization techniques can help to develop domain-agnostic algorithms. For this, multi-scanner datasets with a high variety of slide scanning systems are highly desirable. We present a publicly available multi-scanner dataset of canine cutaneous squamous cell carcinoma histopathology images, composed of 44 samples digitized with five slide scanners. This dataset provides local correspondences between images and thereby isolates the scanner-induced domain shift from other inherent, e.g. morphology-induced domain shifts. To highlight scanner differences, we present a detailed evaluation of color distributions, sharpness, and contrast of the individual scanner subsets. Additionally, to quantify the inherent scanner-induced domain shift, we train a tumor segmentation network on each scanner subset and evaluate the performance both in- and cross-domain. We achieve a class-averaged in-domain intersection over union coefficient of up to 0.86 and observe a cross-domain performance decrease of up to 0.38, which confirms the inherent domain shift of the presented dataset and its negative impact on the performance of deep neural networks.

1 Introduction

Digitizing histological specimens with dedicated slide scanning systems has facilitated machine learning-based image analysis for histopathology. These algorithms have since assisted pathologists in a variety of routine tasks, e.g. mitotic figure detection [1], for which they have been able to outperform trained experts in controlled settings [1, 2]. Still, their performance is highly dependent on the quality and availability of training data [3] and can deteriorate considerably on a test set where the image characteristics differ from the training data [4]. Such differences commonly referred to as "domain shift" can originate not only from different staining and tissue preparation protocols of different pathology laboratories but also from the digitization of histological specimens with different scanning systems. Especially from a clinical perspective, domain-agnostic models are important for generating accurate and reliable predictions.

© Der/die Autor(en), exklusiv lizenziert an
Springer Fachmedien Wiesbaden GmbH, ein Teil von Springer Nature 2023
T. M. Deserno et al. (Hrsg.), *Bildverarbeitung für die Medizin 2023*,
Informatik aktuell, https://doi.org/10.1007/978-3-658-41657-7_46

Previous work has shown that domain generalization techniques, e.g. domain-adversarial training, can help to develop domain-agnostic models [5]. For this, a training dataset composed of a wide range of different domains is highly desirable. So far, the most extensive publicly available multi-scanner histopathology dataset is the training set of the MICCAI MItosis DOmain generalization (MIDOG) 2021 challenge [2]. The dataset consists of $2\,mm^2$-sized cropped regions of 200 breast cancer cases digitized with four scanners. However, the cases were divided between the scanners, and performance differences can therefore not solely be attributed to the slide scanner but also to the case selection. The Mitos & Atypia dataset [6] is the only public multi-scanner histopathology dataset with local image correspondences, i.e. the same case was digitized with multiple slide scanners, however, with 16 cases and two scanners, its extent is limited and it does not leave room for experiments with hold-out test scanners.

In this work, we present a canine cutaneous histopathology dataset, where each of the 44 samples was digitized with five different slide scanning systems. This multi-scanner dataset provides local image correspondences, useful for domain generalization experiments. Accompanied by an annotation database of 1,243 polygon annotations for seven histologic classes (tumor, epidermis, dermis, subcutis, bone, cartilage, and a combined class of inflammation and necrosis), this is the first publicly available multi-scanner segmentation dataset. For each scanner subset, we provide a detailed evaluation of color distributions, sharpness, and contrast. To quantify the extent of the scanner-induced domain shift, we performed a technical validation of the dataset by training a baseline tumor segmentation algorithm on each single scanner domain and then testing the algorithm across all scanners. For some scanners, we observed a considerable performance decrease, which highlights the domain shift inherent in the dataset. The whole slide images (WSIs) and annotation databases are publicly available on Zenodo[1], and code for implementing the baseline architectures can be obtained from our GitHub repository[2].

2 Materials and methods

The dataset presented in this work extends the publicly available CATCH dataset [7], a collection of 350 WSIs of seven of the most common canine cutaneous tumor subtypes

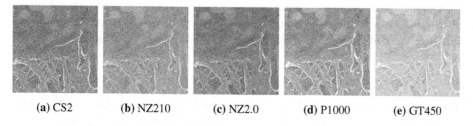

| (a) CS2 | (b) NZ210 | (c) NZ2.0 | (d) P1000 | (e) GT450 |

Fig. 1. Exemplary region of interest of the multi-scanner dataset.

[1]https://doi.org/10.5281/zenodo.7418555
[2]https://github.com/DeepPathology/MultiScanner_SCC

(50 WSIs per subtype). For the CATCH dataset, the specimens were digitized with the Aperio ScanScope CS2 (Leica, Germany) at a resolution of 0.25 μm/pixel using a 40× objective lens. Use of these samples was approved by the local governmental authorities (State Office of Health and Social Affairs of Berlin, approval ID: StN 011/20). For the multi-scanner dataset, we randomly selected one subtype (squamous cell carcinoma) and digitized the samples with four additional slide scanners (Fig. 1):

- NanoZoomer S210 (Hamamatsu, Japan), 0.22 μm/pixel
- NanoZoomer 2.0-HT (Hamamatsu, Japan), 0.23 μm/pixel
- Pannoramic 1000 (3DHISTECH, Hungary), 0.25 μm/pixel
- Aperio GT 450 (Leica, Germany), 0.26 μm/pixel

Due to severe scanning artifacts in at least one of the scans, six specimens were excluded from the dataset, resulting in a total of 220 WSIs (44 samples digitized with five scanners each). The CATCH annotation database provides annotations for the individual tumor subtypes and six additional skin tissue classes (epidermis, dermis, subcutis, bone, cartilage, and a combined class of inflammation and necrosis). We transferred all annotations to the other scanners using the WSI registration algorithm by Marzahl et al. [8] and visually validated them by overlaying the transformed polygon annotations onto the scans. We provide public access to the WSIs on Zenodo[3], licensed under a Creative Commons Attribution 4.0 International License. However, due to storage restrictions, we have converted them to lower-resolution pyramidal TIFFs (4 μm/pixel), which has shown to be adequate for training segmentation tasks on the CATCH dataset [9].

2.1 Dataset validation

For each scanner subset, we evaluated the average RGB color distribution, sharpness, and contrast. For sharpness estimation, we used the cumulative probability of blur detection (CPBD) metric [10], which is a perceptual-based image sharpness metric. It is computed via edge detection, followed by a blur estimation at the detected edges. The CPBD metric then corresponds to the cumulative probability of blur detection, i.e. the percentage of image edges that fall below a threshold of a perceptually noticeable blur. For implementation details, we refer to [10]. For the analysis of RGB distributions and contrast, we used Otsu's adaptive thresholding to separate foreground tissue from white background. For each image, we calculated the average intensities of the color channels I_R, I_G, and I_B in the detected tissue regions. Afterward, we converted the regions to grayscale and computed the Michelson contrast [11] C_M as a measure of global contrast.

2.2 Technical validation

For technical validation of the dataset, we trained a segmentation model on each scanner domain and tested the algorithm across all scanners. For model development, we performed a slide-level split into training (N=30), validation (N=5), and test (N=9) cases.

---

[3]https://doi.org/10.5281/zenodo.7418555

We trained a UNet with a ResNet18 encoder pre-trained on ImageNet for the segmentation into tumor, non-tumor, and background. For this, we combined all skin tissue classes into one non-tumor class and used the automatically detected background areas to train the background class. We trained the networks on image patches sized 512×512 pixels, extracted at a resolution of 4 µm/pixel. During each epoch, we sampled 50 patches per WSI within the annotated polygons. Due to a high class imbalance, we randomly sampled the polygons with a class-weighting of 10 % background and 45 % each of tumor and non-tumor regions. For each scanner, we applied z-score normalization with the training set statistics (mean and standard deviation) and performed data augmentation using random flipping, affine transformations, and random lightning and contrast change. We used the Adam optimizer and trained the networks with a combination of cross-entropy and Dice loss. We trained the models with a batch size of 8 and a cyclic learning rate of 10^{-4} for 100 epochs, after which we observed model convergence. Model selection was guided by the highest intersection over union (mIoU) on the validation set.

3 Results

Figure 2 shows the RGB distribution of the tissue areas for the complete dataset of 44 WSIs per scanner. The distributions match the exemplary patches in Figure 1, where the patches of the Aperio CS2 and the NanoZoomer 210 appear redder, reflected in a shift of the red pixel distributions to higher values. When looking at the distributions of the Aperio GT450, all curves are densely located at the higher color component values, which corresponds to the bright appearance of the patch in Figure 1e. Table 1 summarizes the channel-wise color averages, sharpness, and contrast of the slide scanning systems. These results further underline the visual impression of the patches in Figure 1. When calculating the ratio of the red and the blue color channel I_R/I_B, the NZ210 results in a ratio of 1.12 and the NZ2.0 in a ratio of 1.04, which matches the much redder appearance of the NZ210 patch and the bluer appearance of the NZ2.0 patch. Overall, the CS2, NZ210, NZ2.0, and P1000 show comparable sharpness and contrast values, while the Aperio 450 exhibits a slightly higher sharpness but a considerably lower contrast. Figure 3 visualizes the mIoU when training the segmentation network on one scanner, and testing it on all scanners. The results show high in-domain performance (diagonal) with mIoU values between 0.82 for the P1000 and GT450, and 0.86 for the NZ210. The cross-domain performance highlights the scanner-induced domain shift inherent in our dataset. While the networks trained on the CS2 and the NZ210 generalize considerably

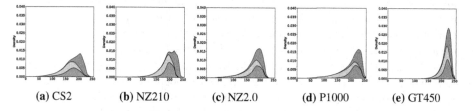

| (a) CS2 | (b) NZ210 | (c) NZ2.0 | (d) P1000 | (e) GT450 |

Fig. 2. Kernel density estimation of RGB values per scanner.

Tab. 1. Channel-wise color distributions I_R, I_G, and I_B, sharpness S_{CPBD} calculated as cumulative probability of blur detection, and Michelson contrast C_M of the scanners ($\mu \pm \sigma$).

	I_R	I_G	I_B	S_{CPBD}	C_M
CS2	202.25 ± 10.22	153.83 ± 20.67	172.45 ± 16.64	0.80 ± 0.02	0.74 ± 0.12
NZ210	219.28 ± 8.12	173.27 ± 15.48	196.21 ± 9.82	0.82 ± 0.03	0.81 ± 0.14
NZ2.0	193.22 ± 10.77	154.34 ± 21.14	185.75 ± 11.58	0.81 ± 0.02	0.81 ± 0.13
P1000	223.56 ± 10.58	165.50 ± 24.80	212.15 ± 11.51	0.80 ± 0.02	0.71 ± 0.14
GT450	226.94 ± 6.65	208.67 ± 11.82	219.39 ± 8.03	0.84 ± 0.04	0.53 ± 0.15

well, with performance decreases of only up to 0.08 and 0.12 compared to the in-domain mIoU, the highest cross-domain performance drop of up to 0.38 was observed when training on the P1000. The segmentation results showed that the network trained on the P1000 misclassified many background areas of the other scanners. A reason might be the integrated tissue detection of the P1000, which sets all pixels outside the tissue bounding box to (255, 255, 255) in order to reduce scanning times. This artificially removes common artifacts, e.g. dust particles, and the network might only look for high pixel values and not learn the morphological characteristics of background areas.

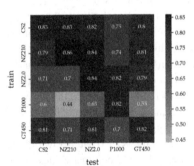

Fig. 3. Scanner-wise performance of segmentation networks. Matrix entry $m_{i,j}$ is the mean intersection over union (mIoU) when training on the scanning system in row i and testing on the scanning system in column j. Diagonal elements indicate in-domain performance, whereas off-diagonal elements represent cross-domain performance.

4   Discussion

Our experiments have demonstrated the negative impact of scanner-induced domain shifts on the performance of neural networks, indicated by a considerable decrease in mIoU on unseen scanners. This confirms the observations of previous works and the need for methods that can tackle this domain shift and adequate datasets to evaluate their generalization capability. The presented dataset exceeds existing multi-scanner datasets regarding sample size and scanning systems. Furthermore, it provides local image correspondences, which isolate the scanner-induced from the morphology-induced domain shift and allow the development of algorithms dependent on these correspondences, e.g. WSI registration algorithms. We have implicitly shown the eligibility of our dataset for this application by successfully transferring the CS2 annotation database to the remaining scanners using WSI registration. The detailed evaluation of our scanner subsets has highlighted considerable differences in color distributions and contrasts present in clinically used scanners. Surprisingly, even though our evaluations resulted in the lowest contrast value for the Aperio GT450, this did not impede segmentation performance, shown by an in-domain mIoU of 0.82, which is comparable to the in-domain mIoUs of the remaining scanners. Our technical validation detected a large cross-domain performance decrease when training on the P1000 scanner. We assume that this can mainly be attributed to the unique pre-processing steps of the scanner vendor, as the P1000 showed similar image statistics to the CS2 but their average cross-domain performance differed considerably. However, we also observed a decrease in cross-domain performance for the remaining scanners, indicating that some of the learned feature representations did not generalize well across scanners. Future work could focus on a closer evaluation of which scanner characteristics hinder the extraction of domain-agnostic features and should therefore be disregarded, e.g. by using specific filters for data pre-processing or using adversarial training to punish the extraction of these features.

Acknowledgement. F.W. gratefully acknowledges the financial support received by Merck Healthcare KGaA and the technical support received by the Clinical Assay Strategy 1 group at Merck Healthcare KGaA during sample digitization. K.B. gratefully acknowledges support by d.hip campus - Bavarian aim in form of a faculty endowment.

References

1. Aubreville M, Bertram CA, Marzahl C, Gurtner C, Dettwiler M, Schmidt A et al. Deep learning algorithms out-perform veterinary pathologists in detecting the mitotically most active tumor region. Sci Rep. 2020;10:16447:1–11.
2. Aubreville M, Stathonikos N, Bertram CA, Klopleisch R, Hoeve N ter, Ciompi F et al. Mitosis domain generalization in histopathology images–The MIDOG challenge. Med Image Anal. 2023;84:102699.
3. Deng S, Zhang X, Yan W, Chang EI, Fan Y, Lai M et al. Deep learning in digital pathology image analysis: a survey. Front Med. 2020;14(4):470–87.
4. Stacke K, Eilertsen G, Unger J, Lundström C. Measuring domain shift for deep learning in histopathology. IEEE J Biomed Health Inform. 2020;25(2):325–36.
5. Wilm F, Marzahl C, Breininger K, Aubreville M. Domain adversarial RetinaNet as a reference algorithm for the MItosis DOmain Generalization challenge. MICCAI 2021 Challenges. Springer. 2022:5–13.
6. Roux L, Racoceanu D, Capron F, Calvo J, Attieh E, Le Naour G et al. Mitos & atypia. IPAL, Agency Sci., Technol. & Res. Inst. Infocom Res., Singapore, Tech. Rep. 2014;1:1–8.
7. Wilm F et al. CAnine CuTaneous cancer histology dataset (version 1). Cancer Imaging Arch. 2022. https://doi.org/10.7937/TCIA.2M93-FX66.
8. Marzahl C, Wilm F, F. DF, Tharun L, Perner S, Bertram CA et al. Robust quad-tree based registration on whole slide images. Comput Pathol (2021). PMLR, 2021:181–90.
9. Wilm F, Fragoso M, Marzahl C, Qiu J, Puget C, Diehl L et al. Pan-tumor CAnine cuTaneous cancer histology (CATCH) dataset. Sci Data. 2022;9:588.
10. Narvekar ND, Karam LJ. A no-reference image blur metric based on the cumulative probability of blur detection (CPBD). IEEE Trans Image Process. 2011;20(9):2678–83.
11. Michelson AA. Studies in optics. Courier Corporation, 1995.

Weakly-supervised Temporal Segmentation of Cell-cycle Stages with Center-cell Focus using Recurrent Neural Networks

Abin Jose[1], Rijo Roy[1], Johannes Stegmaier[1]

Institute of Imaging and Computer Vision, RWTH Aachen University
abin.jose@lfb.rwth-aachen.de

Abstract. Training deep-learning models for biomedical images has always been a problem due to the lack of annotated data. Here we propose using a model and a training approach for the weakly-supervised temporal classification of cell-cycle stages during mitosis. Instead of using annotated data, by using an ordered set of classes called transcript, our proposed approach classifies the cell-cycle stages of cell video sequences. The network design helps to propagate information in time using Recurrent Neural Network and helps to focus the features on the center-cell. The algorithm is evaluated on four datasets from Moreno-Andrés et al. [1] and has a performance close to the supervised approaches, which is impressive, considering that annotated data is not used in training.

1 Introduction

Mitosis is the process by which the cells rearrange and split into two identical daughter cells [2]. It is quite important to study and understand cell division to characterize pathological phenotypes in clinically relevant situations. The cell-cycle is divided into four phases: S, G2, Mitosis, and G1. The G1, S, and G2 phases are referred to as interphase. Mitosis is further classified according to the chromatin morphology into prophase, prometaphase, metaphase, anaphase, and telophase, where the pass to G1 is typically marked at cytoplasmic level by the cytokinetic process, which separates the cell bodies. Here we regard post-mitosis as the period where very gradual changes bring the compact anaphase chromatin to a decondensed G2-like mass in early G1.

In this work, we consider the classification of the cell-cycle stages into three different phases as in [1]: interphase, mitosis, and post-mitosis. Current state-of-the-art methods [1, 3] extract hand-engineered features, which are then classified using clustering methods. Zhong et al. [3] proposed an unsupervised clustering algorithm based on a temporally constrained combinatorial clustering (TC3) method. LiveCellMiner [1] additionally uses conventional convolutional networks to extract image features and uses a long short-term memory (LSTM) network to identify erroneous cell-cycle sequences. K-means clustering, after the feature extraction from fluorescence microscopy images, was proposed by Ferro et al. [4] for classification. Neural networks have strong feature extraction capabilities and are widely used in many computer vision applications [5–8] such as retrieval, hashing, segmentation etc. Many supervised models [9–13] are available for cell-cycle detection and classification. Recently, Jose et al. proposed a recurrent neural network (RNN) based architecture [14] to incorporate time-related propagation

Springer Fachmedien Wiesbaden GmbH, ein Teil von Springer Nature 2023
T. M. Deserno et al. (Hrsg.), *Bildverarbeitung für die Medizin 2023*,
Informatik aktuell, https://doi.org/10.1007/978-3-658-41657-7_47

Fig. 1. Illustration of our proposed architecture [14]. The model consists of two output networks, a focus network to reconstruct the center-cell and a classification network.

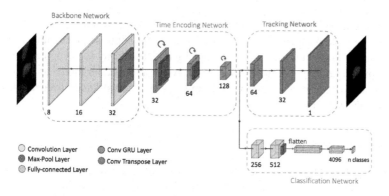

of features for classification. However, this approach is supervised and requires careful annotations by a trained biologist. To overcome this problem, in this paper, we propose a weakly-supervised training scheme. The main advantages of this work are: 1) The network is end-to-end trainable and shallow. 2) The network focuses on the center-cell and occludes neighboring cells. 3) The classification head classifies the different states. 4) The training is weakly-supervised and needs only a transcript, a list of classes in order. For example, the transcript for a cell sequence is represented as : [interphase, mitosis, post-mitosis] as in the order of occurrence of classes, and it does not need dense image-to-image annotations.

2 Materials and methods

Network architecture: For the temporal segmentation of the cell-cycle stages, we propose to use the same architecture as the one we proposed in [14], but the training method varies. The architecture of the model is shown in Figure 1. The model architecture contains four main parts. 1) A backbone network to extract the features, 2) a time encoding network consisting of RNN layers to combine extracted features between the current frame and propagated features from the previous frame, 3) a focus network that helps to focus the extracted features towards the center-cell, and 4) a classification network to classify the cell-cycle stages. We used convolutional gated recurrent unit (GRU) as the type of RNN in our model. The GRU connects connects image sequences temporally and helps to transfer information between images of different time points. The motivation to use convolutions in GRU was because our focus network reconstructs the image from high-level extracted features and focuses the features on the center-cell. The training of the model is explained in detail in the next section.

2.1 Training details

The proposed model architecture contains RNN layers, which help the flow of information through time. Thus, the image at each time frame is dependent on the previous images of the sequence. Inspired by the Neural Network-Viterbi approach proposed in [15], our approach uses the Viterbi decoding method for the weakly-supervised training. For a given input sequence, given the order of occurrence of classes as a constraint, the weakly-supervised method finds the most probable set of labels. This set of labels contains the most probable class for each image in the input sequence under the given constraint. So, following training, the model gains the ability to recognize the classes for an input sequence given the classes' order. As mentioned, our model architecture has two main output networks. The losses from these two networks are trained end-to-end to get the desired output.

2.2 Focus network loss

The output of the focus network has a dimensionality equal to that of the input images. To reconstruct only the center-cell from the input image, the training calculates the loss between the predicted output and a masked image. This network aims to learn the features corresponding only to the center-cell in the input image and thus focuses on the features of the center-cell. The masked image is obtained by using the annotated segmentation mask available with the datasets and setting all pixels that do not belong to the target cell to zero. The last layer of the focus network uses a sigmoid activation layer. The loss between the predicted and the expected input is calculated using binary cross-entropy (BCE) loss [16] and is given by

$$L_{focus} = \frac{1}{W_0 \cdot H_0} \sum_{w \in W_0} \sum_{h \in H_0} BCE\big(y\,(w, h)\,, \hat{y}\,(w, h)\big) \tag{1}$$

where $y\,(w, h)$ and $\hat{y}\,(w, h)$ are the input and predicted values of the network at pixel location (w, h). W_0 and H_0 are the input image dimensions. It is also possible to extract the segmentation mask of unseen images from this dataset using a simple threshold operation on the predicted output of the focus network.

2.3 Classification network loss

The classification network treats the input as a sequence to determine the most probable path of classes. The computation of the most probable path and the loss associated with that path can be calculated only after getting the prediction outputs for all frames in a sequence. The classification network output is the posterior probability. The Viterbi algorithm [15] finds the most probable path using these posterior probabilities and a length model. Our approach used a class-dependent Poisson distribution as the length model as in [15]. Once the Viterbi algorithm finds the most probable path of labels, these labels are used to back-propagate through the network. A negative log-likelihood loss is used to train. Let the most probable path for an input sequence $x^\top$ found by the Viterbi algorithm be given by $c_{n(t)}$. Then the weakly-supervised classification loss is given by

$$L_{clf} = -\sum_{t=1}^{T} \log p\left(c_{n(t)}|x^\top\right) \tag{2}$$

Both losses are computed for a sequence of data as input. A combined focus loss is obtained by summing the focus losses from each frame. The total loss is computed by a weighted sum of the combined focus loss and the weakly-supervised classification loss.

2.4 Datasets and experiments

Datsets: The datasets used for the evaluations are provided by LiveCellMiner [1]. The datasets contain microscopic image sequences of the mitosis process after the cell tracking. The datasets are acquired on human HeLa cells expressing H2B-mCherry transfected with indicated siRNA oligonucleotides in eight-well μ-slide chambers. It contains images that were taken three minutes apart. There are four datasets available from [1], namely LSM710 dataset, LSD1 dataset, RecQL4 dataset, and NikonXLight dataset. The former three datasets are captured using a confocal microscope and the latter is captured using a widefield microscope. Each contained cell is represented by a sequence of 90 frames, cropped from an image containing many cells to a resolution of 96×96 pixels with the target cell at the center. The dataset is annotated into three classes such as interphase class, mitosis class (prophase to early anaphase), and post-mitosis class (late anaphase to interphase). The post-mitosis class also contains cells that have grown into interphase (interphase recovery class) after cell division. Our approach is also able to identify the interphase recovery class, but we do not have a valid ground truth to evaluate. Instead, we qualitatively compared it with the findings from [1].

2.4.1 Experimental setup. For training the weakly-supervised model, a set of ordered labels called transcripts is used instead of the annotated data. The transcripts are simply the list of the classes in their order of occurrence. Our approach finds the number of frames in a sequence belonging to each class, given the transcript. Thus it helps to avoid the task of frame-to-frame annotation for training this model and the time involved for it. Given input sequences, the model trains both losses together with a regularization hyperparameter value of 0.01. We used 85% of the data for training and the remaining 15% of the data for testing, where 10% of the test data were used for validation. The batch size and the learning rate are selected as 4 and 0.01 respectively. The weakly-supervised classification loss is introduced every 20 iterations. The length of the transcript used is 4 considering the interphase recovery class as well. For evaluation, the interphase recovery class is considered a part of the post-mitosis class.

2.4.2 Evaluation criteria. The annotated data is available with the datasets for evaluation. We have calculated the frame-to-frame accuracy for each sequence and then averaged it. We also calculated the confusion matrix to find the correct classification and the misclassification rates. We compared the performance of our approach to the results obtained with the same model architecture trained using supervised methods [14] and the ResNet18 classification model.

3 Results

We plotted the label matrix in which the x-axis represents the length of each cell sequence, and the y-axis represents different sequences selected from the test dataset.

Model	LSM710	LSD1	RecQL4	NikonXLight
Supervised [14]	99.54	99.07	99.32	99.11
ResNet18 [14]	99.30	98.99	98.61	98.70
Ours	96.21	94.82	98.54	96.86

Tab. 1. Frame-to-frame accuracy of our model compared with the supervised approaches [14].

Figure 2 (a) shows the label matrix of the ground truth annotations compared with the label matrix of the predicted output on 50 test sequences of the LSM710 dataset. On closer inspection, it is evident that the predictions by the proposed model are similar to the user annotations.

Figure 2 (b) shows the first three principal components of the embedding space for the three classes of our proposed model. The embedding space contains the characteristics of the input data, in which the three cell-cycle states are clustered and move from blue to red to pink states, which is clearly visible in the feature space. From the figure, it is clear that our proposed weakly-supervised method can cluster the features belonging to different

Fig. 2. Illustration of the a) label matrix of predicted output compared with the ground truth, and b) first three principal components plot of the learned embedding space for the LSM710 dataset.

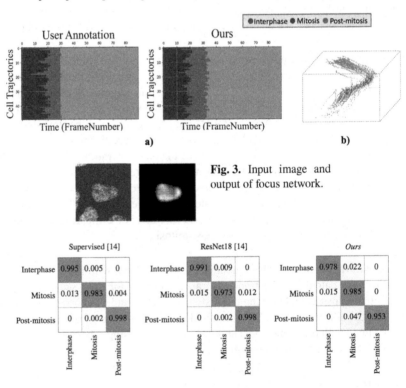

Fig. 3. Input image and output of focus network.

Fig. 4. Normalized confusion matrices for the prediction on the LSM710 test dataset with our proposed model compared to the supervised approaches [14].

Fig. 5. a) Plot from [1] illustrates that the interphase recovery occurs about 20 frames after mitosis. The indicated frame numbers are relative to two manually identified synchronization bars (left bar - interphase to prophase transition, right bar - anaphase onset). The gap between the two transition time points helps to visualize aligned cell tracks irrespective of different durations of mitosis (Details in [1] Fig. S12). b) Our proposed weakly-supervised method when predicting four classes predicted the recovered interphase frames (second set of blue after pink). The post-mitosis class (pink) covers a time span of 20-30 frames and is thus in line with panel a). Note: panel b) shows absolute frame numbers whereas relative frame numbers are used in panel a).

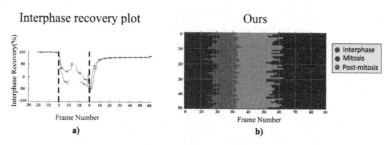

classes without using fully-annotated data for training. Frame-to-frame accuracies can give a better quantitative analysis of the results.

Table 1 shows the accuracies of the proposed model for the four datasets compared to the supervised learning approach [14] and also the ResNet18 classifier. Even though the proposed model has slightly lower (around 3 − 4%) accuracies when compared to the supervised methods, the results are impressive considering that dense ground truth annotations are not required for training. Figure 3 shows the reconstructed image from the focus network for a given input image. The focus network reconstructs only the center-cell and thus helps the features learned in the embedding space to focus on the target cell. A segmentation mask of the target cell can be also predicted from the output of the focus network by using a simple intensity threshold.

Figure 4 illustrates the confusion matrix of the proposed approach compared to the supervised approaches [14]. It is evident from the diagonal elements of the confusion matrix that the correct classification for three different classes is comparable to that of the supervised methods. It is observed that the true positive rate for the mitosis class is higher than that of the other approaches. This indicates that the proposed weakly-supervised method can identify mitosis class images better than supervised approaches. For the other two classes, the misclassification rate is higher for the proposed approach. It is also clear that confusion between unrelated classes does not occur as indicated by the zeros in the top right and the bottom left. Figure 5 (a) demonstrates a plot from [1], which shows interphase recovery for the LSM710 dataset happens around 20 frames after mitosis. Figure 5 (b) illustrates the label matrix of the proposed model when using four class transcripts. Even though there are no ground-truth annotations to evaluate an accurate measure, the qualitative results of the proposed model are in alignment with the findings of Moreno-Andrés et al. [1].

4 Discussion

We propose an automatic method for the identification of cell-cycle stages during mitosis. The proposed weakly-supervised approach only needs the transcript information which indicates the order of occurrence of cell-cycle states. Even though the classification accuracy is slightly lower compared to the supervised RNN model and ResNet18 classifier model, the proposed approach has the advantage that the user needs to provide only the order of occurrence of the states. This avoids the need for the generation of user annotation to train supervised models, which needs the expertise of a trained biologist. In the future, we would like to further extend the experiments to 3D cell datasets. Another interesting research direction is to use unsupervised training methods.

References

1. Moreno-Andrés D, Bhattacharyya A, Scheufen A, Stegmaier J. LiveCellMiner: a new tool to analyze mitotic progression. PloS One. 2022;17(7):e0270923.
2. Araujo AR, Gelens L, Sheriff RS, Santos SD. Positive feedback keeps duration of mitosis temporally insulated from upstream cell-cycle events. Mol Cell. 2016;64(2):362–75.
3. Zhong Q, Busetto AG, Fededa JP, Buhmann JM, Gerlich DW. Unsupervised modeling of cell morphology dynamics for time-lapse microscopy. Nat Methods. 2012;9(7):711–3.
4. Ferro A, Mestre T, Carneiro P, Sahumbaiev I, Seruca R, Sanches JM. Blue intensity matters for cell cycle profiling in fluorescence DAPI-stained images. Laboratory Investigation. 2017;97(5):615–25.
5. Jose A, Ottlik ES, Rohlfing C, Ohm JR. Optimized feature space learning for generating efficient binary codes for image retrieval. Signal Processing: Image Communication. 2022;100:116529.
6. Jose A, Filbert D, Rohlfing C, Ohm JR. Deep hashing with hash center update for efficient image retrieval. ICASSP 2022 - 2022 IEEE International Conference on Acoustics, Speech and Signal Processing (ICASSP). 2022:4773–7.
7. Jose A, Lopez RD, Heisterklaus I, Wien M. Pyramid pooling of convolutional feature maps for image retrieval. 2018 25th IEEE International Conference on Image Processing (ICIP). 2018:480–4.
8. Jose A, Yan S, Heisterklaus I. Binary hashing using siamese neural networks. 2017 IEEE International Conference on Image Processing (ICIP). IEEE. 2017:2916–20.
9. Allehaibi KHS, Nugroho LE, Lazuardi L, Prabuwono AS, Mantoro T et al. Segmentation and classification of cervical cells using deep learning. IEEE Access. 2019;7:116925–41.
10. Narotamo H, Fernandes MS, Moreira AM, Melo S, Seruca R, Silveira M et al. A machine learning approach for single cell interphase cell cycle staging. Sci Rep. 2021;11(1):1–13.
11. Jin X, Zou Y, Huang Z. An imbalanced image classification method for the cell cycle phase. Information. 2021;12(6):249.
12. Saha M, Chakraborty C, Racoceanu D. Efficient deep learning model for mitosis detection using breast histopathology images. Computerized Medical Imaging and Graphics. 2018;64:29–40.
13. Albayrak A, Bilgin G. Mitosis detection using convolutional neural network based features. 2016 IEEE 17th International Symposium on Computational Intelligence and Informatics (CINTI). IEEE. 2016:335–340.
14. Jose A, Roy R, Eschweiler D, Laube I, Azad R, Moreno-Andrés D et al. End-to-end classification of cell-cycle stages with center-cell focus tracker using recurrent neural networks. 2022.

15. Richard A, Kuehne H, Iqbal A, Gall J. Neuralnetwork-viterbi: a framework for weakly supervised video learning. Proceedings of the IEEE Conference on Computer Vision and Pattern Recognition. 2018:7386–95.

16. Ho Y, Wookey S. The real-world-weight cross-entropy loss function: modeling the costs of mislabeling. IEEE Access. 2019;8:4806–13.

Attention-based Multiple Instance Learning for Survival Prediction on Lung Cancer Tissue Microarrays

Jonas Ammeling[1], Lars-Henning Schmidt[2], Jonathan Ganz[1], Tanja Niedermair[3], Christoph Brochhausen-Delius[3], Christian Schulz[4], Katharina Breininger[5], Marc Aubreville[1]

[1]Technische Hochschule Ingolstadt, Ingolstadt, Germany
[2]Medical Department IV, Pulmonary Medicine and Thoracic Oncology, Klinikum Ingolstadt, Ingolstadt, Germany
[3]Institute of Pathology, University of Regensburg, Regensburg, Germany
[4]Department of Internal Medicine II, University Hospital Regensburg, Regensburg, Germany
[5]Department Artificial Intelligence in Biomedical Engineering, Friedrich-Alexander-Universität Erlangen-Nürnberg, Erlangen, Germany
jonas.ammeling@thi.de

Abstract. Attention-based multiple instance learning (AMIL) algorithms have proven to be successful in utilizing gigapixel whole-slide images (WSIs) for a variety of different computational pathology tasks such as outcome prediction and cancer subtyping problems. We extended an AMIL approach to the task of survival prediction by utilizing the classical Cox partial likelihood as a loss function, converting the AMIL model into a nonlinear proportional hazards model. We applied the model to tissue microarray (TMA) slides of 330 lung cancer patients. The results show that AMIL approaches can handle very small amounts of tissue from a TMA and reach similar C-index performance compared to established survival prediction methods trained with highly discriminative clinical factors such as age, cancer grade, and cancer stage.

1 Introduction

Despite advances in medicine over the past two decades, lung cancer remains the leading cause of cancer-related deaths worldwide [1]. Survival prediction methods are used for predicting time-to-event outcomes such as cancer recurrence or death and play an important role in clinical decision making in oncology. Recent survival prediction methods used tissue samples from whole sections [2, 3] to make predictions about a patient's prognosis. However, with the trend toward minimally invasive biopsy techniques in the treatment of lung cancer, approaches that can process smaller amounts of tissue are needed [4]. TMAs provide the opportunity to explore such methods because they typically contain only a very small amount of tissue for each patient from the original tumor sample [5]. Bychkov et al. [6] used a combination of convolutional and recurrent architectures to predict five-year survival as a binary classification problem from TMA cores of colon cancer patients. However, recurrent architectures are more complex than attention-based approaches, which have been shown to be successful for predicting patient prognosis on whole-slide images (WSI) [2, 7]. To investigate the applicability of attention-based methods to TMA slides, we extended an AMIL approach originally developed for weakly supervised classification to the survival prediction task similar to [2] by converting the classification problem into a regression problem by optimizing the modified partial Cox likelihood [8] as our loss function. We applied the model to TMA slides from patients with non-small cell lung cancer (NSCLC) and compared performance with established survival prediction methods trained on prognostically discriminative tabular data. The full code is available online[1].

2 Materials and methods

2.1 Data

Tissue samples, clinicopathologic features, and follow-up information were collected and examined from 379 NSCLC patients in the thoracic department of St. Georgs Klinikum in Ostercappeln, Germany. Clinical TNM staging (including clinical examination, CT scans, sonography, endoscopy, MRI, bone scan) was performed based on UICC/AJCC recommendations. The definite tumor staging was carried out post-surgically by pathological exploration. The histologic grade was determined according to WHO criteria on the original whole section tumor sample. The follow-up time was computed from the date of histological diagnosis to death or censored at the date of last contact. The TMAs were constructed by sampling with a 0.6 mm core needle from the most representative parts of the original tumor block. Three cores per patient were punched from the paraffin-embedded tumor block and assembled into TMA blocks. Multiple (at most 3x) four-micrometer-thick sections were cut from the TMA blocks, stained with hematoxylin and eosin (H&E), and digitized with a whole-slide scanner (Pannoramic P1000, 3D HISTECH Ltd., Budapest, Hungary) at a resolution of 0.24 μm/pixel. The TMA cores were linked to a unique patient identifier and extracted from the whole-slide TMA image. Due to missing values in the tabular data and loss of tissue sections from the TMA blocks, 49 cases were excluded from the analysis. Thus, data from 330 NSCLC patients was included for further analysis.

2.2 Image processing

To compare the use of the patient-level label for different tissue amounts, all cores from the same patient were processed once individually and stitched together once horizontally to create a new patient-level TMA (Fig. 1). All images were processed using the public CLAM [9] repository for WSI analysis. After tissue segmentation, non-overlapping patches of size 256×256 were extracted at full resolution. Then, a ResNet50 model, pre-trained on ImageNet, was used to convert each patch into a 1024-dimensional feature vector by spatial average pooling after the third residual block.

2.3 Attention-based multiple instance learning

In the context of multiple instance learning, each image is viewed as a collection of M patches or instances, known as a bag, with a corresponding bag-level label associated

---

[1]https://github.com/DeepPathology/Cox_AMIL

with it. After image processing, each bag is represented by the patch-level embeddings $\mathbf{H} \in \mathbb{R}^{M \times C}$, where C is the feature dimension from the ResNet50 model. The model consists of three components as shown in Figure 1: the projection layer f_{proj}, the attention module f_{attn}, and the prediction layer f_{pred}. The projection layer f_{proj} is a fully-connected layer with weights $\mathbf{W}_{\text{proj}} \in \mathbb{R}^{512 \times C}$ (all bias terms are implied for notational convenience) that maps the patch-level embedding into a more compact, dataset-specific 512-dimensional feature space. The attention module f_{attn} learns to assign a score to each patch based on its contribution to the patient's predicted prognosis. In particular, f_{attn} consists of three fully connected layers with weights $\mathbf{U} \in \mathbb{R}^{256 \times 512}$, $\mathbf{V} \in \mathbb{R}^{256 \times 512}$, and $\mathbf{Z} \in \mathbb{R}^{1 \times 256}$. After projection, the attention score a_m for the m-th patch embedding $\mathbf{h}_m \in \mathbb{R}^{512}$, is computed by [9]

$$a_m = \frac{\exp\left\{\mathbf{Z}\left(\tanh\left(\mathbf{V}\mathbf{h}_m^{\mathsf{T}}\right) \odot \text{sigm}\left(\mathbf{U}\mathbf{h}_m^{\mathsf{T}}\right)\right)\right\}}{\sum_{m=1}^{M} \exp\left\{\mathbf{Z}\left(\tanh\left(\mathbf{V}\mathbf{h}_m^{\mathsf{T}}\right) \odot \text{sigm}\left(\mathbf{U}\mathbf{h}_m^{\mathsf{T}}\right)\right)\right\}} \tag{1}$$

The computed attention scores for each patch are then used as weight coefficients to aggregate the patch-level embeddings into the bag representation $\mathbf{h}_{\text{bag}} \in \mathbb{R}^{512}$ via attention-pooling [9] by

$$\mathbf{h}_{\text{bag}} = \sum_{m=1}^{M} a_m \mathbf{h}_m \tag{2}$$

The final prediction layer f_{pred} is a single fully-connected layer with weights $\mathbf{W}_{\text{pred}} \in \mathbb{R}^{1 \times 512}$ with a single output node and linear activation. Let θ represent all weights of the network, then the model can be described as a function $h_\theta : \mathbb{R}^{M \times C} \mapsto \mathbb{R}$, where the output is a patient's hazard log risk score, described in more detail in the next section.

2.4 Loss function

The right-censored patient-level survival data for the i-th patient consist of the triple (t_i, δ_i, x_i) and represent the observed time, binary censoring status ($\delta = 0$, death not observed), and image data, respectively. Censoring is assumed to be non-informative, such that for a given x_i, survival time and censoring are independent. Let $t_1 < t_2 < t_D$ be the ordered event times. The risk set $\mathcal{R}(t_i)$ is defined as the set of all individuals

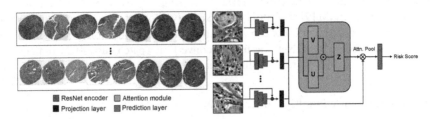

Fig. 1. Data stitching and overall architecture. Left: tissue-cores of the same patient stitched together horizontally. Right: overview of the attention-based multiple instance learning algorithm for survival prediction.

still in the study at a time immediately preceding t_i. The loss function is derived from the common Cox proportional hazards model where the hazard function of the form $\lambda(t \mid x) = \lambda_0(t) \cdot e^{h(x)}$ is composed of the hazard baseline function $\lambda_0(t)$, and a risk score $r(x) = e^{h(x)}$. Our proposed model estimates a patient's log-risk score $\hat{h}_\theta(x)$ parameterized by the weights of the network θ such that the modified Cox partial likelihood becomes [8]

$$L(\theta) = \prod_{i:\delta=1} \frac{\hat{r}_\theta(x_i)}{\sum_{j \in \mathcal{R}(t_i)} \hat{r}_\theta(x_j)} = \prod_{i:\delta=1} \frac{\exp\left(\hat{h}_\theta(x_i)\right)}{\sum_{j \in \mathcal{R}(t_i)} \exp\left(\hat{h}_\theta(x_j)\right)} \tag{3}$$

The loss function which is minimized by the network is then obtained from the average of the negative partial log likelihood with regularization as shown below

$$l(\theta) = -\frac{1}{N} \sum_i \delta_i \left(\hat{h}_\theta(x_i) - \log \sum_{j \in \mathcal{R}(t_i)} \exp\left(\hat{h}_\theta(x_j)\right) \right) + \lambda \cdot \|\theta\|_1 \tag{4}$$

where N is the number of patients with an observable event and λ is the l_1 regularization parameter. Intuitively, the loss function penalizes discordance between the scores of higher-risk and lower-risk patients. Similar loss functions have been used previously by other authors [7, 10]. Details about the training and hyperparameter settings are online[1].

2.5 Baselines

The performance of the proposed model was compared against three established survival analysis methods based on tabular data. The tabular data used to train these baseline methods consist of patient characteristics (age, sex, and smoking status) and clinical characteristics (cancer stage and grade). It should be noted that the latter require elaborate determination and are commonly accepted to be highly prognostic. The first baseline method was a classical linear Cox proportional hazards (CPH) model [8]. The second was a random survival forest (RSF) [11], a non-proportional, flexible and robust alternative to the classical CPH model. The third baseline method was DeepSurv [10], a modern nonlinear, deep learning-based CPH model. Moreover, the proposed model was compared with a MIL method using classical max-pooling, and with the performance of an AMIL model trained on each patient core individually, using the respective patient-level label.

2.6 Evaluation

To evaluate and compare the predictive performance on the survival data, we performed a 10-fold cross-validation and measured Harrell's concordance index (C-index) [12]. The C-index indicates how well a model predicts the ranking of patients' death times, where large values of $\hat{h}_\theta(x_i)$ should be associated with small values of t_i and vice versa. A value of $C = 0.5$ corresponds to the average C-index of a random model, whereas $C = 1$ corresponds to a perfect association. Patient stratification was assessed by assigning patients to either a high-risk or a low-risk group based on the median of the predicted risk score. Kaplan-Meier curves were constructed by pooling the risk predictions of the test folds and plotting them against their survival time. Logrank tests were performed to check for statistically significant differences (P-value < 0.05) between the two survival distributions.

3　Results

The cross-validated C-index values and the Kaplan-Meier curves for the patient stratification results are shown in Figure 2. The classical CPH model achieved the overall best performance with an average C-index of 0.61 ± 0.07 (P-value: 7.98×10^{-4}) and a median C-index of 0.59. Closely similar, the RSF model achieved an average C-index of 0.60 ± 0.06 (P-value: 1.61×10^{-3}) and a median C-index of 0.60. The DeepSurv method performed the worst among all methods with an average C-index of 0.50 ± 0.1 (P-value: 2.20×10^{-1}) and a median C-index of 0.53. Among the image-based methods, the classical MIL model with max-pooling performs the worst with an average C-index of 0.54 ± 0.08 (P-value: 2.90×10^{-1}) and a median C-index of 0.53. The AMIL model performed the best among the image-based methods with an average C-index of 0.61 ± 0.07 (P-value: 1.69×10^{-5}) and a median C-index of 0.63. The AMIL model trained on individual cores performed worse than the AMIL model trained using the patient label for all cores together, with an average C-index of 0.56 ± 0.06 (P-value: 5.72×10^{-11}) and a median C-index of 0.58.

4　Discussion

The results show that the proposed model performed similarly well to established survival prediction methods based on tabular data, such as CPH and RSF, by extracting features directly from the small amount of tissue provided by the TMA. Attention pooling proved to be very effective in this regard for aggregating these features to estimate the patient's risk score. However, the experiments also showed that the prognostically

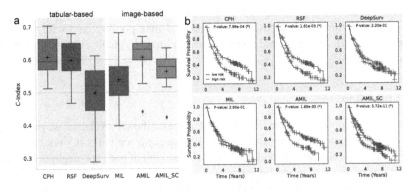

Fig. 2. a) Cross-validated C-index performance. + indicates mean value. b) Kaplan-Meier curves for patient stratification results on the pooled validation splits.

relevant information is not necessarily evenly distributed across a patient's tissue cores when selected from the original sample, as indicated by lower average C-index when trained on individual cores. Thus, performance is highly dependent on tissue core selection, and it is recommended to use all available tissue cores. Nevertheless, the results show that attention-based MIL approaches are applicable to TMA slides where only a small amount of tissue per patient is available to perform reliable patient stratification, as shown by the statistically significant logrank test results. Therefore, in the context of the trend toward minimally invasive biopsy procedures in lung cancer treatment, these methods could become a part of reliable decision support systems in the future.

Acknowledgement. J. A. acknowledges funding by the Bavarian Institute for Digital Transformation (Project ReGInA).

References

1. Wang M, Herbst RS, Boshoff C. Toward personalized treatment approaches for non-small-cell lung cancer. Nat Med. 2021;27:1345–56.
2. Chen RJ, Lu MY, Williamson DF, Chen TY, Lipkova J, Noor Z et al. Pan-cancer integrative histology-genomic analysis via multimodal deep learning. Cancer Cell. 2022;40:865–878.e6.
3. Vale-Silva LA, Rohr K. Long-term cancer survival prediction using multimodal deep learning. Sci Rep. 2021;11:13505.
4. Coley SM, Crapanzano JP, Saqi A. FNA, core biopsy, or both for the diagnosis of lung carcinoma: obtaining sufficient tissue for a specific diagnosis and molecular testing. Cancer Cytopathol. 2015;123:318–26.
5. Schmidt LH, Biesterfeld S, Kümmel A, Faldum A, Sebastian M, Taube C et al. Tissue microarrays are reliable tools for the clinicopathological characterization of lung cancer tissue. Anticancer res. 2009;29:201–9.
6. Bychkov D, Linder N, Turkki R, Nordling S, Kovanen PE, Verrill C et al. Deep learning based tissue analysis predicts outcome in colorectal cancer. Sci Rep. 2018;8:1–11.
7. Yao J, Zhu X, Jonnagaddala J, Hawkins N, Huang J. Whole slide images based cancer survival prediction using attention guided deep multiple instance learning networks. Med Image Anal. 2020;65:101789.
8. Cox DR. Regression models and life-tables. J R Stat Soc Series B Stat Methodol. 1972;34:187–202.
9. Lu MY, Williamson DFK, Chen TY, Chen RJ, Barbieri M, Mahmood F. Data-efficient and weakly supervised computational pathology on whole-slide images. Nat Biomed Eng. 2021;5:555–70.
10. Katzman JL, Shaham U, Cloninger A, Bates J, Jiang T, Kluger Y. DeepSurv: personalized treatment recommender system using a Cox proportional hazards deep neural network. BMC Med Res Methodol. 2018;18:24.
11. Ishwaran H, Kogalur UB, Blackstone EH, Lauer MS. Random survival forests. Ann Appl Stat. 2008;2(3):841–60.
12. Harrell FE, Califf RM, Pryor DB, Lee KL, Rosati RA. Evaluating the yield of medical tests. JAMA. 1982;247:2543–6.

Deep Learning-based Automatic Assessment of AgNOR-scores in Histopathology Images

Jonathan Ganz[1], Karoline Lipnik[2], Jonas Ammeling[1], Barbara Richter[2], Chloé Puget[3], Eda Parlak[2], Laura Diehl[3], Robert Klopfleisch[3], Taryn A. Donovan[4], Matti Kiupel[5], Christof A. Bertram[2], Katharina Breininger[6], Marc Aubreville[1]

[1]Technische Hochschule Ingolstadt, Ingolstadt, Germany
[2]Institute of Pathology, University of Veterinary Medicine Vienna, Vienna, Austria
[3]Institute of Veterinary Pathology, Freie Universität Berlin, Berlin, Germany
[4]The Schwarzmann Animal Medical Center, New York, USA
[5]Department of Pathology and Diagnostic Investigation, Michigan State University, East Lansing, USA
[6]Department of Artificial Intelligence in Biomedical Engineering, Friedrich-Alexander-Universität Erlangen-Nürnberg, Erlangen, Germany
jonathan.ganz@thi.de

Abstract. Nucleolar organizer regions (NORs) are parts of the DNA that are involved in RNA transcription. Due to the silver affinity of associated proteins, argyrophilic NORs (AgNORs) can be visualized using silver-based staining. The average number of AgNORs per nucleus has been shown to be a prognostic factor for predicting the outcome of many tumors. Since manual detection of AgNORs is laborious, automation is of high interest. We present a deep learning-based pipeline for automatically determining the AgNOR-score from histopathological sections. An additional annotation experiment was conducted with six pathologists to provide an independent performance evaluation of our approach. Across all raters and images, we found a mean squared error of 0.054 between the AgNOR-scores of the experts and those of the model, indicating that our approach offers performance comparable to humans.

1 Introduction

Nucleolar organizer regions (NORs) are nucleolar substructures involved in ribosomal RNA transcription [1]. NORs can be visualized in histological tissue sections using silver-based staining because of the silver affinity of two argyrophilic proteins involved in rRNA transcription and processing [1, 2]. The silver-stained argyrophilic NORs are defined as AgNORs [2]. The number of AgNORs per nuclei has been reported to be correlated with cell proliferation in vitro and the rate of tumor growth in vivo, as more malignant neoplasms tend to have more numerous and smaller AgNORs than benign or less malignant tumors [3, 4]. Furthermore, the AgNOR-score was reported to have significant prognostic value for outcome variables like survival [5, 6]. When examining the AgNOR-score in clinical practice, 100 randomly selected nuclei are examined per tissue section under a light microscope, while carefully focusing through the whole thickness of the slide [5]. The mean number of AgNORs per nucleus is then calculated from the assessed nuclei. A limitation of the AgNOR-score is the considerable time effort for the examining pathologists. Deep learning methods are ideal here, as they can accelerate the process. However, there have been only a few attempts in the direction of deep learning based AgNOR scoring. One work in this area comes from Amorim et al., who studied the automatic assessment of AgNORs in cytological samples from cervical cancer using a U-Net architecture [7]. In cytological samples, cells are well separated upon a bright background, however, in histological samples, cell borders are often obscured, with darker intervening stroma, rendering histological samples more difficult for automated AgNOR assessments. This work thus provides a first attempt at automatic scoring of histopathological samples for AgNOR using deep learning. We argue that it is not the segmentation of individual AgNORs within a nucleus that is relevant to determine the AgNOR-score, but their quantity. Therefore, defining this task as a segmentation problem only introduces more unnecessary manual annotation effort for the annotation expert. To circumvent this, we define the problem as an object detection task where the number of AgNORs within a nucleus represents the label. To quantify AgNORs, we used an anchor-free, state-of-the-art object detection algorithm. To evaluate the performance of our approach, we conducted an annotation experiment in which the AgNOR-scores for ten images, all representing individual tumor cases, were assessed by six pathology experts. For this study, we evaluated both AgNOR-scores per image and AgNOR-scores for individual nuclei. The main contributions of this work are:

1. We address the automatic assessment of AgNOR in histopathology using deep learning.
2. We provide a baseline performance using an ensemble of state-of-the-art object detectors and a tailored sampling scheme.
3. We perform extensive evaluations on the results of the human rater experiment.

2   Materials and methods

2.1   Data

In this work, we used 29 images (1569×1177 pixel each) of canine cutaneous mast cell tumor (CCMCT). Each image shows a region of interest selected from a whole slide image by a pathologist. AgNOR histochemical staining was performed using a silver-based stain as described in [3]. The slides were digitized using an Aperio ScanScope CS2 scanner with a spatial resolution of 0.25 microns per pixel. All nuclei present in the images were annotated by a pathologist, with the number of identifiable AgNORs representing the label for each nucleus. This resulted in a total of 23,036 bounding box annotations grouped into twelve classes. The twelfth class includes all nuclei in which more than ten AgNORs are identifiable. The class distribution is strongly skewed toward classes with fewer than four AgNORs per nuclei, as can be seen in Tab. 1. Of these images, ten images are used as a hold-out test set. An overview of samples from different cases of the test set is given in Fig. 1.

Tab. 1. Number of instances in different classes.

Number of AgNORs per nucleus	0	1	2	3	4	5	6	7	8	9	10	>10
Number of cells		5124	9634	4620	1951	886	403	209	78	48	28	26	29

2.2 Human rater experiment

To evaluate the algorithm's performance compared to human experts, we conducted a study with six pathology experts. The experts were asked to determine the number of AgNORs of at least one hundred nuclei for the ten images which are part of the hold-out test set. To reduce inter-rater discordance between the experts, the selection of nuclei to be annotated for the count of AgNORs was modified slightly from the clinical standard. The images used in the study were each divided into 12 fields, which were numbered like in Fig. 1. The experts were asked to process the fields one after another until at least 100 nuclei had been annotated. If the annotation was started in one field, the experts were instructed to annotate all remaining nuclei within this field, even if more than 100 nuclei were annotated in total. The AgNOR-scores for the corresponding image were derived by averaging the annotations of each expert. The mean of the AgNOR-scores per case of all experts for an image was used as the expert value for this image, which is later compared to the algorithmically determined value. To measure the agreement between the algorithm and the experts at the object level, we aggregated ground truth

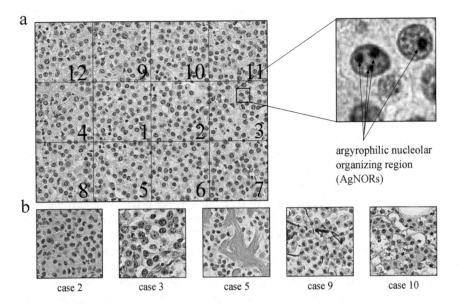

Fig. 1. The left side of Figure a) shows a CCMCT section stained with silver-based staining like described in [3]. The grid used in the experiment is overlaid. On the right side of Figure a), a detailed representation of two nuclei with marked AgNORs is displayed. In Figure b), fields from randomly selected cases of the hold-out test set are shown.

labels from the expert annotations. Since the areas annotated by the experts vary, we only aggregated class-level labels for the first field of the grid in Fig. 1. A nucleus was taken as ground truth if it was annotated by at least two experts and assigned to the same class. If one nucleus was annotated by more than two experts, the class label was determined by a majority vote. To determine the inter-observer agreement, Fleiss's kappa coefficient and the intraclass correlation coefficient (ICC) were used [8, 9]. We report the ICC for a random set of k raters where every instance is rated by all k raters as described by Shrout and Fleiss [9].

2.3 AgNOR-scoring pipeline

To determine the AgNOR-score, we consider the problem an object detection task, where nuclei are discriminated based on the number of identifiable AgNORs. For detection, we used the fully convolutional one-stage object detector (FCOS) by Tian et al. [10], which is a state-of-the-art object detector that does not use anchor boxes like previous approaches and thus comes with a reduced set of hyperparameters to tune. To account for imbalances in the training data, we ensembled five detection models which were trained on five random subsets of the training data. Each of the five models produced its own AgNOR-score by averaging the class labels of all nuclei detected in one image. We used the median to aggregate the results of the ensemble of models per image. During training, we oversampled classes with lower support because of the class imbalance present in the training data. For the same reason, we used a small patch size of 128 × 128 pixels for training since this gave us better control over the classes present on each patch. All models were trained until convergence as observed by the validation loss with a learning rate of 10^{-4} and Adam as optimizer. To ensure comparability between the results of the study and those of the algorithm, the inference of the detectors was performed analogously to the annotation of the experts described before. The respective image was divided into the same 12 fields, which needed to be processed in the same order as in the study until at least 100 nuclei were detected and classified.

3 Results

Figure 2 shows the individual AgNOR-score for each rater, as well as the mean label for each case. The highest mean AgNOR-score across raters was 2.774 with a standard deviation of 0.500 and found for the third case in the set. The lowest mean AgNOR-score across raters was 1.075 with a standard deviation of 0.119. The average of these mean AgNOR-scores of all experts when calculated across all cases is 1.550 with a standard deviation of 0.441. Between the nucleus-level annotations made by the experts, we found a Fleiss' kappa value of 0.545 and an ICC value of 0.390. According to the verbal description by Landis et al. [8] the Fleiss' kappa value corresponds to a moderate agreement. In general, we found a slight disagreement between the AgNOR values determined by the algorithm and the experts' AgNOR-scores. The mean squared error between the algorithm-determined AgNOR-scores and those of the experts was 0.054, the mean absolute error was 0.201. Evaluating the model using the object level labels derived from the expert annotations, we found satisfactory performance in detecting classes of up to 2 AgNORs per nucleus, with mean F1-scores greater than 60%. All classes with more than 2 AgNORs per nucleus were not detected as accurately, with mean F1 values of less than 40%. Since there were only three nuclei within the ground truth with greater than or equal to six AgNORs, we combined the results from these classes into one box in Fig. 2.

4   Discussion

The results of the annotation experiment show that there are individual tendencies in assigning higher or lower AgNOR-scores among raters. The results of the experiment for case three suggest that the inter-rater concordance degrades with the average AgNOR-score per nucleus, and thus might coincide with proliferation speed. A reason for this might be that more malignant neoplasms have more numerous and smaller AgNORs as previously described. Therefore, the AgNORs in case three might also be smaller, making it harder for the experts to distinguish them from each other and leading to a higher variance in the assessed AgNOR-scores. The moderate Fleiss' kappa and ICC values show that the experts had difficulty arriving at a consistent result for different nuclei.

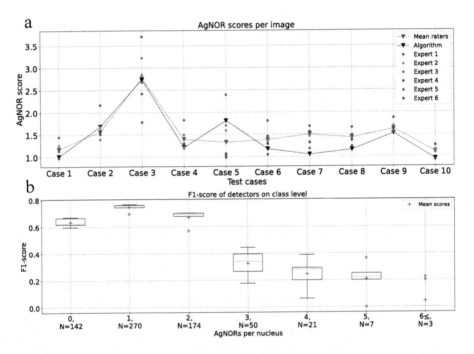

Fig. 2. The AgNOR-scores of the different raters across the cases of the test data set are shown in Figure. a). The green triangles represent the image label formed from the mean of the AgNOR-scores of the pathologists. The black triangles depict the AgNOR-scores of the algorithm. Figure b) shows the performance of the individual object detectors of the ensemble at object level. The number of instances per class in the ground truth labels is specified by N.

Since we performed the experiment with digital slides using a single z plane, focusing through each cell individually, as stated in [5], was not possible. One possible solution to mitigate this issue might be the use of stacks of images at multiple focus lengths. In this process, a slide is scanned in its entirety at various levels of focus and the multiple images are stitched together to form a three-dimensional image that allows for digital post-hoc focusing. Moreover, the use of higher scans with severely increased resolution could help experts to better separate individual AgNORs. Overall, the low error between the algorithmically determined values and those of the experts shows that the algorithm is able to determine AgNOR-scores with human-like performance. Its tendency to predict lower AgNOR-scores is presumably a consequence of the considerable class imbalance in the training data set. As a result, the algorithm confuses the higher classes, which is also reflected in the detection scores of the individual detectors in Fig. 2. Here, the detectors of the ensemble achieve favorable F1 scores on the three most dominant classes, whereas from three AgNORs per nucleus on, the performance decreases significantly. Nevertheless, this only has a minor effect on the estimation error on image-level due to the distribution of AgNORs per nucleus (Tab. 1). We encourage the use of fully automated pipelines such as this to investigate the utility and prognostic significance of AgNOR in future clinical tumor research.

References

1. Ploton D, Menager M, Jeannesson P, Himber G, Pigeon F, Adnet J. Improvement in the staining and in the visualization of the argyrophilic proteins of the nucleolar organizer region at the optical level. Histochem J. 1986;18(1):5–14.
2. Derenzini M. The AgNORs. Micron. 2000;31(2):117–20.
3. Webster JD, Yuzbasiyan-Gurkan V, Miller RA, Kaneene JB, Kiupel M. Cellular proliferation in canine cutaneous mast cell tumors: associations with c-KIT and its role in prognostication. Vet Pathol. 2007;44(3):298–308.
4. Crocker J, Boldy DA, Egan MJ. How should we count AgNORs? Proposals for a standardized approach. J Pathol. 1989;158(3):185–8.
5. Kiupel M, Bostock D, Bergmann V. The prognostic significance of AgNOR counts and PCNA-positive cell counts in canine malignant lymphomas. J Comp Pathol. 1998;119(4):407–18.
6. Pich A, Chiarle R, Chiusa L, Palestro G. Argyrophilic nucleolar organizer region counts predict survival in thymoma. Cancer. 1994;74(5):1568–74.
7. Amorim JGA, Macarini LAB, Matias AV, Cerentini A, Onofre FBDM, Onofre ASC et al. A novel approach on segmentation of AgNOR-stained cytology images using deep learning. Proc IEEE CBMS. 2020:552–7.
8. Landis JR, Koch GG. The measurement of observer agreement for categorical data. biometrics. 1977:159–74.
9. Shrout PE, Fleiss JL. Intraclass correlations: uses in assessing rater reliability. Psychol Bull. 1979;86(2):420.
10. Tian Z, Shen C, Chen H, He T. Fcos: A simple and strong anchor-free object detector. IEEE Trans Pattern Anal Mach Intell. 2020.

Unsupervised detection of Small Hyperreflective Features in Ultrahigh Resolution Optical Coherence Tomography

Marcel Reimann[1,2], Jungeun Won[1], Hiroyuki Takahashi[1,3], Antonio Yaghy[3],
Yunchan Hwang[1], Stefan Ploner[1,2], Junhong Lin[1], Jessica Girgis[3], Kenneth Lam[3],
Siyu Chen[1], Nadia K. Waheed[3], Andreas Maier[2], James G. Fujimoto[1]

[1]Department of Electrical Engineering and Computer Science, Research Laboratory of
Electronics, Massachusetts Institute of Technology, USA
[2]Pattern Recognition Lab, Friedrich-Alexander-Universität Erlangen-Nürnberg, Germany
[3]New England Eye Center, Tufts Medical Center, USA
marcel.reimann@fau.de

Abstract. Recent advances in optical coherence tomography such as the development of high speed ultrahigh resolution scanners and corresponding signal processing techniques may reveal new potential biomarkers in retinal diseases. Newly visible features are, for example, small hyperreflective specks in age-related macular degeneration. Identifying these new markers is crucial to investigate potential association with disease progression and treatment outcomes. Therefore, it is necessary to reliably detect these features in 3D volumetric scans. Because manual labeling of entire volumes is infeasible a need for automatic detection arises. Labeled datasets are often not publicly available and there are usually large variations in scan protocols and scanner types. Thus, this work focuses on an unsupervised approach that is based on local peak-detection and random walker segmentation to detect small features on each B-scan of the volume.

1 Introduction

Age-related macular degeneration (AMD) ranks fourth on the leading causes of vision loss worldwide [1]. To develop new potential treatments, trial endpoints need to be defined based on early markers of disease progression. New systems such as the ultrahigh resolution spectral domain OCT (UHR SD-OCT) enable the detection of smaller hyperreflective features in the human retina, such as specks (HRS), which have been suggested as indicators for cellular activities associated with visual dysfunction in AMD [1].

For the detection of conventional, but larger, hyperreflective foci (HRF) multiple algorithms already exist [2–5]. They can be divided into algorithms that work on volumes, B-scans or on enface projections of specific retinal layers. Most approaches focus on intensity based thresholds applied to 8-bit images as they are available in commercial OCT instruments. More recent methods utilize optical attenuation coefficients or deep learning. However, most of these algorithms do not utilize the full dynamic range of the OCT signal, suffer from limited resolution scanners, or do not consider the limited amount of available labeled data. [2–5]

To overcome these issues, we propose an unsupervised algorithm that is able to detect features in anisotropic high-definition volumetric OCT datasets by applying a

© Der/die Autor(en), exklusiv lizenziert an
Springer Fachmedien Wiesbaden GmbH, ein Teil von Springer Nature 2023
T. M. Deserno et al. (Hrsg.), *Bildverarbeitung für die Medizin 2023*,
Informatik aktuell, https://doi.org/10.1007/978-3-658-41657-7_50

combination of out-of-the-box image analysis tools. In addition, we show that the algorithm is applicable to different scan patterns, including anisotropic high-definition scans and isotropic motion corrected data from multiple merged scans.

2 Materials and methods

2.1 Data acquisition and preprocessing

Studies were performed under an IRB approved protocol at MIT and the NEEC. Written informed consent was obtained. Data was collected by a UHR SD-OCT prototype with an axial resolution of ~2.7 µm. The anisotropic high-definition volumetric scan was acquired over a 9 × 6 mm field with an A-scan spacing of 5 µm and a B-scan spacing of 25 µm. No B-scan or volumetric averaging was performed and the data was stored using 32 bit floating point values. After resampling, the pixel size is 0.89 µm in axial direction and the B-scan dimensions are 1600 × 1800 pixels.

For evaluation of the algorithm, a total of 49 B-scans from 10 different eyes diagnosed with early (3) and intermediate (7) AMD were selected based on potential appearences of HRS/HRF. Three expert readers independently labeled HRF and HRS and their results were combined using STAPLE [6] with a threshold of $\frac{2}{3}$ and used as ground truth. Of all annotated feature instances 32.2 % were labeled by all readers. After STAPLE was applied, 49.24 % of all previously labeled feature instances remained as ground truth.

To test the applicability of the algorithm on different imaging protocols, on the same device, 4 isotropic scans with 500×500 A-scans were acquired over a 6×6 mm field with alternating horizontal and vertical B-scan directions. The transverse and (resampled) axial pixel spacings were 12 µm and 1.78 µm, respectively. The scans were motion corrected and merged using the approach of Ploner et al. [7]

2.2 Algorithm description

The algorithm is separately applied to each B-scan of the volumetric scan. An essential requirement is the availability of retinal layer segmentation for the posterior of the outer plexiform layer (OPL), external limiting membrane (ELM) and the inner segment/outer segment border (IS/OS), as detecting HRF and HRS in the outer nuclear layer and external to ELM was our priority. For simplification, we refer to this combined region as ONL. As a first step, the layer boundaries are smoothed and the ONL mask eroded to account for possible inaccuracies in the provided layer segmentation. Next, varying illumination (OCT signal) within the ONL was equalized by dividing with a bias field. The field was computed using the axial mean projection of the ONL without considering zero values, and then smoothed by a 30 pixels standard deviation Gaussian kernel following the implementation by Kraus et al. [8] To prevent false positives on the highly reflective ELM, each pixel value in the area of 5 pixels above and below was adjusted so that their axial mean is just below the axial mean of the ONL. For the detection of high intensity features, we utilize local maxima detection. Very isolated maxima are deleted using a hit-or-miss transform with a single pixel structuring element to prevent false positives. After defining the detected local maxima as foreground pixels, the gray scale values of the B-scan are re-scaled to a range of [-1,1], based on the minimum and maximum values of the B-scan, and background pixels are defined to be below a threshold of -0.9. Random walker segmentation is then applied to expand the regions around the local maxima [9].

In the end, multiple thresholds are applied to eliminate false positives by constraining the results to optical properties of the system and clinically relevant features. The minimum size of the detected features is set to be at least 4 pixels in axial dimension and 3 pixels transverse, corresponding to laser beam spot size and optical resolution. The pixel intensities of the feature are compared to a threshold derived from all ONL values covering the same transverse span. The threshold requires the maximum intensity to be larger than the mean plus two times the standard deviation of the ONL values. In addition, the axial mean position of the feature should be within a relative position of 0.25 to 0.8 between the IS/OS (0.0) and OPL (1.0). If the positional requirement is not fulfilled, but the maximum intensity of the detected feature is twice as high as the mentioned threshold, the feature is still considered as detected in the evaluation. Another hard requirement is that the features must be detached from the IS/OS and OPL to be considered as detection, as defined by a previous study by Echols et al. [1] All of these constraints were also applied to the ground truth after labeling.

3   Results

The evaluation is based on binary classification metrics, in which labeled hyperreflective features were considered positives. Because only very few pixels per B-scan were labeled as positives we chose metrics that take high class imbalances into account. Precision and

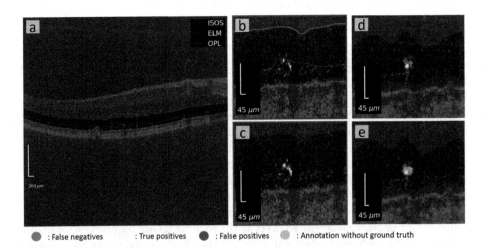

Fig. 1. a) Annotated B-scan from 9 × 6 mm volume including layer segmentation and algorithm results b)-c) Zoomed in version of a reference without annotations and including annotations by algorithm and expert reader d)-e) Zoomed in version of a corresponding frame in the merged 6 × 6 mm volume without and with algorithm annotations.

recall were calculated based on accumulated confusion matrix values over all B-scans. Results are shown in table 1 and figure 1. The per instance results are calculated based on 66 true positives out of 93 labeled features and 44 false positives. A detection was considered as true positive, if there is at least one pixel overlap with an area in the ground truth mask. Also shown in table 1 are results reported by Schlegl et al. [2] for the detection of large conventional HRF. Their deep learning method was trained on 1051 B-scans acquired on Cirrus HD-OCT and Spectralis OCT and evaluated for Cirrus and Spectralis images separately. They include cases with AMD, diabetic macular edema and retinal vein occlusion. They harmonized the different scan protocols by re-sampling the images achieving unified pixel dimensions of ~6 μm axial and ~11.5 μm transverse.

In our case, the average dimensions of the labeled features are 5.0 pixels in transverse dimension and 9.8 pixels axial corresponding to 25 μm transverse and ~8.7 μm axial based on the pixel spacing. The features cover an average area of 36 pixels or ~160.2 μm². Unfortunately, Schlegl et al. do not provide average sizes of their features. However, on their figures, they appear to be much larger, corresponding to conventional HRF. In addition, they also include features in different retinal layers. Due to the difference in sizes and scale, the performance of their algorithm is not directly comparable to our results, yet their results show the performance of a different algorithm on a similar task. A more detailed comparison of our algorithm and the ground truth yields the following observations (Fig. 2). Labeled features with slightly higher intensity values than the background are difficult to detect and the reader agreement on these is not high.

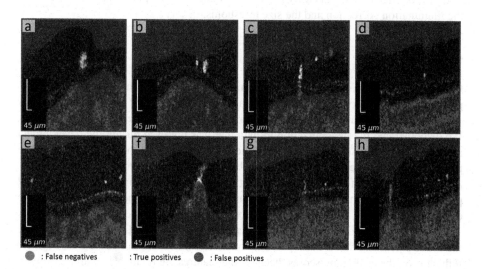

Fig. 2. a)-d) Example images of well segmented hyperreflective features. e) False positive on ELM with high intensity. f) Ground truth annotations in contact with the OPL and algorithm annotations in contact with the IS/OS are, because of the defined constraints, deleted and not shown. Inaccurate layer segmentation is also visible. g) False negative feature appears clearly in neighboring scan, but has low intensity in the current B-scan. h) Ground truth in contact with IS/OS and, therefore, not considered or shown.

Tab. 1. Per pixel and per instance evaluation for the detection of small hyperreflective specks and foci in comparison to pixel-wise results for larger conventional hyperreflective foci reported by Schlegl et al. [2] for data acquired on a Cirrus/Spectralis OCT scanner.

	Evaluation per pixel	Evaluation per instance	Schlegl et al. per pixel
Precision	49.00 %	60.00 %	66.55 % / 55.98 %
Recall	63.25 %	70.97 %	64.01 % / 73.32 %
F1 score	55.22 %	65.03%	65.26 % / 63.49 %

This also applies to boundary regions of the features because of the smooth transition to background intensities and a missing consensus of where to delineate feature boundaries. Another situation of disagreement can occur on much higher intensity values on the ELM compared to the rest of the ELM. They are usually detected by the algorithm, but usually not annotated by the human experts. In addition, for features that are close to IS/OS and OPL, it is sometimes unclear, if they are detached from these layers. It occurs that only either the algorithm or the readers include or exclude them, which has a high impact on the scores as the regions are comparably large. Also, features that clearly appear in neighboring B-scans, but are not clearly visible in the current frame, are occasionally annotated by human readers and not by the algorithm.

In figure 1 we show, that the algorithm is also applicable to data acquired with a different scan protocol and averaged scans. The algorithm only requires the adjustment of hyperparameters that can easily be converted based on the pixel sizes. These include the illumination correction and the size thresholds.

4   Discussion

Compared to previous work, this algorithm has the advantage that it is inherently explainable and does not require labeled data. For the deployment on new datasets only certain parameters have to be converted to match the pixel spacing of the new input. We demonstrated the generalization to data that was not used during the development and hyperparameter selection. Although the study data can, at this point, not be made publicly available, the method can readily be re-implemented and used out of the box. Another advantage of the algorithm is that it utilizes depth information, which is not possible for algorithms that only work on enface projections of the volume. By this, we exploit one of the big strengths of our prototype, namely the high resolution.

We choose thresholds based on the optical properties of the OCT system and include the smallest features that are still possible to detect. As a result, this has a great negative influence on the evaluation scores, because the features are relatively small and single-pixel misclassifications have a large impact on pixel-wise metrics. However, it is not proven that the exact size of the feature is of clinical relevance. In contrast, studies suggest that the number of detected HRF and HRS might be of clinical relevance and can be associated with delayed rod-mediated dark adaptation, which is linked to AMD progression [1]. Therefore, we propose to rather look at detected feature instances instead of semantic segmentation, which is a measure used by Echols et al. [1]. Comparing the algorithm to other state-of-the-art methods is very difficult and we only report the results of Schlegl et al. [2] to give an idea about the performance of most recent methods on similar tasks. However, most of the datasets are collected with different devices and scan protocols and differ in resolution, dynamic range and image sizes. For example, Schlegl et al. cannot report on features as small as ours because of a lower resolution. In addition, there is not yet a clinical consensus on what HRS exactly are and how to label them. HRS sizes are usually below or close to the resolution of commercial systems and have not been investigated on a larger scale. Our work will provide a tool for larger clinical studies on HRF and HRS distributions close to optical resolution and can potentially be used on datasets collected at different sites with different devices. The only requirement is the availability of layer segmentation for the IS/OS, OPL and ELM. However, the ELM scaling is an optional step in the processing and can be omitted. In the future, the algorithm could be adapted to other retinal layers. For now, the focus lies on the ONL, as we expect more HRF and HRS in this layer during the early stages of AMD. In addition, an extension for isotropic volumes should be considered that operates in 3D to, for example, overcome the issue of detached or non-detached features from the ONL mask boundaries. At the time of submission only limited data for isotropic volumes was available. More clinical studies with larger patient cohorts will follow.

Acknowledgement. We acknowledge funding by the National Institutes of Health, project 5-R01-EY011289-36, and the German Research Foundation, project 508075009.

References

1. Echols BS, Clark ME, Swain T, et al. Hyperreflective foci and specks are associated with delayed rod-mediated dark adaptation in nonneovascular age-related macular degeneration. Ophthalmol Retina. 2020;4(11):1059–1068.
2. Schlegl T, Bogunovic H, Klimscha S, et al. Fully automated segmentation of hyperreflective foci in optical coherence tomography images. 2018.
3. Nassisi M, Fan W, Shi Y, et al. Quantity of intraretinal hyperreflective foci in patients with intermediate age-related macular degeneration correlates with 1-year progression. Invest Ophthalmol Vis Sci. 2018;59(8):3431–3439.
4. Okuwobi IP, Ji Z, Fan W, et al. Automated quantification of hyperreflective foci in SD-OCT with diabetic retinopathy. IEEE J Biomed Health Inform. 2020;24(4):1125–1136.
5. Zhou H, Liu J, Laiginhas R, et al. Depth-resolved visualization and automated quantification of hyperreflective foci on OCT scans using optical attenuation coefficients. Biomed Opt Express. 2022;13(8):4175.
6. Warfield SK, Zou KH, Wells WM. Simultaneous truth and performance level estimation (STAPLE): an algorithm for the validation of image segmentation. IEEE Trans Med Imaging. 2004;23(7):903–921.
7. Ploner S, Chen S, Won J, et al. A spatiotemporal model for precise and efficient fully-automatic 3D motion correction in OCT. Medical Image Computing and Computer Assisted Intervention – MICCAI 2022. Cham: Springer Nature Switzerland, 2022:517–527.
8. Kraus MF, Liu JJ, Schottenhamml J, et al. Quantitative 3D-OCT motion correction with tilt and illumination correction, robust similarity measure and regularization. Biomed Opt Express. 2014;5(8):2591–2613.
9. Grady L. Random walks for image segmentation. IEEE Trans Pattern Anal Mach Intell. 2006;28(11):1768–1783.

Comparison of CNN Architectures for Detecting Alzheimer's Disease using Relevance Maps

Devesh Singh, Martin Dyrba

Deutsches Zentrum für Neurodegenerative Erkrankungen (DZNE), Rostock, Germany
devesh.singh@dzne.de

Abstract. Alzheimer's disease (AD) is a neurodegenerative disorder which can be detected using T1-weighted MRI scans. Recent developments in convolutional neural networks (CNN) achieved promising results in various image classification tasks. Specifically, four CNN architectures are widely used: AlexNet, VGG, ResNet, and DenseNet. Feature attribution methods such as layer-wise relevance propagation allow to trace back the information flow in CNNs to derive relevance heatmaps, which approximate the contribution of the input image regions on the model decision. We addressed the open question, which of these CNN architectures is best suited for medical image detection, i.e. AD classification based on MRI data. We adapted the CNN architectures to be used with 3D brain MRI data and trained the models on a heterogeneous dataset with N>2200 from four large studies. We applied tenfold cross-validation and additionally validated results in an independent test dataset. DenseNet and ResNet provided best results, although the overall differences in accuracy did not reach statistical significance. DenseNet provided the most focused relevance maps best matching a-priori expectations of brain regions contributing to the detection of AD, i.e. atrophy in medial temporal lobe.

1 Introduction

In 2020, it was reported that approximately 1.8 million people suffer from dementia in Germany. The most common reason for dementia is Alzheimer's disease (AD), which accounts for almost 60-70% of all the dementia cases. The pathophysiological development of AD begins almost a decade before the first symptoms of the disease appear. AD is a neuro-degenerative disease, which causes gradual and irreversible damage to the brain. Specifically, this damage includes accumulation of the protein beta-amyloid (also called plaques), deaths of neurons caused by neurofibrillary tangles, and gray matter volume reduction (atrophy) in hippocampus, medial temporal lobe, and later-on more widespread cortical areas. These reductions in brain volume are visible in T1 weighted MRI scans, already in early stages of AD [1]. AD causes behavioural changes like memory loss, deteriorating orientation and executive functioning, deregulated emotions, motor control loss and speech impairment. Due to the gradual nature of AD, it is difficult to clinically diagnose its early stages. The first symptomatic stage of AD is called mild cognitive impairment (MCI). It is reported that approximately 10%-15% of the people with MCI will convert into dementia each year[1].

---

[1] https://alz.org/facts

T. M. Deserno et al. (Hrsg.), *Bildverarbeitung für die Medizin 2023*,
Informatik aktuell, https://doi.org/10.1007/978-3-658-41657-7_51

State of the art research shows that deep convolutional neural networks (CNN) have been successfully applied for detecting AD using brain MRI scans [2–6]. Notably, CNNs have solved a variety of machine vision problems like image classification, image segmentation and object detection, within and outside the medical domain. Some of the most widely applied CNN architectures are: AlexNet, VGG, ResNet, Inception-net and DenseNet. Though, due to the black box nature of CNNs, it is difficult to include them in clinical decision support systems, as they lack transparency and comprehensibility. To address this issue, attribution methods have been proposed to produce relevance maps highlighting key features from input samples which contributed to a particular model decision. Few studies systematically compared attribution methods for CNN models for AD classification [4–6], proposing the layer-wise relevance propagation (LRP) or Integrated Gradients methods as most useful.

Notably, to our knowledge, the studies mentioned above compared attribution methods for a single CNN model architecture, but little is known about the influence of the different CNN architectures on the derived relevance maps. In this study we address this gap by i) the comparison of four different CNN architectures with respect to model performance, and ii) the face to face comparison of derived relevance maps.

2 Materials and methods

In our study, T1-weighted volumetric MRI scans were obtained from five study sources: The Alzheimer's disease neuroimaging initiative (ADNI)[2] study phases ADNI2 and ADNI3, the Australian imaging, biomarker & lifestyle Flagship Study of Ageing (AIBL)[3], the DZNE Longitudinal Study on cognitive ampairment and dementia (DEL-CODE)[4], and the European DTI study on dementia (EDSD)[5]. Data obtained from ADNI2, AIBL, DELCODE, and EDSD was used as training data and ADNI3 was used as independent test data. Sample characteristics are listed in Tab. 1. The image preparation pipeline included the N4ITK bias field correction and the SyN algorithm from ANTs to perform an affine registration of each scan to the MNI space. The brain scans were segmented into the compartments gray and white matter, and cerebrospinal fluid using ANTs Atropos. Only the normalized gray matter segments were used as model input. Finally, each gray matter map was cropped to the size of 169 × 208 × 179, with 1 mm isotropic voxel size. Notably, only one (the first) MRI scan from each participant was considered in our study, in case scans from multiple timepoints were available.

Four different convolutional neural network (CNN) architectures were tested in this study, which were chosen because of their successful application across various machine vision problems: AlexNet, VGG, ResNet and DenseNet (Fig. 1). The shallower and simpler network AlexNet was successfully applied before in [3]. Recent studies additionally applied more sophisticated model architectures such VGG [2], ResNet, and DenseNet. We hypothesized that more complex CNNs - ResNet and DenseNet, which use skip connections, should perform better than other simpler CNNs - VGG and

---

[2]More information about the ADNI can be found on https://adni.loni.usc.edu/
[3]https://aibl.csiro.au/ for further details
[4]https://www.dzne.de/en/research/studies/clinical-studies/delcode/
[5]https://www.gaaindata.org/partner/EDSD

Tab. 1. Sample statistics per diagnosis state. The training dataset is an aggregation of ADNI2, AIBL, DELCODE, and EDSD study datasets, while independent ADNI3 study data is used for testing. CN: a cognitively normal, MCI: mild cognitive impairment, AD: dementia due to Alzheimer's disease, MMSE: mini-mental state examination score, F: female, M: male.

	CN	MCI	AD
Training dataset N	1109	640	487
Age (SD)	71.8 ± 6.6	73.0 ± 7.3	74.1 ± 7.7
MMSE (SD)	29.0 ± 1.2	27.3 ± 2.1	22.0 ± 4.3
Education (SD)	14.9 ± 3.3	14.5 ± 3.5	13.4 ± 3.9
Sex (F/M)	610 / 499	287 / 353	253 / 234
Testing dataset N	325	185	62
Age (SD)	70.2 ± 6.4	72.2 ± 7.5	74.8 ± 7.7
MMSE (SD)	29.1 ± 1.1	27.8 ± 2.0	23.1 ± 3.3
Education (SD)	16.6 ± 2.2	16.6 ± 2.5	16.5 ± 2.4
Sex (F/M)	210 / 115	84 / 101	27 / 35

Alexnet, which use linear feature processing steps. Our implementation of these models is available via GitHub[6].

To train these models, a ten-fold cross-validation approach was used, which allowed unbiased comparison of these model architectures. The samples aggregated from ADNI2, AIBL, DELCODE, and EDSD were used as training dataset and ADNI3 study data was used as independent test dataset. We hypothesized that learning from a mixed cohort of pooled mdatasets should help the model learn more general features. Below we report two model performance estimates, first, on the left out validation sets of the cross-validation and second, on the independent test set (ADNI3).

The models were trained with a binary classification target, where Alzheimer's dementia (AD) patients and patients with amnestic mild cognitive impairment (MCI) were merged into one disease-positive class, which was compared to the cognitively normal (CN) participants as the control class. Categorical cross-entropy was chosen as the loss function. An early stopping regularization method was applied, monitoring the training set accuracy as performance metric over epochs, to reduce model over-fitting. The models were optimised using Adam optimiser with the default parameter settings.

It has been previously shown that feature attribution visualisation methods can improve clinical users' understanding of a model's prediction. Specifically, relevance propagation methods help in explaining the neural network's prediction by propagating activation backwards and eventually highlighting features from the input sample as heatmaps or relevance maps. In the context of AD, Böhle et al. [4] showed that the layer-wise relevance propagation (LRP) method highlights neuro-anatomically specific and stable input features and should be preferred over other relevance propagation methods like guided backpropagation (GB). Here, we also applied the compositional LRP$_{\alpha=1,\beta=0}$ rule as shown by Dyrba et al. [3] to produce clinically valuable relevance maps. To choose signal over noise while visualising the relevance maps, we first re-scaled the relevance intensities using their $q = 0.9999$ quantile value and clipped values between

---

[6]Source code is available via GitHub. URL: https://github.com/martindyrba/VisualAiD

the range $[-1, 1]$. Then, the relevance values were smoothed using a Gaussian blur with a kernel size of 6 mm. We used Keras/Tenserflow 1.15 for our implementation of the CNN models and the iNNvestigate[7] library for deriving the relevance maps.

3 Results

Tab. 2 shows the mean accuracy obtained from the various CNN models. ResNet and DenseNet achieved the highest mean accuracy levels on the tasks of AD vs CN and MCI vs CN, respectively.

The mean relevance maps of the AD dementia patients group and MCI patients were very similar to each other, both in the training sample as well as in the independent test dataset. Comparing different CNN architectures, the mean relevance maps for the MCI group of the ADNI3 test dataset were plotted (Fig. 2). These maps were calculated only for a single CNN model of each architecture, namely the second cross-validation iteration which had the highest average accuracy among all ten iterations.

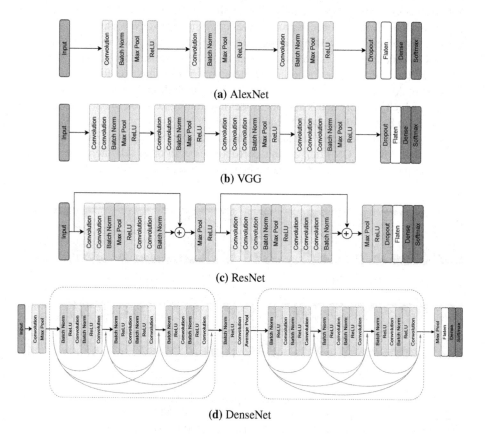

(a) AlexNet

(b) VGG

(c) ResNet

(d) DenseNet

Fig. 1. CNN model architectures used for classifying dementia.

---

[7]https://github.com/albermax/innvestigate

Tab. 2. Mean and standard deviation of accuracy obtained for the cross-validation dataset (top) and independent ADNI3 test data (bottom). AD: Alzheimer's dementia, CN: a cognitively normal state, MCI: mild cognitive impairment.

	AlexNet	VGG	ResNet	DenseNet
Validation-set accuracy				
AD vs CN	0.68 ± 0.12	0.70 ± 0.04	0.75 ± 0.09	0.71 ± 0.05
MCI vs CN	0.63 ± 0.08	0.64 ± 0.03	0.67 ± 0.06	0.65 ± 0.05
Independent test-set accuracy				
AD vs CN	0.72 ± 0.18	0.76 ± 0.08	0.81 ± 0.14	0.76 ± 0.07
MCI vs CN	0.64 ± 0.08	0.66 ± 0.03	0.66 ± 0.05	0.67 ± 0.03

4   Discussion

The mean accuracy levels revealed a consistently higher test accuracy than the validation accuracy (Tab. 2). This suggests that separating the classes for the pooled and more heterogeneous study datasets is more challenging for the models than performing this task on a relatively homogeneous prospective cohort such as ADNI3. This is in agreement with our hypothesis that training on pooled heterogeneous datasets from different study cohorts is beneficial and improves robustness of the models. Though these accuracy levels are lower than those found in AD literature [5, 6], which could be attributed to combining AD dementia and MCI groups into a single disease-positive group during training, which possibly needs another model fine-tuning iteration to optimize different thresholds to better demarcate CN, MCI, and AD.

The accuracy levels also suggest that the group separation task of AD vs CN was simpler than MCI vs CN (Tab. 2), this corroborates with other AD literature findings. Upon comparing the different CNN architectures with each other, we found that complex

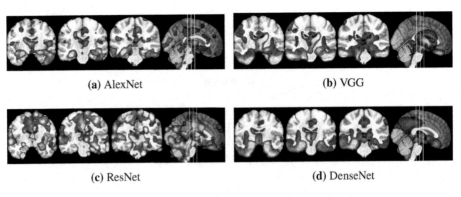

(a) AlexNet   (b) VGG

(c) ResNet   (d) DenseNet

Fig. 2. Mean relevance maps for the MCI group of the ADNI3 dataset obtained using the $LRP_{\alpha=1,\beta=0}$ relevance propagation method overlaid on the MNI brain template. Coronal slices show Y=[-10,-20,-30] mm in MNI reference space are shown. Bright yellow represent the most relevant regions while the dark red regions are of lower relevance. Relevance maps were created following proportional scaling of the activations.

architectures with skip connections - ResNet and DenseNet, performed slightly better than the two other models. This is in agreement with our other hypothesis that more complex models perform better. Notably, the differences in performance did not reach statistical significance overall.

From the relevance maps derived from all the models (Fig. 2), we see that DenseNet mainly focuses on medial temporal lobe and posterior cingulate cortex, also highlighted in [1]. The relevance map for the ResNet model is more noisy and heterogeneous, suggesting that the model's relative high test accuracy for AD vs CN is achieved by considering more widespread brain atrophy or potential artifacts. In contrast to AlexNet and ResNet, the DenseNet model seems to be less sensitive to noise. Its dense connections between layers enabled a highly efficient information flow at various scales.

In future, we will test the CNN models on each individual study dataset (AIBL, EDSD etc.) to replicate previous studies, and investigate the gap between our reported accuracy levels and other studies' accuracy levels. It will also be of interest to examine relevance maps of individuals and the gain of relevance values for specific brain regions.

In this study, we showed that having a pooled training dataset from different study cohorts is beneficial. We also showed that DenseNet utilised an efficient information flow at various scales to generate relevance maps which focused on clinically relevant features. While ResNet derived its high accuracy levels from learning heterogenerous patterns or potential artifacts. This demonstrated the added value of a holistic evaluation of models where relevance maps are being used in combination with classical performance metrics like accuracy, F1-score or ROC-AUC.

References

1. Bernard C, Helmer C, Dilharreguy B, et al. Time course of brain volume changes in the preclinical phase of Alzheimer's disease. Alzheimers Dement. 2014;10(2):143–51.
2. Dyrba M, Hanzig M, Altenstein S, et al. Improving 3D CNN comprehensibility via interactive visualization of relevance maps: evaluation in Alzheimer's disease. Alzheimers Res Ther. 2021:1–18.
3. Dyrba M, Pallath AH, Marzban EN. Comparison of CNN visualization methods to aid model interpretability for detecting Alzheimer's disease. Proc BVM. 2020:307–12.
4. Böhle M, Eitel F, Weygandt M, et al. Layer-wise relevance propagation for explaining deep neural network decisions in MRI-based Alzheimer's disease classification. Front Aging Neurosci. 2019;11:194.
5. Qiu S, Joshi PS, Miller MI, et al. Development and validation of an interpretable deep learning framework for Azheimer's disease classification. Brain. 2020;143(6):1920–33.
6. Wang D, Honnorat N, Fox PT, et al. Deep neural network heatmaps capture Alzheimer's disease patterns reported in a large meta-analysis of neuroimaging studies. Neuroimage. 2023:119929.

Abstract: Deep Geometric Supervision Improves Spatial Generalization in Orthopedic Surgery Planning

Florian Kordon[1,2,3], Andreas Maier[1,2], Benedict Swartman[4], Maxim Privalov[4], Jan S. El Barbari[4], Holger Kunze[3]

[1]Pattern Recognition Lab, Friedrich-Alexander Universität Erlangen-Nürnberg (FAU), Erlangen
[2]Erlangen Graduate School in Advanced Optical Technologies (SAOT), Friedrich-Alexander Universität Erlangen-Nürnberg (FAU), Erlangen
[3]Siemens Healthcare GmbH, Forchheim
[4]Department for Trauma and Orthopaedic Surgery, BG Trauma Center Ludwigshafen, Ludwigshafen
florian.kordon@fau.de

Careful planning of the individual surgical steps is an indispensable tool for the orthopedic surgeon, elevating the procedure's safety and ensuring high levels of surgical precision [1]. A surgical plan for routine interventions like ligament reconstruction describes several salient landmarks on a 2D X-ray image and relates them in a geometric construction. Previous attempts to automate this planning type typically separate automatic feature localization with a learning algorithm and geometric post-processing. The separation allows us to mimic the manual step-wise workflow and enables granular control over each planning step. However, this approach comes with the drawbacks of optimizing a proxy criterion different from the actual planning target, limiting generalization to complex image impressions and the positioning accuracy that can be achieved. We address this problem by translating the geometric steps to a continuously differentiable function, enabling end-to-end gradient flow. Combining this additional objective function with the original proxy formulation improves target positioning while preserving the geometric relation of the underlying anatomical structures. We name this concept Deep Geometric Supervision. The developed method is evaluated for graft fixation site identification in medial patellofemoral ligament (MPFL) reconstruction surgery on (1) 221 diagnostic and (2) 89 intra-operative knee radiographs. Using the companion objective reduces the median Euclidean Distance error for MPFL insertion site localization from (1) 2.29 mm to 1.58 mm and (2) 8.70 px to 3.44 px, respectively. Furthermore, we empirically show that our method improves spatial generalization for strongly truncated images where only a small part of the relevant anatomy is visible.

References

1. Kordon F, Maier A, Swartman B et al. Deep Geometric Supervision improves spatial generalization in orthopedic surgery planning. Proc MICCAI. 2022:615–25.

© Der/die Autor(en), exklusiv lizenziert an
Springer Fachmedien Wiesbaden GmbH, ein Teil von Springer Nature 2023
T. M. Deserno et al. (Hrsg.), *Bildverarbeitung für die Medizin 2023*,
Informatik aktuell, https://doi.org/10.1007/978-3-658-41657-7_52

Abstract: Deep-learning on Lossily Compressed Pathology Images
Adverse Effects for ImageNet Pre-trained Models

Maximilian Fischer[1,2], Peter Neher[1,2,11], Michael Götz[1,3], Shuhan Xiao[1,4], Silvia Dias Almeida[1,5], Peter Schüffler[6], Alexander Muckenhuber[6], Rickmer Braren[7], Jens Kleesiek[8,9], Marco Nolden[1,10], Klaus Maier-Hein[1,4,5,10,11]

[1]Division of Medical Image Computing, German Cancer Research Center (DKFZ), Heidelberg, Germany
[2]German Cancer Consortium (DKTK), partner site Heidelberg
[3]Clinic of Diagnostics and Interventional Radiology, Ulm University Medical Centre, Ulm, Germany
[4]Faculty of Mathematics and Computer Science, Heidelberg University, Heidelberg, Germany
[5]Medical Faculty, Heidelberg University, Heidelberg, Germany
[6]School of Medicine, Institute of Pathology, Technical University of Munich, Munich, Germany
[7]Department of Diagnostic and Interventional Radiology, TU Munich, Germany
[8]Institute for AI in Medicine (IKIM), University Medicine Essen, Essen, Germany
[9]German Cancer Consortium (DKTK), partner site Essen
[10]Department of Radiation Oncology, Heidelberg University Hospital, Germany
[11]National Center for Tumor Diseases (NCT), Germany
maximilian.fischer@dkfz-heidelberg.de

Digital whole slide imaging (WSI) systems allow scanning complete probes at microscopic resolutions, making image compression inevitable to reduce storage costs. While lossy image compression is readily incorporated in proprietary file formats as well as the open DICOM format for WSI, its impact on deep-learning algorithms is largely unknown. We compare the performance of several deep learning classification architectures on different datasets using a wide range and different combinations of compression ratios during training and inference. We use ImageNet pre-trained models, which is commonly applied in computational pathology. With this work, we present a quantitative assessment on the effects of repeated lossy JPEG compression for ImageNet pre-trained models. We show adverse effects for a classification task, when certain quality factors are combined during training and inference. This work was published on the International Workshop on Medical Optical Imaging and Virtual Microscopy Image Analysis [1].

References

1. Fischer M, Neher P, Götz M, Xiao S, Almeida SD, Schüffler P et al. Deep-learning on lossily compressed pathology images: adverse effects for ImageNet pre-trained models. Medical Optical Imaging and Virtual Microscopy Image Analysis. Ed. by Huo Y, Millis BA, Zhou Y, Wang X, Harrison AP, Xu Z. Cham: Springer Nature Switzerland, 2022:73–83.

Contrastive Representations for Unsupervised Anomaly Detection and Localization

Carsten T. Lüth[1], David Zimmerer[2], Gregor Koehler[2], Paul F. Jaeger[2], Fabian Isenensee[3], Klaus H. Maier-Hein[4]

[1]Interactive Machine Learning Group, German Cancer Research Center (DKFZ)
[2]Helmholtz Imaging, German Cancer Research Center (DKFZ)
[3]Medical Image Computing Group, Deutsches Krebsforschungszentrum (DKFZ)
carsten.lueth@dkfz.de

Abstract. Unsupervised anomaly detection in medical imaging aims to detect and localize arbitrary anomalies without requiring labels during training. Often, this is achieved by learning a data distribution of normal samples and detecting anomalies as regions in the image which deviate from this distribution. In the medical imaging domain, most current state-of-the-art methods use latent variable generative models operating directly on the images. However, generative models have been shown to mostly capture low-level features s.a. pixel-intensities instead of rich semantic features, which also applies to their representations. We circumvent this problem by proposing CRADL whose core idea is to model the distribution of normal samples directly in the low-dimensional representation space of an encoder which has been trained with a contrastive pretext-task. By utilizing the representations of contrastive learning we aim to fix the over-fixation on low-level features and aim to learn more semantic-rich representations. Our experiments on the task of anomaly localization on three distinct datasets show that 1) the contrastive representations are superior to generative latent variable models and 2) the CRADL framework shows competetive or superior performance to state-of-the-art.

1 Introduction

The task of anomaly detection is a long-standing task in the medical domain with many diseases being defined by their deviation from what is considered to be normal. In medical image analysis detecting and localizing anomalies is therefore also often the general goal. With powerful deep learning algorithms this task is often tackled using supervised machine learning, which can be extremely effective given that enough diseased cases are avalaible and annotated during the training process. However, most supervised models are not explicitly designed to handle out-of-distribution data and thus might struggle to extrapolate the heterogenity of a disease beyond the training distribution. As a consequence, each new class of pathology or imaging modality necessitates the creation of new annotated datasets—a process that scales poorly with the large number of existing pathologies and the ever-increasing amount of image acquisition methods. Here, unsupervised anomaly detection promises to deliver predictions in the absence of annotated diseased data. Thus, overcoming the need for cumbersome manual annotations, this class of methods could offer a far greater breadth of applications. In principle, this can be realized by learning the distribution of healthy samples. Images (or rather some voxels in the images) 'deviating' from this distribution are then defined as outliers. The problem of detecting these deviations can be posed as an out-of-distribution (OoD) detection problem similar to a blood screening. In the medical imaging domain, the current state-of-the-art methods for anomaly detection are latent variable generative models operating directly in pixel space, mainly different subtypes of and scoring methods based on variational autoencoders (VAEs) and generative adversarial networks (GANs) [1–3]. It has been shown, however, that the likelihoods these methods return tend to focus on low-level features such as background characteristics [4–7] and that their representations have problems capturing semantic information [4, 8]. This makes the anomaly scores of these methods heavily dependent on background statistics such as brightness and contrast. Driven by the hypothesis that more discriminative features are superior to low-level features, we wanted to investigate if self-supervised contrastive learning can aid unsupervised anomaly localization. For this, we propose CRADL, a simple unsupervised representation-based OoD framework consisting of a feature extractor and a generative model. These semantically rich and low dimensional representations obtained with a feature extractor trained with a contrastive self-supervised task [9] allow to fit a wide variety of generative models, e.g. gaussian mixture models (GMMs). We show that anomalies can be localized by back-propagating the negative log-likelihood of representations into the sample. Finally, in our experimental evaluation, we find that the representations of CRADL can yield improvements over reconstruction-based representations for anomaly localization and show competitive performance to state-of-the-art methods like the VAE and context encoding VAE.

2 Method

We propose CRADL, a method using *Contrastive Representations for unsupervised Anomaly Detection and Localization*. CRADL is comprised of two stages (Fig. 1). During the first stage, the encoder f, which maps from the image space X to a learned feature/representation space $Z : z = f(x)$, is trained. In the second stage, a generative model p is fitted on the representations of healthy samples, defining the probability distribution $p(z)$. The anomaly-score as sample is given by the negative-log-likelihood (NLL) of its representation: $s(x) = -\log(p(f(x)))$. Pixel-level anomaly scores for a sample are obtained by back-propagating the gradients of the representation NLL into the sample. Implicitly this approach assumes that regions with large gradients exhibit anomalies.

2.1 Contrastive training

Our contrastive pretext task is conceptually identical to SimCLR [9], where positive pairs are obtained by using data augmentations t drawn randomly from a set of augmentations $\mathcal{T}$ and negative pairs being all other samples. To this end, each sample x_i in a minibatch of N examples is transformed twice, yielding two different views which make up the positive pair. The representations produced by feeding the views through the encoder and projection head, $\tilde{u}_i = g(f(\tilde{t}(x_i)))$ and $\hat{u}_i = g(f(\hat{t}(x_i)))$, are encouraged to be similar by optimizing the NT-Xent contrastive loss

$$l(x_i) = -\log \frac{\exp(\mathrm{sim}(\tilde{u}_i, \hat{u}_i)/\tau)}{\sum_{\tilde{u} \in \Lambda^-} \exp(\mathrm{sim}(\tilde{u}_i, \tilde{u}))/\tau)} \qquad (1)$$

Here the set Λ^- are the negative pairs for sample x_i consists of all examples except $\tilde{u}_i$, which are all other $2N - 1$ examples in the minibatch. The loss over the whole minibatch is obtained by summing all positive pairs.

2.2 Generative model

In general, an arbitrary generative model can be fitted on the representations. In our experiments, we use a Gaussian mixture model (GMM) as the generative model since it is one of the simplest generative models used for anomaly detection. The probability distribution of a GMM with K components is noted in equation 2. We fit the GMM with the expectation-maximization (EM) Algorithm [10] with K being the number of components (specified before the fit).

$$p(z) = \sum_{k=1}^{K} \mathcal{N}(z; \mu_k, \Sigma_k) \cdot \pi_k \qquad (2)$$

3 Experiments

3.1 Data

In our experiments, we used T2-weighted brain MRI datasets. For *training* we used a subset of the HCP dataset [11], which purely consists of 'normal' MRI Scans, using 894 scans split into training and validation sets. For *evaluation of anomaly localization* we

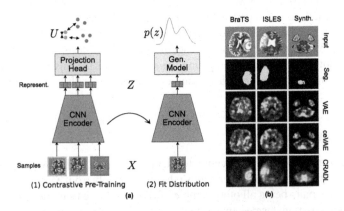

Fig. 1. (a) Visualization of the fitting pipeline, from contrastive pretext (SimCLR) (1) to fitting of the generative model (2). (b) Pixel-wise scores - clamped and normalized for visual inspection.

used the following three datasets. 1) a synthetic anomaly dataset (similar to [12]) from 100 HCP separate scans (*HCP Synth.*) by rendering real-world objects into brain regions. This allows the test set to have the same original distribution (i.e., same scanner, site, ...) as the training set, with only the anomalies differing. We split HCP Synth. dataset into two distinct parts with 49 scans each, one for model development (i.e., to choose our hyperparameter settings and setting of K) and one for testing only. 2) the BraTS-2017 (tumor segmentation) [13] and 3) ISLES-2015 (stroke lesion segmentation) [14] datasets to test the approach in real-world settings with different pathologies. Our BraTS-2017 and ISLES test sets consist of 266 and 20 scans, respectively, as well as validation sets comprised of 20 and 8 scans for selecting K. All datasets were preprocessed similarly, with a patient-wise z-score normalization and slice-wise resampling to a resolution of 128 x 128, followed by clipping the range of intensities from -1.5 to 1.5.

3.2 Model

We used a unified model architecture for our experiments which is based on the deep convolutional architecture from [15], so our encoder solely consists of 2D-Conv-Layers and our decoder (for the VAE models) of 2D-Transposed-Conv-Layers (for more details, please refer to the Suppl.). We chose an initial feature map size of 64 and a latent dimension of 512. For the projection head, we use a simple 2-layer MLP with ReLU non-linearities, a 512 dim. hidden layer, and 256 dim. output.

3.3 Training

All models work on 2D-slices of the data. The contrastive pretext training of the encoder is performed for 100 epochs on the HCP training set using the Adam Optimizer, a learning rate of 1e-4, Cosine Annealing [16], 10 Warm-up Epochs and a weight decay of 1e-6, the temperature of the contrastive loss is 0.5. As transformations for generating different views for the contrastive task, we used a combination of random cropping, random scaling, random mirroring, rotations, and multiplicative brightness, and Gaussian noise.

We fitted the GMM on representations of the encoder from all samples in the HCP training set without any augmentation. The means of the components were randomly initialized, and the convergence limit for the EM algorithm was set to 0.1. We pick the optimal K based on a small validation set where we observe the best AUPRC score. We believe this is a clinically very reasonable approach since the fit of the GMM takes only 10 minutes on a GPU compared to more than 8 hours for the VAE and ceVAE. The post-processing pipeline for the pixel-level scores is identical for all methods evaluated and, based on the approach from Baur et al. [1]. As a performance measure for the final test sets, we used the pixel-wise AUROC and AUPRC metrics with pixel-level scores, as is common practice.

4 Results and discussion

First, we analyze the discriminative power of the representations obtained with contrastive learning to that of generative models in the context of anomaly localization

Tab. 1. Pixel-level anomaly localization metrics for different datasets.

Dataset	Metric	CRADL	VAE	ceVAE
HCP Synth.	AUROC	**0.978(01)**	0.955(01)	0.921(04)
HCP Synth.	AUPRC	**0.325(08)**	0.249(06)	0.172(15)
ISLES	AUROC	**0.898(03)**	0.875(06)	0.879(02)
ISLES	AUPRC	**0.186(39)**	0.077(12)	0.145(13)
BraTS	AUROC	0.942(01)	0.925(01)	**0.948(03)**
BraTS	AUPRC	0.380(16)	0.298(04)	**0.483(03)**

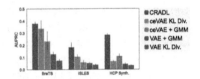

Fig. 2. Pixel-level anomaly localization performance comparison purely using representations and gradients.

and further compare the anomaly localization with the VAE and ceVAE state-of-the-art methods [1, 8, 17].

4.1 Discriminative power of representations for anomaly localization

The discriminative power of the representations obtained with CRADL and generative model, here VAE and ceVAE are compared by using GMM on their representations in an identical scheme to CRADL (Sec. 3). We depict the anomaly localization performance in Fig. 2, where it becomes apparent that CRADL-based representations outperform both VAE and ceVAE-based representations: for both ISLES and HCP Synth. significantly, while on BraTS the KL-Divergence of the ceVAE showed performance within 1σ, however, with lower mean performance. This strengthens the hypothesis that the self-supervised representations of CRADL carry more semantic information, enabling a better localization of fine semantic differences between anomalous and normal brain volumes. A further supporting fact is that the ceVAE, which also employs a self-supervised task, outperforms the VAE.

4.2 Comparison to state-of-the-art anomaly localization

Here, we compare CRADL with our re-implementations of the state-of-the-art methods VAE and ceVAE in the context of anomaly localization both quantitatively (Tab. 1) and qualitatively (Fig. 1b). For the HCP Synth. dataset and ISLES-2015, CRADL obtained the best AUROC and AUPRC metrics by a large margin, followed by the presented baselines. On the BraTS dataset, the ceVAE outperforms the other methods. However, for the BraTS and ISLES datasets, there is a domain gap between the training dataset and test dataset, i.e., different scanners, image quality, and the patient's overall health. This leads to a change in the pixel intensities of the overall pixel distribution. Further, the HCP Synth. dataset includes more varied anomalies and no domain gap, and thus its result could receive more importance.

5 Conclusion

In this work, we propose CRAL, a simple framework for unsupervised anomaly detection and localization based on representations obtained with a contrastive pretext task that shows competitive anomaly localization performance compared to a VAE and ceVAE. We show that the representations obtained with this contrastive framework outperform representations obtained with latent variable generative models for anomaly localization. Other self-supervised tasks [18, 19] might also be worth investigating. The next steps are a generalization to 3D inputs and improve methodology to obtain scores with iterative techniques s.a. image restoration [2].

Acknowledgement. Part of this work was funded by the Helmholtz imaging platform (HIP), a platform of the Helmholtz Incubator on Information and Data Science and the Helmholtz Association under the joint research school HIDSS4Health – Helmholtz Information and Data Science School for Health.

References

1. Baur C, Denner S, Wiestler B, Navab N, Albarqouni S. Autoencoders for unsupervised anomaly segmentation in brain MR images: a comparative study. Med Image Anal. 2021;69:101952.
2. Chen X, You S, Tezcan KC, Konukoglu E. Unsupervised lesion detection via image restoration with a normative prior. Med Image Anal. 2020;64:101713.
3. Schlegl T, Seeböck P, Waldstein SM, Langs G, Schmidt-Erfurth U. F-AnoGAN: fast unsupervised anomaly detection with generative adversarial networks. Med Image Anal. 2019;54:30–44.
4. Nalisnick E, Matsukawa A, Teh YW, Gorur D, Lakshminarayanan B. Do deep generative models know what they don't know? arXiv:1810.09136. 2019.
5. Ren J, Liu PJ, Fertig E, Snoek J, Poplin R, DePristo MA et al. Likelihood ratios for out-of-distribution detection. arXiv:1906.02845. 2019.
6. Xiao Z, Yan Q, Amit Y. Likelihood regret: an out-of-distribution detection score for variational auto-encoder. arXiv:2003.02977. 2020.
7. Meissen F, Kaissis G, Rueckert D. Challenging current semi-supervised anomaly segmentation methods for brain MRI. 2021.
8. Zimmerer D, Kohl SAA, Petersen J, Isensee F, Maier-Hein KH. Context-encoding variational autoencoder for unsupervised anomaly detection. arXiv:1812.05941. 2018.
9. Chen T, Kornblith S, Norouzi M, Hinton G. A simple framework for contrastive learning of visual representations. arXiv: 2002.05709. 2020.
10. Dempster AP, Laird NM, Rubin DB. Maximum Likelihood from incomplete data via the *EM* Algorithm. Journal of the Royal Statistical Society: Series B (Methodological). 1977;39(1):1–22.
11. Van Essen D, Ugurbil K, Auerbach E, Barch D, Behrens T, Bucholz R et al. The human connectome project: a data acquisition perspective. NeuroImage. 2012;62(4):2222–31.
12. Zimmerer D, Petersen J, Köhler G, Jäger P, Full P, Roß T et al. Medical out-of-distribution analysis challenge. 2020.
13. Bakas S, Akbari H, Sotiras A, Bilello M, Rozycki M, Kirby JS et al. Advancing the Cancer Genome Atlas Glioma MRI collections with expert segmentation labels and radiomic features. Sci Data. 2017;4(1):170117.
14. Maier O, Menze BH, von der Gablentz J, Häni L, Heinrich MP, Liebrand M et al. ISLES 2015 - a public evaluation benchmark for ischemic stroke lesion segmentation from multispectral MRI. Med Image Anal. 2017;35:250–69.

15. Radford A, Metz L, Chintala S. Unsupervised representation learning with deep convolutional generative adversarial networks. arXiv:1511.06434. 2016.

16. Loshchilov I, Hutter F. SGDR: stochastic gradient descent with warm restarts. arXiv: 1608.03983. 2017.

17. Zimmerer D, Isensee F, Petersen J, Kohl S, Maier-Hein K. Unsupervised anomaly localization using variational auto-encoders. arXiv:1907.02796. 2019.

18. Li CL, Sohn K, Yoon J, Pfister T. CutPaste: self-supervised learning for anomaly detection and localization. CVPR. 2021:9659–69.

19. He K, Chen X, Xie S, Li Y, Dollár P, Girshick R. Masked autoencoders are scalable vision learners. 2021.

Abstract: AUCMEDI

Von der Insellösung zur einheitlichen und automatischen Klassifizierung von Medizinischen Bildern

Dominik Müller[1,2], Dennis Hartmann[1], Iñaki Soto-Rey[2], Frank Kramer[1]

[1]IT-Infrastructure for Translational Medical Research, University of Augsburg
[2]Medical Data Integration Center, Institute for Digital Medicine, University Hospital Augsburg
dominik.mueller@uni-a.de

Klinische Anwendungsstudien offenbaren, dass die Integration von Pipelines für die Bildklassifizierung in eine Krankenhausumgebung erhebliche Schwierigkeiten bereitet aufgrund von sogenannten Inselloesungen, welche für einen einzelnen Datensatz entwickelt und optimiert wurden. Durch die fehlende Generalisierbarkeit stehen Klinker vor dem Problem, dass keine Wiederverwendbarkeit auf eigene Datensätze und somit kein praktischer Einsatz in der klinischen Forschung möglich ist. Das Open-Source Python Framework AUCMEDI bietet für die beschriebenen Herausforderungen eine Lösung. Das Softwarepaket bietet nicht nur eine Bibliothek als „High-Level" API für den standardisierten Bau von modernen medizinischen Bildklassifizierung-Pipelines an, sondern auch die reproduzierbare Installation und direkte Anwendung mittels Dockerisierung und automatischer Hyperparameter Erkennung. Mit AUCMEDI ist es Forschern möglich, mit nur wenigen Codezeilen eine vollständige, als auch leicht zu integrierende Pipeline für die medizinische Bildklassifizierung aufzusetzen. AUCMEDI ist als Python-Paket über PyPI und als Repository über GitHub verfügbar mit ausführlicher Dokumentation, Beispielen und Anbindungen an moderne DevOps (CI/CD) Techniken: https://frankkramer-lab.github.io/aucmedi/. AUCMEDI wurde bei der 67. Jahrestagung der GMDS (2022) präsentiert [1]. Ein Tutorial zur Anwendung von AUCMEDI ist aktuell bei der 68. Jahrestagung der GMDS (2023) eingereicht. Ein Anwendungsfall wurde im Band der 31. Jahrestagung der MIE (2021) veröffentlicht [2].

References

1. Müller D, Hartmann D, Soto-Rey I, Kramer F. AUCMEDI: Von der Insellösung zur einheitlichen und automatischen Klassifizierung von medizinischen Bildern. 67. Jahrestagung der Deutschen Gesellschaft für Medizinische Informatik, Biometrie und Epidemiologie e. V. (GMDS). Kiel: German Medical Science GMS Publishing House, 2022.
2. Müller D, Soto-Rey I, Kramer F. Multi-disease detection in retinal imaging based on ensembling heterogeneous deep learning models. Studies in Health Technology and Informatics. Vol. 283. (March). IOS Press BV, 2021.

Cavity Segmentation in X-ray Microscopy Scans of Mouse Tibiae

Mingxuan Gu[1], Mareike Thies[1], Fabian Wagner[1], Sabrina Pechmann[2], Oliver Aust[3], Daniela Weidner[3], Georgiana Neag[3], Zhaoya Pan[1], Jonas Utz[1], Georg Schett[3], Silke Christiansen[2], Stefan Uderhardt[3], Andreas Maier[1]

[1]Pattern Recognition Lab, FAU Erlangen-Nürnberg, Germany
[2]Fraunhofer Institute for Ceramic Technologies and Systems IKTS, Germany
[3]Department of Rheumatology and Immunology, FAU Erlangen-Nürnberg, Germany
mingxuan.gu@fau.de

Abstract. Osteoporosis is a chronic disease that causes lower bone density and makes bones fragile. This severely impairs patient life qualities and increases the burden on the social and health care system. X-ray microscopy (XRM) allows tracking of osteoporosis-related changes at a microstructural level in the bone, entailing the characterization of osteocyte lacunae and blood vessel canals. Unfortunately, no segmentation methods for micro-structures in XRM images have yet been established. In this work, we compare the performance of a traditional thresholding-based method with three deep learning networks including 2D and 3D models in both binary and multi-class segmentation. We further propose a clustering method to automatically distinguish blood vessels from lacunae for the binary methods. The performance is evaluated with Dice score (F1 score). The thresholding-based method reaches a mean Dice score of 0.729, which the deep learning models improve by 0.129 - 0.168.

1 Introduction

Osteoporosis is a systematic disorder of the skeleton system which leads to a great reduction in bone mass. Various causes have been linked to the pathogenesis of osteoporosis including menopause and aging [1]. The prevalence of fall-related fractures in osteoporotic patients is massively increased compared to healthy controls and can even occur in response to minor trauma rendering patients immobile and frail, thus laying a severe burden on the social and health care system [1]. As a result, a highly effective diagnosis and treatment system is eagerly desired to be established.

Osteocytes, the main regulator cells of bone homeostasis, reside in bone cavities called lacunae, and account for around 95% of all bone cells. They are distributed through the entire bone matrix and range in sizes from $8 - 15\,\mu m$, this makes their study via conventional μCT difficult [2]. Osteocytes are critical for mechanotransduction and bone turnover [3], while their role in bone remodelling diseases like osteoporosis remains unclear. As a first step toward understanding this relationship, we investigate the shape of the lacunae where the osteocytes reside. X-ray microscopy (XRM) achieves resolution down to 700 nm [4] which makes it suitable for the investigation of lacunae. Besides, XRM is capable of producing volumetric scans without complicated sample preparation, This makes XRM even a candidate for in-vivo acquisition in the future [5].

To investigate the micro-structures in XRM, segmentation is first required. As manual segmentation is time-consuming and expensive, automatic segmentation is more desirable. Previous studies have mainly focused on thresholding-based methods for lacunae segmentation [3, 6, 7]. However, thresholding methods are sensitive to the shifts of the histogram across the samples, as well as the global intensity inconsistency within the same sample. These negative effects could be introduced unintentionally during scanning. In addition, previous studies either do not consider the blood vessels or remove the blood vessels manually which severely increases the labour burden [3, 6, 7].

Recent studies have confirmed the great potential of deep learning methods on bone segmentation [8]. In this work, we present the performance of deep learning networks on XRM lacunae and blood vessel segmentation in a 2D and 3D binary model, as well as a 3D multi-class model. For the binary models, we propose a method to automatically split the segmentation into lacunae and blood vessels with Isolation Forest [9]. We also compare the model performance qualitatively and quantitatively with a baseline thresholding-based method. To the best of our knowledge, this is the first work presenting a complete measurement on lacunae and blood vessel segmentation in XRM.

2 Materials and methods

2.1 Dataset

Samples were retrieved from seventeen 11-14 weeks old C57BL/6 mice, in which four were control mice, and the rest thirteen mice were ovaries-removed to induce osteoporosis. All the operations were conducted in compliance with all the ethical regulations for organ removals in this study and were approved by the local animal ethics committees.

XRM scans were acquired by a Zeiss Xradia Versa 620. The resulting scans have an isotropic pixel spacing of $1.4\,\mu m$, and each volume has around 2000^3 voxels. Among the scans, two slices (2×2000^2) from one sample are used for training the 2D model. Two crops ($2 \times 32 \times 256^2$) from the same sample are used for training the 3D models. One slice from another sample is used for validation. Three slices (each from one different sample) are used for testing. The ground truth annotation is generated by manually correcting the segmentation predicted by the baseline thresholding method and the proposed automatic classification method between lacunae and blood vessels.

The two 2D training slices are cropped into patches of size 256^2 during training. All the samples are normalized with min-max normalization and clipped to range from 0 to 1. Furthermore, affine transformation, random scale, random crop, Gaussian blur, Gaussian noise, and elastic deformation are applied for augmentation.

2.2 Thresholding-based method

We follow the implementation of previous works [3, 7]. First, bone mask is extracted by applying a threshold at 0.35. Then closing operation is applied to close the holes in the bone mask. To extract the cavities, we invert the intensity of the image so that the cavities have a higher intensity than the bone mask. Then a hysteresis threshold is applied, setting the lower threshold and higher threshold as 0.3 and 0.35 respectively. After that, the results are masked by the previously calculated bone mask so that the background is excluded. Finally, the objects with less than 20 voxels are removed since the size of these objects is way less than the majority of the lacunae in this study.

2.3   Lacuane and blood vessel classification

We consider the classification of the lacunae and blood vessels as an anomaly detection problem, as blood vessels occupy only around 1% of the segmented objects in this work. To distinguish vessels from lacunae, we use Isolation Forest [9], taking eigenvalues, stretch, oblateness, vesselness, and sizes of the segmented objects as the features.

The eigenvalues are calculated as the eigenvalues of the covariance matrix of the object. Stretch describes the difference between the largest and the smallest eigenvalue compared with the largest eigenvalue of the segmented object, and oblateness describes how flat the object is. We follow the implementation in [3] and define the stretch as

$$S = \frac{\lambda_3 - \lambda_1}{\lambda_3} \tag{1}$$

where $\lambda_{1/2/3}$ are the eigenvalues of the object in ascending order in magnitude. The oblateness is defined as

$$O = 2\frac{\lambda_2 - \lambda_1}{\lambda_3 - \lambda_1} - 1 \tag{2}$$

The vesselness is defined as the mean value of the result of the Frangi filter [10] on the segmented object. The sizes are the number of voxels occupied by the segmented objects.

After all the features are calculated, we set the contamination rate in the Isolation Forest as 0.01, which produces the best result on the validation data.

2.4   Deep learning-based method

We trained the 2D model for the binary segmentation task where only cavities are segmented, and the lacunae and blood vessels are afterward classified with the Isolation Forest [9]. We trained two more 3D models for comparison. One is a binary 3D model, which is a replacement of all the 2D layers in the 2D model with the corresponding 3D layers. The other is a multi-class 3D model, which directly generates the segmentation for lacunae and blood vessels for comparison with binary models in performance and time consumption.

DR-UNet [11] is used as the segmentation network. The number of encoder and decoder blocks is set to 4, and the number of bottleneck blocks is set to 3. We adjust the number of features in each model so that they have enough parameters to optimize the loss function, meanwhile they do not overfit too early during training. The number of parameters in the 2D binary model, 3D binary model, and 3D multi-class model is 11M, 8M, and 0.5M, respectively.

The Adam optimizer is used for optimization. The learning rate is set to 1.2e-3 for all the models and no learning rate decay is applied. (Binary) cross entropy loss and

Jaccard (intersection-over-union) loss are used as loss functions. We trained all three models for 1500 epochs, and the model with the best performance on the validation set is used for inference.

During inference, the scans are first cropped into patches (256×256 for 2D model, and 32×256×256 for 3D models) and forwarded to the networks, then reconstructed into the original shape after prediction.

3   Results and discussion

Qualitative results are demonstrated in Figure 1. All the wrongly classified objects are circled. The hysteresis threshold and the 2D model are prone to misclassification of lacunae. The thresholding-based method is highly dependent on intensity shifts in local position, and the 2D model is not able to determine whether a small low bone density region is at the margin of a lacuna or just an artifact in the scan, since it does not have the view into the third dimension. Besides, the thresholding-based method tends to produce coarser segmentation (see arrows) which may harm the downstream analysis tasks.

Over-segmentation can be observed at the border of the bone in the prediction of all the deep learning models. During inference, we split the volume into patches, and patches at the border may have a limited view around the border. This makes the borders look like lacunae or blood vessels. The 3D multi-class model predicts some of the objects as a mixture of lacunae and blood vessels which is shown in the third row within

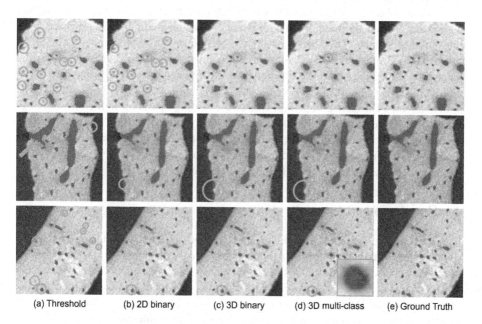

| (a) Threshold | (b) 2D binary | (c) 3D binary | (d) 3D multi-class | (e) Ground Truth |

Fig. 1. Qualitative comparison among the thresholding-based method, 2D binary network, 3D binary network and 3D multi-class network. Green objects represent the lacunae and the red ones are the blood vessels (better in color mode). All the misclassified objects are circled or pointed.

Method	Lacunae	Vessels	Mean	Std
Threshold	0.729 ± 0.016	0.728 ± 0.047	0.729	0.0315
2D Binary	0.899 ± 0.048	0.895 ± 0.056	0.897	0.052
3D Binary	0.907 ± 0.02	0.885 ± 0.015	0.896	0.0175
3D Multiclass	0.868 ± 0.008	0.848 ± 0.037	0.858	0.0225

Tab. 1. Quantitative comparison of Dice score the methods. The best results are emphasized.

a zoom window. The reason might be that there is a severe class imbalance problem as only around 1% of the objects are blood vessels. This makes the 3D multi-class model easy to overfit in the blood vessel segmentation.

We measure the Dice score (F1 score) for performance comparison as shown in Table 1. We first measure the Dice score of each model on the three test slices for lacunae and blood vessels individually, then the average Dice and the standard deviation (Std) are calculated for each class respectively. Finally, the mean and standard deviation of the Dice scores of both lacunae and blood vessels are averaged. The thresholding-based method generates the worst performance for both lacunae and blood vessels. The 3D binary network achieves the highest Dice score for lacunae while the 2D binary network reaches the best Dice score for blood vessels. This is in line with the observation on the qualitative results where the 3D models tend to predict extra blood vessels on the boundary and the 2D model sometimes ignores part of the lacunae. Despite the outstanding performance on the blood vessels, the 2D model has the largest Std, which implies that the performance of the 2D model is unstable, while on the contrary, the 3D models are more robust across different samples.

During inference, we splitted the whole volume into crops with 256 slices, so that we did not exceed the memory. The inference time for predicting one such crop for thresholding method, 2D binary, 3D binary, and 3D multi-class model was 6.5 + 15 mins, 6 + 15 mins, 5 + 15 mins, and 2 + 6 mins, respectively, in which the first value represented the time used for model prediction, and the second value referred to the time used for classification plus 6 mins of operation to remove the small artifacts with connected component labeling. Due to the closing operation in the thresholding-based method, it unexpectedly takes the maximum inference time. As having fewer parameters and no demand for an additional classification, the 3D multi-class model requires the minimum time for inference, which makes it beneficial for practical use. All the inferences are operated on an RTX3000 and an intel i7 with 32G RAM.

4 Conclusion

In this work, we presented the performance of four different segmentation models, showing that the thresholding-based method is sensitive to the intensity shift and is prone to generate coarse predictions. On the contrary, deep learning models are more desirable for the task as they have outstanding segmentation performance on the lacunae and the blood vessels. The 3D models perform even better than the 2D model on the performance stability across the samples, and less time is required for inference. Additionally, we proposed an automatic method to classify lacunae and blood vessels. This approach makes it possible to generate accurate lacunae and blood vessel segmentation from the cavity segmentation, and it dramatically reduces labour burden during labeling.

To further improve the performance of the 3D models, a cortical bone segmentation could be applied to remove the over-segmentation at the boundary of the bone. Another patching method could be introduced as well to intentionally bring the model a larger view at the boundary of the bone. Furthermore, more samples could be used to tackle the lack of blood vessels in the training set or even a synthetic data set with less class imbalance could be used for auxiliary training. Despite the shortages of the current 3D models, the high performance of the segmentation obtained is sufficient for the subsequent measurement of the characteristics of the lacunae and blood vessels.

Acknowledgement. The authors gratefully acknowledge the support from European Research Council (ERC Grant No. 810316) and HPC resources provided by the Erlangen National High Performance Computing Center (NHR@FAU) of the Friedrich-Alexander-Universität Erlangen-Nürnberg (FAU). The hardware is funded by the German Research Foundation (DFG).

References

1. Marcus R, Dempster DW, Cauley JA, Feldman D. Osteoporosis. Academic Press, 2013.
2. Bonewald LF. The amazing osteocyte. J Bone Miner Res. 2011;26(2):229–38.
3. Mader KS, Schneider P, Müller R, Stampanoni M. A quantitative framework for the 3D characterization of the osteocyte lacunar system. Bone. 2013;57(1):142–54.
4. Thies M, Wagner F, Huang Y, Gu M, Kling L, Pechmann S et al. Calibration by differentiation–self-supervised calibration for X-ray microscopy using a differentiable cone-beam reconstruction operator. J Microsc. 2022;287(2):81–92.
5. Wagner F, Thies M, Karolczak M, Pechmann S, Huang Y, Gu M et al. Monte Carlo dose simulation for in-vivo X-Ray nanoscopy. Proc BVM 2022. Springer, 2022:107–12.
6. Gauthier R, Langer M, Follet H, Olivier C, Gouttenoire PJ, Helfen L et al. 3D micro structural analysis of human cortical bone in paired femoral diaphysis, femoral neck and radial diaphysis. J Struct Biol. 2018;204(2):182–90.
7. Heveran CM, Rauff A, King KB, Carpenter RD, Ferguson VL. A new open-source tool for measuring 3D osteocyte lacunar geometries from confocal laser scanning microscopy reveals age-related changes to lacunar size and shape in cortical mouse bone. Bone. 2018;110:115–27.
8. Aust O, Thies M, Pechmann S, Mill L, Andreev D, Miyagawa I et al. Tibia cortical bone segmentation in micro-CT and X-ray microscopy data using a single neural network. Bildverarbeitung für die Medizin 2022. Springer, 2022:333–8.
9. Liu FT, Ting KM, Zhou ZH. Isolation forest. 2008 Eighth IEEE International Conference on Data Mining. 2008:413–22.
10. Frangi AF, Niessen WJ, Vincken KL, Viergever MA. Multiscale vessel enhancement filtering. International conference on medical image computing and computer-assisted intervention. Springer. 1998:130–7.
11. Vesal S, Ravikumar N, Maier A. Automated multi-sequence cardiac MRI segmentation using supervised domain adaptation. STACOM. 2020:300–8.

Abstract: A Spatiotemporal Model for Precise and Efficient Fully-automatic 3D Motion Correction in OCT

Stefan B. Ploner[1,2], Siyu Chen[2], Jungeun Won[2], Lennart Husvogt[1],
Katharina Breininger[1], Julia Schottenhamml[1], James G. Fujimoto[2], Andreas K. Maier[1]

[1]Pattern Recognition Lab, Friedrich-Alexander-Universität Erlangen-Nürnberg, Germany
[2]Department of Electrical Engineering and Computer Science, Research Laboratory for
Electronics, Massachusetts Institute of Technology, Cambridge, MA, USA
stefan.ploner@fau.de

Optical coherence tomography (OCT) is a micrometer-scale, volumetric imaging modality that has become a clinical standard in ophthalmology. OCT instruments image by raster-scanning a focused light spot across the retina, acquiring sequential cross-sectional images to generate volumetric data. Patient eye motion during the acquisition poses unique challenges: Non-rigid, discontinuous distortions can occur, leading to gaps in data and distorted topographic measurements. We present a new distortion model and a corresponding fully-automatic, reference-free optimization strategy for computational motion correction in orthogonally raster-scanned, retinal OCT volumes. Using a novel, domain-specific spatiotemporal parametrization of forward-warping displacements, eye motion can be corrected continuously for the first time. Parameter estimation with temporal regularization improves robustness and accuracy over previous spatial approaches. We correct each A-scan individually in 3D in a single mapping, including repeated acquisitions used in OCT angiography protocols. Specialized 3D forward image warping reduces median runtime to < 9 s, fast enough for clinical use. We present a quantitative evaluation on 18 subjects with ocular pathology and demonstrate accurate correction during microsaccades. Transverse correction is limited only by ocular tremor, whereas submicron repeatability is achieved axially (0.51 μm median of medians), representing a dramatic improvement over previous work. This allows assessing longitudinal changes in focal retinal pathologies as a marker of disease progression or treatment response, and promises to enable multiple new capabilities such as supersampled/super-resolution volume reconstruction and analysis of pathological eye motion occuring in neurological diseases. This paper was accepted and presented at medical image computing and computer assisted intervention (MICCAI) 2022 [1].

References

1. Ploner S, Chen S, Won J, Husvogt L, Breininger K, Schottenhamml J et al. A spatiotemporal model for precise and efficient fully-automatic 3D motion correction in OCT. Medical Image Computing and Computer Assisted Intervention – MICCAI 2022:517–527.

© Der/die Autor(en), exklusiv lizenziert an
Springer Fachmedien Wiesbaden GmbH, ein Teil von Springer Nature 2023
T. M. Deserno et al. (Hrsg.), *Bildverarbeitung für die Medizin 2023*,
Informatik aktuell, https://doi.org/10.1007/978-3-658-41657-7_57

Label Efficient Classification in Liquid Biopsy Data by Self-supervision

Hümeyra Husseini[1], Maximilian Nielsen[1], Klaus Pantel[2], Harriet Wikman[2], Sabine Riethdorf[2], René Werner[1]

[1]Department of Computational Neuroscience, University Medical Center Hamburg-Eppendorf
[2]Institute of Tumor Biology, University Medical Center Hamburg-Eppendorf
h.husseini@uke.de

Abstract. A cut-off of 5 circulating tumor cells (CTCs) per 7.5 ml of blood in metastatic breast cancer patients is highly predictive of progression-free survival and overall survival. These rare events potentially reflect the disease and heterogeneity of the tumor and therefore need to be isolated and characterized from liquid biopsy samples. Identification of CTCs in peripheral blood samples is only partially automated by the rule-based commercially available Cellsearch® system. However, the system still requires manual post-processing and selection of CTCs from a large number of proposed cell image candidates. We propose a self-supervised (DINO), label-efficient combination of deep learning (DL) and support vector machine (SVM) to reliably identify CTCs. We evaluate the label data efficiency of our method in comparison to supervised DL and show that it consistently outperforms supervised state of the art models in terms of F1 score for different balanced subsets as well as for all available data.

1 Introduction

A liquid biopsy is performed by a blood draw from which microscopy images are generated to analyse therapeutic targets that are released into the peripheral blood of metastatic patients. Here, one of the critical liquid biopsy markers is the presence of CTCs [1], but they are extraordinarily heterogeneous and rare in the background of millions of hematopoietic cells in patients' blood. At the present time, CellSearch® is the only FDA-approved technology for CTC isolation and enumeration. The system consists of a rule-based algorithm with the following defined criteria for a CTC: a cell with a round to oval morphology over 4 μm in diameter that is DAPI+ (nucleus, located in and smaller than the cytoplasm), CK+ (cytokeratin, covers approx. part of the nucleus) and CD45- (marker for leukocytes) [1]. Based on that, CellSearch® presents candidate cells to the reviewer who has to manually identify CTCs [2] which is not trivial because of the shine-through effect of signals, ambiguous cells, artefacts etc. In practice, sometimes several hundreds of false positive candidate cells or artefacts are shown.

As the importance and research of the automatic recognition of CTCs are increasing and accelerating [3], DL has been shown to address and overcome some of the aforementioned challenges [2]. In the context of supervised DL, Zeune et al. introduced a framework by the use of CNNs for CTC identification based on the pre-selection of

CellSearch® candidate cells [2] and the system's uncertainties. However, this framework requires extensive labeling, which is time-consuming and tedious.

In computer vision and partly in the medical domain, self-supervision is an emerging approach to reduce the number of required train labels [4]. Unlike labelled data sets, unlabelled data are usually plentiful. Building on the promising power of trending self-supervision methods [4], our work can be summarized by the following main highlights:

- we apply the principle of self-supervision to the liquid biopsy field and exceed the performance of supervised state of the art DL models for binary classification of "CTC" and "Non-CTC",
- we analyse the performance of both approaches with limited labelled train data, and
- we explore the latent space of the learned cell representations and show that the self-supervision approach depicts distinct clusters for CTCs and Non-CTCs without incorporating labels in the training process.

2 Materials and methods

2.1 Data set

The standard data for a patient from a liquid biopsy sample are 175 3-channel (DAPI, CK, CD45) images with a size of 1384 × 1036 px. We used the data of 12 metastatic breast cancer patients, resulting in a total of 69,297 cells. An exemplary image (channel: CK) is depicted as a "raw image" in Fig. 1. Segmentation of objects in CK channel images was done by StarDist [5] with the default parameters and the pretrained model 2D_versatile_fluo. The segmented objects (green outlines, Fig. 1) were then used to create square-cropped images of size 48 × 48 px.

To generate a ground truth, two experts labeled by consensus rating 1,101 cells as CTCs across all patients and 2,333 as Non-CTCs, leaving 65,863 unlabeled cells.

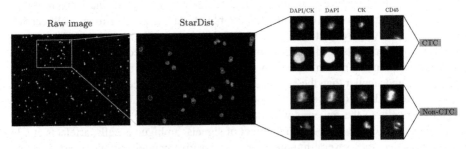

Fig. 1. Overview of the segmentation and labeling framework. A CK channel image of size 1384 × 1036 px is input to the StarDist model, which generates outlines (green) for segmented objects. Right: exemplary cropped images of CTCs and Non-CTCs. From left to right column: composite image of DAPI and CK, DAPI, CK, and CD45 channel.

2.2 Methods

Input to all networks were min-max-normalized (between 0 and 1) 3-channel images (fluorescent channel order: DAPI, CK, CD45) that were resized from 48×48 px (Sec. 2.1) to a size of 224×224 px to adjust to the input dimensions of the pre-trained models (see model details below).

2.2.1 Supervised learning: XCiT and EfficientNetB0.
The supervised learning setup encompassed two baseline models and was realized by training the pre-trained (on ImageNet) XCiT model [6] `xcit_nano_12_p8_224_dist` and the pre-trained base model B0 of the EfficientNet family [7].

Similar to Zeune et al., we subtracted in each channel image the lowest 10 % of the intensity values present [2]. As for data augmentation, we randomly rotated and flipped the images on the vertical and horizontal axis. We used the binary cross entropy (CE) loss and trained the respective networks for a maximum of 600 epochs but applied early stopping to prevent overfitting on the train set.

2.2.2 Self-supervision: DINO.
For self-supervision, we deployed the DINO approach [8], a form of self-distillation, to work on unlabeled image data during the training process. The core of DINO are two networks with identical architecture, one student and one teacher network. The teacher parameters are the running mean of the student ones. Each network consists of a backend, which can be any domain applicable network, and a projection head. To be consistent with supervised learning baseline, we utilised the XCiT network as backend. Settings and parameters were chosen similarly to those reported by Caron et al. [8]. The key idea of DINO is to minimize the cross entropy (CE) between the output distributions of the student and the teacher network. We trained DINO to a maximum of 300 epochs but stopped the training when a loss value < 3 was reached. As input to the networks, different augmentations of the same image are used: mainly global (> 50 % of the image area) and local (< 50 % of the image area) cropping, where the teacher only receives global crops and the student all crops, respectively. The CE is calculated between all possible student and teacher output combinations.

2.3 Experiments

Two main experiments were conducted: the first one covers the assessment of the general performance of supervised learning versus self-supervision on all train data whereas the performance of both approaches on limited label sets is analysed in the second experiment setup.

2.3.1 General performance in comparison.
To conduct the first experiment, we divided the labeled data set into a train set consisting of 2,824 samples (CTCs: 816, Non-CTCs: 2,008), a validation set of 200 samples (CTCs: 100, Non-CTCs: 100), both derived from 8 patients, and a test set of 410 samples (CTCs: 185, Non-CTCs: 225). The test samples are from 4 patients that are not present in the train or validation set. The labeled validation and test set remained the same for the self-supervision setup. The

train set for DINO consists of all unlabeled objects (including ambiguous cells, artifacts etc.; $n = 61,865$) except for the test patients.

After the training process of DINO, we extracted its learned features to fit a classifier, more precisely a SVM (standard sklearn parameters; radial basis function kernel), henceforth denoted as DINO+SVM, to perform a classification and to draw a comparison between the self-supervision approach and the supervised baseline models. Additionally, 4 EfficientNets and 4 XCiTs were trained on all labeled train samples by performing a 4-fold cross validation and were ensembled, henceforth referred to as Ensemble-DL.

Evaluation of the binary classification of CTCs and Non-CTCs was carried out by calculating the F1 score for the test data.

2.3.2   Label data efficiency. Our working hypothesis is that self-supervised feature extraction without any labels allows for classification with accuracy (here: in terms of the F1 score) similar to classical supervised learning - but with a significantly smaller number of available labels. To study the impact of the availability of only a limited set of label data, we formed smaller and balanced data sets based on the pool of the available labeled train set: 50 (CTCs: 25, Non-CTCs: 25), 100, 200, 500, and 1000 samples. The supervised XCiT model was trained 3 times and the SVM for the DINO+SVM approach was fitted 100 times. The train samples were randomly drawn from the entire pool of labeled train samples ($n = 2,824$ samples) for each run. The repeated runs were performed to estimate the variability of the F1 scores. Fitting the SVM to new data sets is computationally not expensive - in comparison to re-training the end-to-end-trained XCiT model. Therefore, the XCiT model was only re-trained 3 times.

In addition to the experiments, we analysed the latent space of the learned cell representations. Therefore, the features of the respective model were extracted and used to fit a UMAP (after PCA) on all labeled train samples. The transformation was applied to the labeled test data.

3   Results

A comparison of the general performance on all labeled data, measured by the F1 score, was drawn between the self-supervision (DINO+SVM) and the standard supervised DL approach. Here, DINO+SVM achieved a higher F1 score (F1: 0.965) than the baseline model XCiT (F1: 0.943) and the Ensemble-DL (F1: 0.944) (Fig. 2).

Based on the analysis of the performance on smaller labeled data sets, DINO+SVM starts at a higher F1 score: 0.865 ± 0.043 (supervised XCiT: 0.687 ± 0.025) for 50 train samples, continuing with 0.910 ± 0.033 (XCiT: 0.747 ± 0.021) for 100 samples, 0.925 ± 0.023 (XCiT: 0.837 ± 0.011) for 200, 0.959 ± 0.004 (XCiT: 0.854 ± 0.012) for 500, hereby crossing the Ensemble-DL (reference) line and 0.963 ± 0.01 (XCiT: 0.871 ± 0.026) for 1000 samples (Fig. 2). Thus, DINO+SVM performs consistently better for the same number of samples than the supervised approach and with 500 labeled samples better than the best supervised approach of our setup trained on all available labeled data.

The latent space of DINO and supervised trained XCiT after feature extraction and the observed clustering according to the cell classes CTCs (orange) and Non-CTCs (purple) is visualised in Fig. 2. We then analysed the behavior of the cell cluster regarding supervised training over the limited size train sets. By inspecting the CTC clusters near to the decision boundary, as illustrated in Figure 3, a trend of the cells from having a heterogeneous distribution at 50 train samples to a more homogeneous one is visible when more labeled data is included. DINO, however, which is trained without labeled data, shows distinct clusters for CTCs and Non-CTCs and a homogeneous distribution of cells within the respective cell clusters whereas the supervised model, comparable to the supervised XCiT model trained on 1000 train samples (Fig. 3).

4   Discussion

Building on recent developments and success in the field of self-supervision [8], we deployed DINO for processing of liquid biopsy microscopy images and demonstrated that, combined with a standard SVM classifier, it exceeds the F1 score for CTCs and Non-CTCs differentiation compared to classical end-to-end supervised DL. We thereby demonstrate that label-efficient classification of cells by self-supervision is also feasible and promising for the liquid biopsy field.

When analysing the latent space of the extracted feature maps, we not only observed distinct clusters for the cell classes for the supervised but also for the self-supervised approach, even though DINO extracted the features of the cells without any annotation

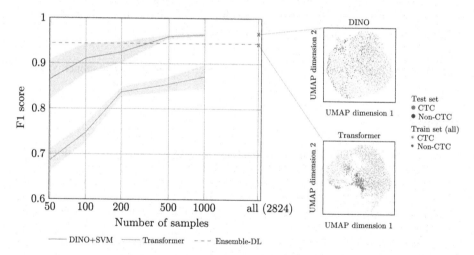

Fig. 2. Performance of DINO+SVM and XCiT models on different train sample sizes. Mean and standard deviations are visualised. Magenta: DINO+SVM, green: XCiT, red: ensemble-DL (our reference). Evaluation metric: F1 score. Because the Transformer (=XCiT) achieved better results than the EfficientNet model, only the XCiT performance is shown. There is no line drawn from 1000 to 2824 samples since the latter does not represent a balanced sample size but rather all available train data. On the right: UMAP clustering of the two cell classes is depicted. Latent space analysis of DINO was performed without incorporating labels during training. Orange: CTCs, purple: non-CTCs; greater dots: ground truth (GT) test samples, smaller dots: GT train samples (all).

Fig. 3. Latent space visualization of the learned cell representations. The self-supervision (DINO) approach depicts distinct clusters for CTCs and Non-CTCs without incorporating labels during training. For supervised learning (XCiT): the more train samples (50 to 1000) are used the more distinct and homogeneous clusters are formed. Orange: CTCs, purple: non-CTCs; GT greater dots: test samples, GT smaller dots: train samples (all).

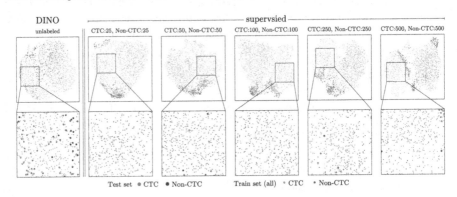

information during training. Even though latent space visualization is always to be interpreted with caution, it supports the quantitative results and the above statement.

In the future, usage of unlabeled data of more patients is planned to improve the performance of the self-supervision approach and to become more robust. Further, it would be interesting to apply it to different tumor entities.

Acknowledgement. The work is funded by the Erich und Gertrud Roggenbuck-Stiftung.

References

1. Andree K, Dalum G van, Terstappen LW. Challenges in circulating tumor cell detection by the CellSearch system. Mol Oncol. 2016;10(3):395–407.
2. Zeune LL, Boink YE, Dalum G van, et al. Deep learning of circulating tumour cells. Nat Mach Intell. 2020;2(2):124–33.
3. Guo Z, Xiaoxi L, Hui Y, et al. Circulating tumor cell identification based on deep learning. Front Oncol. 2022:359.
4. Singh P, Sizikova E, Cirrone J. CASS: cross architectural self-supervision for medical image analysis. ArXiv preprint arXiv:2206.04170. 2022.
5. Schmidt U, Martin W, Broaddus C, et al. Cell detection with star-convex polygons. Proc MICCAI. 2018:265–73.
6. Ali A, Touvron H, Caron M, et al. XCiT: cross-covariance image transformers. Proc NeurIPS. 2021;34:20014–27.
7. Mingxing T, Le QV. EfficientNet: rethinking model scaling for convolutional neural networks. Proc ICML. 2019:6105–14.
8. Caron M, Touvron H, Misra I, et al. Emerging properties in self-supervised vision transformers. Proc ICCV. 2021:9650–60.

Motif Analysis of Resting-state and Stimulus-driven fMRI Networks with Special Focus on Neurotransmitter-specific Subnetworks 2023

Drăgălina Dulea[1], Isabel Wank[1], Claudiu Ivan[1], Tanja Niedermair[2,3],
Susanne Grässel[3], Andreas Maier[4], Andreas Hess[1]

[1]Friedrich-Alexander Universität Erlangen-Nürnberg, Experimental Pharmacology and Toxicology
[2]University of Regensburg, Institute of Pathology
[3]University of Regensburg, Department of Orthopaedic Surgery
[4]Friedrich-Alexander Universität Erlangen-Nürnberg, Department of Pattern Recognition
dragalina.d.dulea@fau.de

Abstract. Complex large scale brain networks can be broken down to small, repetitive building blocks, termed motifs. Here, motif-compositions were investigated in functional brain networks of different mouse models of A) resting state (RS) corresponding to brain function in absence of a specific task, and B) peripheral heat stimulation with warm and hot temperatures. The brain-wide networks obtained were decomposed to subnetworks of different neurotransmitters (NT): glutamate, acetylcholine, serotonin, dopamine, noradrenaline, substance P and α-CGRP based on expression data of neurotransmitters and their receptors from Allen Mouse Brain Atlas (ABA), a genome-wide, high-resolution database of gene expression. Those NT-specific subnetworks and their motif composition allow for deeper insight into specific brain functions.

1 Introduction

A motif is considered to be any commonly used network architecture or recurring, "significant" pattern of inter-connections, even if that subgraph structure has unknown computational properties. Identifying motifs is one motivation for the field of connectomics, the study of the brain through the lens of its connectivity [1]. The aim of this work is to assess how motif composition of the neurotransmitter (NT)-specific subnetworks changes depending on the experimental condition and mouse model.

For this purpose, the distribution of different motifs was investigated in functional brain networks obtained from different mouse models lacking various NT. Networks of resting state (RS) - brain function in absence of a specific task, and brain activity evoked by peripheral heat stimulation with warm (40°C + 45°C) and hot temperatures (50°C + 55°C) were analyzed. First, brain-wide networks obtained after the two types of functional (f)MRI measurements were characterized by their motif distribution in wild type mice. The term brain-wide network refers to functional networks based on functional connectivity between all regions of the brain. Second, subnetworks of different neurotransmitters and their motif respective decomposition were generated to allow for deeper insight into specific brain functions. Neurotransmitters are fundamental and

T. M. Deserno et al. (Hrsg.), *Bildverarbeitung für die Medizin 2023*,
Informatik aktuell, https://doi.org/10.1007/978-3-658-41657-7_59

Tab. 1. The analyzed mouse models with the corresponding number of animals.

Mouse model	Number of animals
Wild type (WT)	13
α-CGRP-KO (CGRP)	9
Tachykinin1-KO (TAC)	9
Sympathectomy (SYX; 80mg/kg 6-OHDA i.p.)	8

endogenous chemicals that enable neurons to communicate with each other. In this way, the brain provides multiple but very specific functions, due to the process of synaptic transmission by the different NT (see below), done primarily through the release of NT's from presynaptic neurons binding to postsynaptic receptors [2]. Motif decomposition was generated using DotMotif Python library for undirected motif search. The currently used motif search methods depend on closed-form matrix algebra subgraph-counting techniques, established only for very specific types of motifs [1]. The main advantage of the DotMotif library is that the user can create complex motif queries of arbitrary size which incorporate graph, node, and edge attributes. Finally, this workflow was applied to different partially genetically modified mouse models which lack known important NT highly relevant to orchestrate bone fracture healing.

2   Materials and methods

Using female mice, 3 groups with deficits in the abundance of sensory and sympathetic NT [3] were compared with wild type (Tab. 1). 10 min RS BOLD-fMRI and 50 min stimulation with either warm perception (T12: 40°C + 45°C) or hot noxious heat perception (T34: 50°C + 55°C) (at left paw) were acquired (BRUKER 4.7 T; GE EPI, TR = 2000 ms; TEef = 25.3 ms; matrix 64*64, 22 slices 500 my each; array head coil). Brain networks were constructed based on functional connectivity - temporal synchronicity of the functional BOLD-signal between pairs of brain regions, i.e. nodes. For more details on data acquisition, data pre-processing and analysis see Wank et al. [4].

The NT subnetworks were constructed using data from the ABA mouse gene expression database: mean expression data of genes encoding A) the NTs (source) and B) the corresponding receptors (target) were calculated for summarized brain regions matching the mouse brain atlas used for fMRI analysis [5]. Information from ABA database was used to select only those nodes from the entire network and to create subgraphs using NetworkX library [6]. This step was performed for the NT glutamate, acetylcholine, serotonin, dopamine, noradrenaline, substance P and α-CGRP. We analyzed NT subnetworks of A) T12, T34 and RS networks of WT mice, and B) significant NBS (network-based statistics) [7] differences between T12 and T34 stimulus-driven networks in CGRP, SYX, TAC, and WT.

NetworkX Python library (visualize and compare the networks), which offers features for the creation, manipulation, and study of the structure, dynamics, and functions of complex networks [6] and DotMotif (undirected motif search with 3, 4, and 5 nodes) were used as network analysis tools. Resulting NT subnetworks (Fig. 1) contain information about the structure such as number of edges, number of nodes, and anatomical positions of each node in frontal (coronal) plane. The nodes are color-coded according to the anatomical brain area they belong to (see legend Fig.1). The shape of the node was used to encode if the brain region is expressing the NT (source: triangle pointing to the right ">") or is expressing the receptors and can therefore be modulated by the NT (target: triangle pointing to the left "<"). The node size is determined by the mean gene expression coefficients extracted from the ABA database.

After displaying the general information about NT subnetworks, subnetwork motif decomposition was performed to analyze connectivity in more detail. In this regard, DotMotif Python library was used for undirected motif search. DotMotif [1] is an intuitive graph tool designed for interrogating biological graphs of any size and acts as an interface to common graph management systems such as the NetworkX. The search was performed for motifs with 3, 4, and 5 nodes (Fig.2) in the brain-wide networks and NT subnetworks. Given two graphs, one is isomorphic to another if there exists a bijection. In case of a monomorphism the bijection requirement is reduced to simply injection, meaning that the match in the host graph may contain extra edges [8]. The results of a motif search with DotMotif are all the subgraphs that match a query graph in a search graph. Matching means that one of the mappings exists. By default, a search is performed for all subgraphs that are monomorphic to the query subgraph.

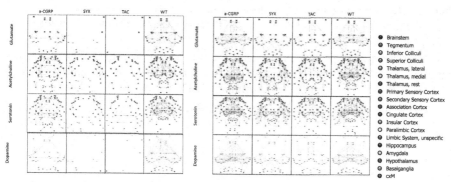

(a) Innocuous temp. T12: average brain networks evoked by stimulation with 40°C + 45°C.

(b) Noxious temp. T34: average brain networks evoked by stimulation with 50°C + 55°C.

Fig. 1. Example of NT subnetworks. The color-coded nodes represent the single brain regions, involved in the respective NT signaling, connected by edges indicating functional connectivity averaged over the animals of each group. The size of the nodes represents the gene expression coefficient for this node, derived structure-wise from the ABA database. Arrangement of the nodes represent grossly the anatomical location of the brain structures in coronal sections. NT source regions are displayed as right-pointing triangle, target regions expressing the corresponding receptors as left-pointing triangle.

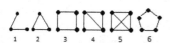

Fig. 2. Motif representation.

For each type of graph General (brain-wide network) and Glutamate, Acetylcholine, Serotonin, Dopamine, Noradrenaline, Substance P, α-CGRP (corresponding subnetworks of each NT) the number of motifs for each defined motif (Motif1 - Motif6, Fig. 2) was calculated. To analyze the relationship between number of motifs and the structure of the network, the number of edges was calculated.

At the end, all functions created to realize different operations such as: reading json files corresponding to each analyzed network, reading the information from the atlas, create the subnetworks, plotting the networks and subnetworks, perform the motif search, and show the results were added to the GenNet Python library, and made user-accessible via Jupyter notebook.

3   Results

Comparison of motif distribution for NT subnetworks in WT mice (Fig. 3) revealed that all NT showed a higher number of motifs in RS data compared to stimulus-driven data, especially for serotonin. The highest incidence in both cases (RS and stimulus-driven data) was found for motif 6, a closed pentagon with 5 nodes and 5 edges.

Dopamine and Substance P networks showed substantial impact of the stimulation, with lower temperatures leading to higher motif count. Overall, stimulation was found to have differential impact on motif count for the different NT subnetworks. Graphs show that in case of high temperature stimulation the number of motifs decreased compared with low temperature stimulation.

Assessing phenotype-specific percentage motif distribution per NT-subnetwork (fingerprints Fig. 4) revealed a strong phenotype influence: WT: dopamine, α-CGRP, substance P; SYX: glutamate and dopamine; TAC: acetylcholine, serotonin and noradrenaline; CGRP: α-CGRP. Highest percentages were obtained for motifs 1, 2, and

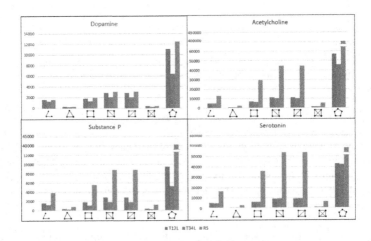

Fig. 3. WT mice motif distribution averaged across animals: warm and hot stimulation as well as RS subnetworks of Dopamine, Substance P (similar distribution for α-CGRP and Glutamate) and Acetylcholine, Serotonin (similar distribution for Noradrenaline).

6. Depending on the mouse phenotype, the motif that had the maximum percentage in most of the subgraphs differed: for TAC and CGRP the most frequent motif was motif 6 and in case of WT and SYX it was motif 1. It could be observed that a high incidence of motif 6 was obtained in highly connected networks compared to the sparser ones, where motif 1 was the most present (data not shown).

Finally, we investigated how the number of motifs is influenced by the network density. Past analyzes had revealed that most dramatic changes in the small world index, a measure for network efficacy, occur, when a network is reduced to 4-7 % of its original

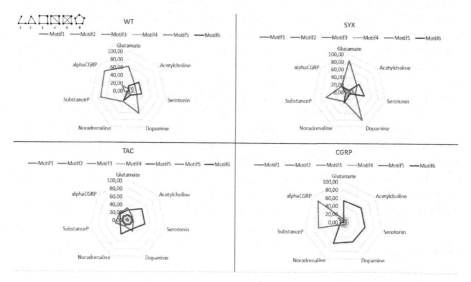

Fig. 4. Fingerprints of motif percentages in neurotransmitters subgraphs obtained from significant differences in functional connectivity between warm and hot temperature networks for the different mice phenotypes (SYX - chemically induced adrenaline/noradrenaline knock-down, TAC - substance P knock-out , CGRP – α-CGRP knock-out).

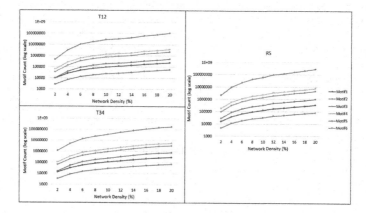

Fig. 5. Comparison between different network densities for WT mice mean networks.

density. Therefore, the density of the networks was increased in 2 % steps from 2 % to 20 %, each separate. In order to increase the density, edges were added gradually. Exemplified for WT, the number of motifs grew linearly with the network densities (Fig. 5) for both, the mean stimulus-driven networks as well as in the RS networks.

4 Discussion

Analyzing brain networks by different NT systems and motifs allow a specific decomposition. Motif incidences for NT systems were similar for RS and stimulus driven networks demonstrating the underlying importance of NT networks. In case of WT mice, RS networks differed in motif incidence and had overall more motifs. Increased stimulus intensity decreased the motif incidence. The reason behind might be a strong focusing effect due to the highly salient sensory input, that leads to more efficient information processing and therefore sparser networks with less brain regions involved. Moreover, NT-related mouse phenotypes were characterized by motif-specific fingerprints.

Further improvement includes a user-friendly GUI for NetworkX and DotMotif, to make the access easier for physicians or neurobiologists not familiar with Python. To obtain the desired result knowledge about the correct name and parameters of the function is mandatory. Another useful improvement will be to adapt the program to work also with human and rat fMRI data. Finally, this workflow allows now to investigate probably larger motifs, derived directly from the brain networks and defined by their functional uniqueness.

References

1. J. K. Matelsky E. P. Reilly ea. DotMotif: an open-source tool for connectome subgraph isomorphism search and graph queries. Scientific Reports volume. 2021;(13045).
2. Sheffler ZM Reddy V PL. Physiology, Neurotransmitters. StatPearls Publishing. 2022.
3. Niedermair Tanja ea. Impact of the sensory and sympathetic nervous system on fracture healing in ovariectomized mice. Int J Mol Sci. 2020:405.
4. Wank Isabel ea. Central amygdala circuitry modulates nociceptive processing through differential hierarchical interaction with affective network dynamics. Commun Biol. 4.1 (2021):1–10.
5. Allen Institute for Brain Science(2004). Allen Mouse Brain Atlas [dataset]. 2011:mouse.brain-map.org.
6. Aric A. Hagberg DAS, Swart PJ. Exploring network structure, dynamics, and function using NetworkX. Proceedings of the 7th Python in Science Conference (SciPy2008), Gäel Varoquaux, Travis Vaught, and Jarrod Millman (Eds), (Pasadena, CA USA). 2008:11–5.
7. Zalesky Andrew ea. Network-based statistic: identifying differences in brain networks. Neuroimage. 53.4 (2010):1197–207.
8. West DB. Introduction to Graph Theory Vol. 2. Prentice Hall, 2001.

Detection of Arterial Occlusion on Magnetic Resonance Angiography of the Thigh using Deep Learning

Tri-Thien Nguyen[1,2], Folle Lukas[1], Thomas Bayer[2], Andreas Maier[1]

[1]Fakultät für Pattern Recognition, FAU Erlangen-Nürnberg
[2]Insitut für Radiologie und Neuroradilogie, Klinikum Fürth
tri-thien.nguyen@fau.de

Abstract. Magnetic resonance angiography (MRA) is an imaging tool used to evaluate arterial steno-occlusions in the lower limbs of patients with peripheral artery disease (PAD). This study aimed to train a deep learning method for the detection of arterial occlusions in the Superficial Femoral- and Popliteal Artery using radial maximum intensity projections (MIP) of contrast-enhanced MRA. A retrospective study was performed with 500 MRA exams included, using only the radial MIP of the thigh. Stenosis labeling was performed based on severity, considering only significant stenosis, and differentiating between no stenosis, focal stenosis, mid-length stenosis, and long stenosis. Class labels were combined to form four-class, three-class, and binary-class scenarios. An EfficientNet-B0 was trained and tested using a six-fold cross-validation for the right and left sides separately. The neural network (NN) achieved decent results with an area under the receiver operating characteristic curve (AUROC) of 0.917 ± 0.040 and accuracy of 0.851 ± 0.043 in the binary class case for the left side. The results degraded slightly for the three- and four-class cases and were overall minimally worse for the right side. The trained NN showed promising results in detecting arterial stenosis on MRA, which could potentially be a helpful tool for objectifying findings and reducing the workload of radiologists in the future.

1 Introduction

Arterial occlusions block the flow of oxygenated blood to the tissues. If the arteries in the lower extremities are affected, it results in peripheral arterial disease (PAD) of the lower limbs. Symptoms can range from pain while walking to gangrenous tissue and even amputation. Although PAD is uncommon in people under 40 years of age, it is more frequent in older age groups and is estimated to affect 202 million people worldwide in 2010 [1].

The disease is initially diagnosed through anamnesis, physical examination, and the ankle-brachial index. For further localization and evaluation of the severity of vessel occlusions, additional medical imaging can be used. Different imaging techniques are available, including magnetic resonance angiography (MRA). MRA images are reviewed by radiologists, and the results are documented in radiology reports, which are often written in free text form and can vary in quality between personnel [2].

Therefore, a deep learning (DL) based method to detect arterial occlusions could help reduce the workload of radiologists and improve the objectivity of findings. Only a few studies have been performed using DL techniques for PAD [3]. Additionally, to the best

T. M. Deserno et al. (Hrsg.), *Bildverarbeitung für die Medizin 2023*,
Informatik aktuell, https://doi.org/10.1007/978-3-658-41657-7_60

of our knowledge, only one study focused on the detection of arterial occlusions of the lower limbs on the comparable case of computed tomography angiography (CTA) [4].

In this study, a private and labeled database of MRA was used to train and test a convolutional neural network (CNN) for the detection and classification of arterial steno-occlusions in the superficial femoral- and popliteal artery.

2   Materials and methods

This study was conducted as a retrospective single-center study and received written approval from the responsible ethics committee of the Friedrich-Alexander-Universität Erlangen-Nürnberg (application number 21-366-Br).

2.1   Image acquisition

This study included 500 examinations of patients who underwent contrast-enhanced MRA for PAD between 2018-2021 at the Klinikum Fürth. Three different magnetic resonance machines from different vendors were used (1.5 T Symphony TIM/ 3 T Skyra, Siemens, Forchheim, Germany; 1.5 T Philips Ingenia Ambition X, Philips, Amsterdam, Netherland). All patient data was anonymized and handled only by staff from the originating hospital.

Radial maximum intensity projections (MIP) are created by summing up images along vectors from different viewing angles (Fig. 1a). Only radial MIPs of the thigh, which depict the Superficial Femoral- and Popliteal Artery, were used (Fig. 1b).

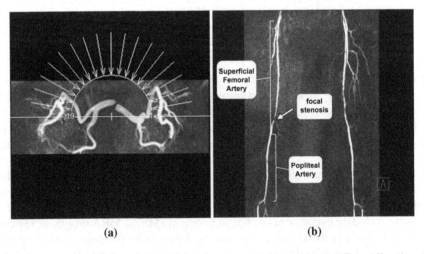

(a)   (b)

Fig. 1. Exemplary MIP of the thigh: (a) shows a transversal view with the different directions for the radial reconstruction indicated by arrows; (b) shows an exemplary frontal view of the radial MIP reconstruction with denoted arteries and an exemplary focal stenosis.

2.2 Labels

Labeling was performed by a radiologist in training with more than four years of clinical experience, based on radiological reports and image data. Steno-occlusions of the Superficial Femoral- and Popliteal Arteries were recorded on both the right and left sides, according to length. Four classes were used to differentiate between no stenosis, focal stenosis, mid-length stenosis, and long stenosis. Only stenoses greater than 50 % of the diameter were considered significant. In the three-class problem, focal and mid-length stenoses were combined into one class. In the binary-class case, no and focal stenosis were merged, as were mid-length and long stenosis.

The class distribution was skewed towards the class label denoting no stenosis, with more than 50 % of all labels. This was the case for both the right and left sides (Fig. 2). Note that the absolute numbers do not add up to 500, as samples that showed stents or bypasses were excluded.

2.3 Neural network and training

A pre-trained EfficientNet-B0, which is a CNN optimized in width, depth, and resolution [5], was used for classification within a PyTorch Lightning framework [6]. The radial MIP projections were fed into the CNN as grayscale images as channels.

The radial MIP acquisitions varied between the different machines and had to be homogenized. The direction of rotation was manually equalized to a counterclockwise direction for all samples, and the resolution was re-scaled to 224 x 224 pixels. The images were normalized.

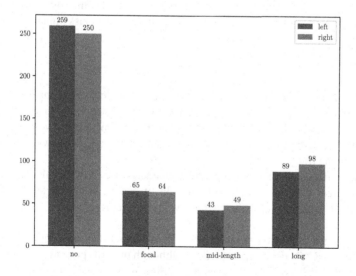

Fig. 2. The charts depict the absolute number of samples in the different denoted classes of the left and right sides.

Tab. 1. Tabular results for the left and right side with the different class scenarios. Stated values are rounded to $1 * 10^{-3}$.

Side	#Classes	Accuracy	AUROC	F1 score
Left	Two	0.851±0.043	0.917±0.040	0.851±0.043
Right	Two	0.818±0.030	0.885±0.039	0.818±0.030
Left	Three	0.810±0.024	0.838±0.027	0.711±0.040
Right	Three	0.814±0.056	0.837±0.067	0.707±0.090
Left	Four	0.863±0.015	0.803±0.060	0.717±0.032
Right	Four	0.836±0.022	0.771±0.038	0.655±0.049

In preliminary testing, it was noted that the results of the CNN did not benefit from the most lateral views from the right and left sides, and the number of MIP angles also varied from 15 to 19. As a result, the most lateral views were left out, and only 13 MIPs around the frontal views were included.

To avoid overfitting, data augmentation was applied during the training process. The same augmentation techniques were applied to all input channels with a certain chance and degree of expression, including Gaussian blur, cropping, translation of the image, and changes in contrast. The training was performed using a stochastic gradient descent optimizer with a learning rate of 0.01 and cross-entropy as the loss function.

The CNN was trained for 400 epochs with a batch size of four, using the validation loop loss as a metric to checkpoint the best models. Six-fold cross-validation was used, and the database was separated into six data blocks using a stratified method to preserve class distribution. Six CNNs were trained, with a different data block used as the test data each time, and the remaining data were split randomly into a 0.85/0.15 ratio for training and validation loops. A weighted random sampler that oversamples the less frequent class was applied during training to counteract the class imbalance.

3   Results

The CNN achieved slightly better average results for the left side compared to the right side, as shown in (Tab. 1). The area under the receiver operating characteristic curve (AUROC) was 0.917± 0.040, 0.838± 0.027 and 0.803± 0.060 for the two-, three- and four class case respectively. Due to the skewed data distribution, AUROC was considered the most reliable metric.

For the left side, the receiver operating characteristic (ROC) of the two-class case for the different folds is plotted in Figure 3a. It can be seen that all trained CNNs outperformed a random classifier, which would be represented by a linear diagonal curve.

The averaged confusion matrices (Fig. 3b, 4) depict that most miss-classifications are made by the CNN denoting no stenoses although one was present. Note that the sum of the absolute values of the samples may differ by one between the matrices due to rounding. ROC and Confusion Matrices are slightly worse but similar in composition for the right side so these results are not explicitly shown.

4   Discussion

Several limitations were encountered during the implementation of this study. The radial MIP reconstruction was used due to hardware limitations and it provided the best balance between image information and data size. The thigh region, including the Superficial Femoral- and Popliteal Arteries, was selected to simplify the problem. The classification was chosen based on clinical significance in order to evaluate endovascular and surgical treatment options. Labeling was only performed by one reader, but was based on radiological reports from other readers.

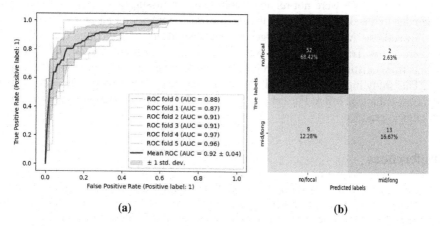

Fig. 3. Results from the binary class case from the left side: a) receiver operator characteristic (ROC) for the left side with zero denoting no/focal stenosis and one mid-length/long stenosis; b) averaged Confusion Matrix, each field shows the number of samples and percentage. Denoted number of samples are rounded to absolute numbers and percentage values to $1 * 10^{-2}$.

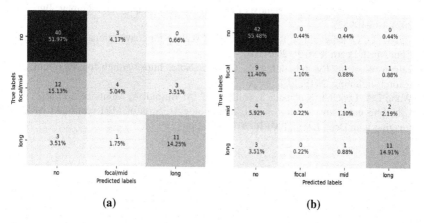

Fig. 4. Averaged confusion matrix from all folds for the a) three- and b) four class case for the left side. Each field shows the number of samples and the percentage. Denoted number of samples are rounded to absolute numbers and percentage values to $1 * 10^{-2}$.

This study demonstrated decent results in the detection and classification of stenoses in the Superficial Femoral- and Popliteal Arteries depicted on radial MIP reconstructions of contrast-enhanced MRA, with an AUROC of up to 0.917 ± 0.040 in the binary class case. In comparison, Dai et al. [4] achieved a higher AUROC of 0.987 in detecting above-knee stenosis on CTA. However, they used small segmented areas of single axial slices depicting contrast enhanced arteries. In this study, the whole three-dimensional volume was used, and steno-occlusions could therefore also be evaluated by their length.

The results of this study decreased with a more finely-grained class separation, which differ between more degrees of stenosis. To be feasible for use in clinical practice, even more sophisticated class separation would be necessary. Additionally, the predictions made by the CNN were not reliable enough, often missing stenosis, which may have been due to the skewed class distribution towards samples with no stenosis.

To address these issues, a larger database could alleviate the data dependency of DL processes. Transformer-based Neural Network can be used to automatically extract labels from existing radiological reports [7] and increase the amount of labeled data.

This study highlights the feasibility of automatic detection of arterial occlusions in contrast-enhanced MRA. Further research is needed before this technique can be applied in clinical practice.

References

1. Fowkes FGR, Rudan D, Rudan I, Aboyans V, Denenberg JO, McDermott MM et al. Comparison of global estimates of prevalence and risk factors for peripheral artery disease in 2000 and 2010: a systematic review and analysis. Lancet. 2013;382(9901):1329–40.
2. Pool F, Goergen S. Quality of the written radiology report: a review of the literature. J Am Coll Radiol. 2010;7(8):634–43.
3. Lareyre F, Behrendt CA, Chaudhuri A, Lee R, Carrier M, Adam C et al. Applications of artificial intelligence for patients with peripheral artery disease. J Vasc Surg. 2022.
4. Dai L, Zhou Q, Zhou H, Zhang H, Cheng P, Ding M et al. Deep learning-based classification of lower extremity arterial stenosis in computed tomography angiography. Eur J Radiol. 2021;136:109528.
5. Tan M, Le Q. Efficientnet: Rethinking model scaling for convolutional neural networks. Int Conf Mach Learn. PMLR. 2019:6105–14.
6. Falcon W et al. Pytorch lightning. GitHub. Note: https://github.com/PyTorchLightning/pytorch-lightning. 2019;3(6).
7. Wood DA, Lynch J, Kafiabadi S, Guilhem E, Al Busaidi A, Montvila A et al. Automated Labelling using an attention model for radiology reports of MRI scans (ALARM). Med Imaging with Deep Learn. PMLR. 2020:811–26.

Localizable Instruments for Navigated Treatment of Ischemic Stroke

Lena Stevanovic[1], Ramona Bodanowitz[1], Benjamin J. Mittmann[2],
Ann-Kathrin Greiner-Perth[1], Eva Marschall[1], Tobias Kannberg[1], Timo Baumgärtner[2],
Michael Braun[3], Bernd Schmitz[3], Alfred M. Franz[1,2]

[1]Institute for Medical Engineering and Mechatronics, Ulm University of Applied Sciences
[2]Institute for Computer Science, Ulm University of Applied Sciences
[3]Neuroradiology Section, Günzburg District Hospital
alfred.franz@thu.de

Abstract. Mechanical thrombectomy as a therapeutic option for ischemic stroke can possibly be supported by localizing the used catheters and guidewires during the intervention. In this study we equipped a probing catheter and a guidewire with electromagnetic (EM) sensors that can be localized in real time by means of an EM field generator. These instruments were tested regarding tracking accuracy and handling in laboratory and clinics. While accuracy was better than 0.4 mm in all cases and the probing catheter showed promising handling and robustness, we observed handling problems and a sensor defect in case of the guidewire. We further demonstrated 3D navigation of the tracked catheter by probing 10 targets inside a vascular phantom with an average error of 1.8 mm.

1 Introduction

Ischemic stroke is a common disease worldwide. If left untreated it can lead to severe disability or death, but there is a chance of full recovery if treatment is provided quickly within a few hours. Besides the standard drug therapy, mechanical thrombectomy is a therapeutic option that has shown promising results in several large clinical trials [1]. In this intervention the stroke causing blood clot is removed by using a system of guidewires and catheters. These instruments are positioned in the vessel tree at the location of the clot with the help of fluoroscopy. However, there are still cases, where thrombectomy is not successful or reperfusion of the vessels is too late. A challenge during the procedure is the navigation of the instruments, e.g. caused by vascular tortuosity. Research should therefore focus on maximizing first-pass success and complete reperfusion [2].

There is potential for improvement of navigation through instrument localization and registration of preinterventional computed tomography (CT) data to the interventional scene. A possible implementation is the use of electromagnetic (EM) tracking of instruments and anatomy. Position and rotation can be determined by EM sensors within a magnetic field created by a field generator. In thrombectomy the use of EM tracking would allow a continuous 3D localization of instruments equipped with EM sensors and visualize them together with a vessel tree extracted from a registered CT image. This would provide additional information for the radiologist and may enable an easier and faster navigation.

The attachment of EM sensors to catheters and guidewires has already been demonstrated for other medical fields like endovascular and cardiac surgery [3][4]. Furthermore, the commercial electromagnetically trackable catheter ThermoCool SmartTouch of Biosense Webster Inc. (California, US) exists for the treatment of cardiac arrhythmias. Due to the larger diameter it cannot be used for thrombectomy.

In a previous study we showed that accurate tracking in a thrombectomy setting is possible with the right setup [5]. This work aims to equip a catheter and a guidewire used in thrombectomy with EM sensors and investigate if the handling of the instruments can be maintained despite sensor integration. Evaluation is performed by an experienced neuroradiologist in a vascular phantom. The accuracy of the sensors is determined by the measurement protocol of Hummel et al. [6] under laboratory conditions and in a clinical setting. Furthermore the reachability of targets inside a cerebral vessel phantom by using the tracked instruments with a prototype of a navigation system for thrombectomy is demonstrated.

2 Methods

2.1 Trackable catheter and guidewire prototypes

For the development of the trackable catheter the commercial catheter Cordis Tempo™ (Cardinal Health, Dublin, Ireland) with a diameter of 1.35 mm was picked. The guidewire prototype was based on a micro guidewire with 0.2 mm diameter (ev3 Mirage.008 Hydrophilic Guidewire, Medtronic plc, Dublin, Ireland). Catheter and guidewire with a comparably small diameter were chosen to keep the overall diameter after sensor integration as small as possible. An Aurora sensor (SN: 610099) from Northern Digital Inc. (NDI) (Waterloo, Canada) with 5 degrees of freedom (DoF) and a diameter of 0.55 mm was selected as EM sensor for the prototypes. It can give information about its xyz-position and two rotational axes. 6-DoF EM sensors, that could provide additional rotation information are not used due to their larger diameter which is problematic for the probing of small vessels and catheters.

For the catheter two sensors were attached to it (Fig. 1). By tracking the shape of the catheter tip using both sensors the rotation around the catheter axis, i.e. the missing degree of freedom when using a single 5 DoF sensor, can be visualized. The sensors were attached to the catheter with medical glue Vitralit® 473 from Panacol-Elosol GmbH (Steinbach, Germany). Afterwards a thin-walled (0.01 mm) polytetrafluoroethylene (PTFE) tube from Zeus Industrial Products, Inc. (Letterkenny, Ireland) was pulled over the probing catheter including the EM sensors. The openings of the tube at the tip and the end of the catheter were sealed with the glue to prevent contact with liquid.

For the guidewire prototype (Fig.2) the sensor was inserted in a PTFE tube which was then glued to the wire. It was developed with regards to the inner diameter of the catheter prototype to enable insertion. The outer diameter of the prototypes were 1.8 mm for the catheter and 0.94 mm for the guidewire.

For tracking the EM sensors a NDI Aurora system (Waterloo, Canada) with table-top field generator was used together with the open-source software Medical Imaging Interaction Toolkit (MITK) (www.mitk.org).

2.2 Assessment of accuracy and handling

To assess the accuracy of the prototypes, the measurement protocol of Hummel et al. [6] was used to determine the position and rotation errors of the EM sensors. The instruments were placed in a planar grid of 3 x 4 poses, which is a smaller subset of the 9 x 10 grid of the original protocol [7]. The reference distance between the poses is 5 cm. On each of the 12 poses, 150 samples were recorded and the root mean square error (RMSE) on each pose was calculated as a measure for the jitter. In addition, the distance between the mean positions of pairs of adjacent poses were compared to the reference of 5 cm leading to 8 vertical and 9 horizontal = 17 distance errors as a measure for accuracy. To assess orientational accuracy, a circle of 32 holes spaced 11.25° apart was used. The measured angles were compared to the reference of 11.25° and the average error was determined over all 32 measurements. This was repeated for both orientational degrees of freedoms (Rot 1, Rot 2, c.f. [6]) for the used 5 DoF EM sensors.

The measurements were performed under laboratory conditions and in a clinical environment of a stroke unit. To ensure comparability, the measurement setup of Greiner-Perth et al. was used [5]. In this setup, the angiography device was placed directly above the area to be measured. With the sensors used in the prototypes, no measurement results could be generated with this setup. It was necessary to move the angiography device to the side to enable the determination of the sensor position.

A cerebral vessel phantom, that was developed in a previous work, was used for the evaluation of the prototype handling [8]. The instruments were inserted in the fluid-filled phantom by an experienced neuroradiologist. This involved placing the catheter prototype into a guiding catheter and testing its capabilities to move it inside the vessel tree. The guidewire prototype was inserted into a probing catheter and its handling was compared to a conventional guidewire.

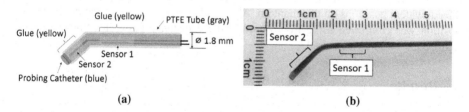

Fig. 1. Catheter prototype in schematic structure (a) and the real prototype (b).

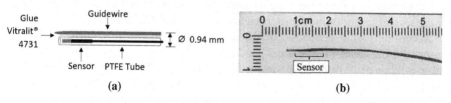

Fig. 2. Guidewire prototype in schematic structure (a) and the real prototype (b).

Tab. 1. Position error of EM sensors attached to the catheter and guidewire in laboratory and clinics averaged over 17 measured 5 cm distances, jitter averaged over 12 root mean square errors of 150 measurements per position, rotation error of both orientational DoFs averaged over 32 measurements of 11.25°.

	Laboratory			Clinc		
	pos. error [mm]	jitter [mm]	rot. error [°]	pos. error [mm]	jitter [mm]	rot. error [°]
Sensor 1	0.20	0.04	Rot 1: 0.12	0.33	0.04	Rot 1: 0.65
			Rot 2: 0.13			Rot 2: 0.65
Sensor 2	0.23	0.12	Rot 1: 0.10	0.36	0.13	Rot 1: 0.16
			Rot 2: 0.10			Rot 2: 0.15
Guidewire	0.10	0.04	Rot 1: 0.19	0.34	0.15	Rot 1: 0.17
			Rot 2: 0.12			Rot 2: 0.11

2.3 Thrombectomy navigation experiment

In addtion, a custom software based on MITK was used to test navigation with the instruments inside the vessel phantom. The software allows for automatic registration of a preinterventional CT data set to the intraoperative scene with a reattachable fiducial marker that we presented in a previous study [9]. This enables visualization of the instrument position in a 3D scene with a vessel tree segmentation from the CT data set.

The navigation experiment with the catheter prototype was performed by a experienced neuroradiologist in the stroke unit of the district hospital Guenzburg (BV, Germany). Ten predetermined targets inside the vessel tree were to be reached three times each with exclusively the navigation visualization while the (transparent) phantom was not visible to the operator. The targets to be reached were within the left and right *Arteria carotis externa* and *Arteria carotis interna*. As shown in Fig. 3, the target positions were defined in the digital vessel tree and marked with radiopaque lines at the equivalent positions on the phantom. After each experimental run, the final catheter position was controlled using fluoroscopy and the distance between catheter tip and radiopaque line was measured.

3 Results

The averaged results of the accuracy assessment are shown in Tab. 1. In lab and clinics the mean values of position error and jitter for catheter and guidewire prototype stayed in the submilimeter range. Average rotation errors were below 0.2° in all cases except for the second sensor of the catheter with an error up to 0.65° in clinics.

According to the evaluation of the neuroradiologist, the attachment of the EM sensors did not change the original handling of the probing catheter. The localization and orientation of the catheter tip was easily identifiable in MITK (Fig.3a). The guidewire prototype showed a reduced range in the vascular phantom compared to a conventional guidewire. In contrast to the catheter, handling of the guidewire had changed noticeably, in particular the special behavior of the tip could not be maintained with the sensor.

Although an initial test with the navigation software prototype showed the movement of the guidewire in relation to the catheter in a 3D scene, we observed a sensor defect after the guidewire prototype was pushed through the bend at the tip of the catheter several times. Therefore we focussed on the promising catheter prototype with a conventional guidewire for the thrombectomy navigation experiment shown in Fig.3. In all 30 experimental runs, the catheter prototype could be placed successfully under the use of the navigation software with a measured mean error of 1.8 mm (standard deviation: 1.6 mm, maximum error: 4.9 mm) between catheter tip and target. In 8 of these runs (26 %), the catheter tip was positioned exactly at the target (error: 0 mm).

4 Discussion

With the aim of localizing and navigating instruments in thrombectomy by EM tracking, a guidewire and a catheter were equipped with sensors and evaluated. We observed average position errors of up to 0.36 mm in the clinical environment which is lower compared to the determined position error of Greiner-Perth et al. of 1.64 mm, with the same tracking system but a different EM sensor [5]. This can be explained by the different placement of the angiography device. By placing it outside the area to be measured, the interference is reduced and lower position errors are obtained. The performed accuracy measurements for tracking of the sensors resulted in a slightly higher error in a clinical setting than under laboratory conditions both for guidewire and catheter prototype.

The original characteristics of the probing catheter were not changed by the integration of two EM sensors. The determined position and rotation errors in the submillimeter or subdegree range are comparable to typical values of EM trackers known from related work [7]. The navigation experiment showed that probing the vessels and turning at branches was performed succesfully. This indicates a sufficient accuracy to help facilitate the procedure and reducing radiation exposure. During preparation of the experiments, recalibration of the marker [9] with a static offset became necessary for registration,

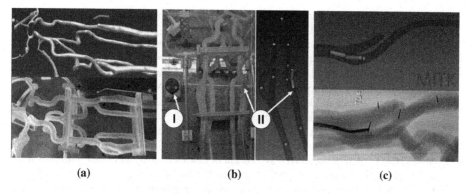

(a)　　　　　　(b)　　　　　　(c)

Fig. 3. Catheter prototype: a) Outside the phantom showing the shape of the tip by means of two EM sensors. b) Photograph with registration sensor (I)[9] and 3D visualization of the registered vessel tree with 10 targets (yellow) and catheter (II). c) Visualisation and fluoroscopic image with reference (radiopaque lines) after an experimental run. Note: The radiopaque lines were applied after the photos in (a) and (b) were taken.

which we did not expect. Nevertheless, during the experiments registration worked automatically and accurately. Altogether the catheter prototype seems to be promising for further investigations and research.

By attaching the EM sensor to the guidewire its flexibility was limited and the diameter was enlarged resulting in increased stiffness and worsened handling. We observed a defect of the sensor attached to the guidewire which was most likely due to the necessary bending to pass the curved catheter tip. It is worth mentioning that we had a second prototype without the PTFE tubing which showed the same behaviour. Related work showed the sensors' ability to bend once up to 40°[10], but defects can occur after bending it multiple times as our study shows. Even though the tracking accuracy is promising and defects are frequently observed with conventional guidewires as well, it appears difficult to implement tracked guidewires because of the worsened handling.

In this work a trackable probing catheter prototype for the use in thrombectomy was presented. Its handling and measurement accuracy were successfully validated. In addition the reachability of 10 targets inside a cerebral vessel phantom by using the tracked catheter and a prototype of a navigation system for thrombectomy was shown with an average error of 1.8 mm. Future research can focus on the preservation of handling in guidewires despite sensor integration.

Acknowledgement. This work was funded by the Federal Ministry for Economic Affairs and Climate Action (BMWK, Funding Code: ZF4640301GR8).

References

1. Goyal M, et al. Endovascular thrombectomy after large-vessel ischaemic stroke: a meta-analysis of individual patient data from five randomised trials. Lancet. 2016;387(10029):1723–31.
2. Yoo AJ, Andersson T. Thrombectomy in acute ischemic stroke: challenges to procedural success. J Stroke. 2017:121–30.
3. Condino S, et. al. Electromagnetic navigation platform for endovascular surgery: how to develop sensorized catheters and guidewires. Int J Med Robot. 2012;8(3):300–10.
4. Jäckle S, et al. Instrument localisation for endovascular aneurysm repair: comparison of two methods based on tracking systems or using imaging. Int J Med Robot. 2021;17(6):1–14.
5. Greiner-Perth AK, et al. Elektromagnetisches Instrumententracking für die Schlaganfallbehandlung mittels Thrombektomie. Proc BVM. 2022:121–30.
6. Hummel JB, et al. Design and application of an assessment protocol for electromagnetic tracking systems. J Med Phys. 2005;32(7):2371–9.
7. Maier-Hein L, et al. Standardized assessment of new electromagnetic field generators in an interventional radiology setting. Med Phys. 2012;39(6):3424–34.
8. Stevanovic L, et al. Open-Science Gefäßphantom für neurovaskuläre Interventionen. Proc BVM. 2021:172–7.
9. Mittmann BJ, et al. Reattachable fiducial skin marker for automatic multimodality registration. Int J CARS. 2022;17(11):2141–50.
10. Piazza R, et al. Towards electromagnetic tracking of J-tip guidewire: precision assessment of sensors during bending tests. Proc. SPIE Medical Imaging. 2020;1131506.

Needle Tip Tracking During CT-guided Interventions using Fuzzy Segmentation

Gino Gulamhussene[1], Arnab Das[1], Jonathan Spiegel[1], Daniel Punzet[2], Marko Rak[1], Christian Hansen[1]

[1]Faculty of Computer Science, Otto von Guericke University, Magdeburg, Germany
[2]Institute for Medical Engineering, Otto-von-Guericke-University Magdeburg, Magdeburg, Germany
hansen@isg.cs.uni-magdeburg.de

Abstract. CT-guided interventions are standard practice for radiologists to treat lesions in various parts of the human body. In this context, accurate tracking of instruments is of paramount importance for the safety of the procedure and helps radiologists avoid unintended damage to adjacent organs. In this work, a novel method for the estimation of 3D needle tip coordinates in a CT volume using only two 2D projections in an interventional setting is proposed. The method applies a deep learning model for the fuzzy segmentation of the region containing the tip on 2D projections and automatically extracts the position of the tip. A simple UNet achieves a Dice score of 0.9906 for the fuzzy segmentation and an average euclidean distance of 2.96 mm for the needle tip regression task.

1 Introduction

CT scans are an important and indispensable part of interventional radiology, which includes a wide range of lesion treatments in various parts of the human body. However, depending on the size, location, and visibility of lesions, the process of diagnostic and therapeutic intervention becomes challenging for radiologists. Radiologists rely on imaging and tracking data that show the exact position of the needle in real time to guide insertion. Hence, for these image-guided procedures to be accurate and safe, it must be possible to precisely track the needle's path and identify crossing structures [1]. In addition, technical units used during CT-guided interventions, such as automatically moving gantries or robotic ultrasound, could benefit from needle tip tracking data in the future [2]. In addition to accuracy, the tracking should also be (near) real-time. Therefore, this work introduces a novel and fast method of tracking the needle tip in interventional CT scans.

As a result of decades of research and developments, AI-based technologies, especially deep learning-based methods are becoming very successful in a wide range of image or vision-related tasks. Medical image-based procedures are no exception either. There is numerous research where deep learning methods have significantly outperformed traditional image analysis techniques in various modalities like MRI, US, CT, and PET scan when applied to diverse problem-solving tasks of segmentation, classification, detection/localization, registration, and many more [3].

A Convolution Neural Network (CNN) based approach was proposed in [4] for real-time detection of needles in 2D US images. The proposed method tracks the needle based on the concept of "region of interest" and bounding boxes like general object detection algorithms. The authors of the paper employed a fully convolutional network (FCN) along with a region-based convolutional neural network (R-CNN) to achieve the desired goal, where the former network proposes candidate regions from the 2D ultrasound image and fed to the latter for fine-tuning and producing the final bounding boxes. In [5] an innovative approach is taken by the researchers for needle trajectory and tip Localization in real-time 3D Ultrasound. The 3D needle localization task is converted into a 2D problem by using 2D projections and then an automatic image analysis technique was used to capture the changes in the appearance of the movement of the needle stylus. A 3D CNN architecture is applied for a similar task of needle segmentation and tip localization by [6]. The CNN network is inspired by the 3D UNet model [7], but the authors made some improvements to capture the anisotropic nature of MRI volumes before it can be applied to a needle segmentation problem. The authors claimed that the computational efficiency of the asymmetric network design resulted in the feasibility of the network training using full T2-weighted in gantry MRI volumes. Research around deep learning approaches for needle-tracking problems can also be noted in [8–10].

Although the deep learning-based approaches show a remarkable result, the training of these networks requires a huge amount of annotated data. While acquiring medical domain data is a very challenging task in itself, annotating the same poses a far greater deal of challenge.

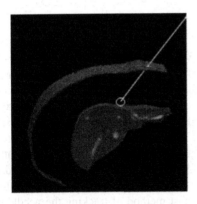

Fig. 1. An iCT volume with a needle.

Figure 1 depicts an iCT volume of the abdomen scanned from a phantom with an inserted needle. The green circle marks the needle tip, whose coordinate we are interested in. This paper proposes a pipeline/scheme for simple and fast needle tip localization, which has several contributions to the research community:

- Conversion of the 3D needle tip localization and coordinate regression task to a 2D problem by taking only two maximum intensity projections per CT volume.
- Automatic fuzzy segmentation [11] of the circular region of interest around the needle tip using CNN, and from that automatically regressing the 3D coordinates.
- Semi-automatic annotation of the training and test data using Hough transform to ease lengthy and time-consuming completely manual annotation overhead.

A detailed description of the proposed method is provided in section 2. Subsection 2.1 highlights the data, annotation mechanism, and training setup. An in-depth discussion along with results can be found in Section 3.

2 Methodology

In this paper, we apply a CNN network that segments a circular region of interest around the needle tip. Here, a fuzzy segmentation technique is chosen instead of hard segmentation. Section 3 shows that a simple UNet model is enough for the fuzzy segmentation task. For comparison, a relatively complex model, inspired by the TransUNet model [12], is also applied to the same task. Along with convolutional layers, the later network consists of a few multi-head self-attention (MHA) layers [13]. [12] applied the TransUNet model for multi-organ segmentation tasks on CT images and showed that it performs better for segmenting small regions.

In the context of the paper, the region of interest is defined as a circular region in which the needle tip is present in the image. Directly regressing the coordinate of the needle tip voxel is extremely difficult even for a human. And for a network to learn to automatically detect the voxel in a huge CT volume is also extremely challenging, if not impossible, for various reasons [14]. Often, the CT scan taken in CT-guided intervention procedures is of low dose and large slice thickness, immensely affected by moving and metal artifacts [15, 16]. Moreover, the intensity of the needle in the CT image varies around the needle body and edges and also due to the angle of penetration. Hence, segmenting a circular area of a certain pre-defined radius around the needle tip is a far more sensible, efficient, and less error-prone approach compared to regressing the tip coordinate itself.

An alternate way of direct regression was proposed in [11]. The authors showed that when compared to a direct coordinate regression work, a fuzzy segmentation task produces localizations that are more reliable and accurate. To prepare the ground truth mask for the fuzzy segmentation task, a circular binary mask of radius 10 pixels is considered around the tip pixel. Then a Gaussian filter of a predefined standard deviation of 5 is applied to the mask. Hence the center pixel of the mask always has the highest intensity and the intensity slowly decreases towards the edge of the mask. One could argue that a hard segmentation mask can also be a potent but fuzzy segmentation masks come with an inherent benefit. Regressing the center of the segment, as the underlying task of the needle tip coordinate localization demands, can be very easily and cheaply done just by taking the Argmax of the predicted segmentation mask, whereas a complex computation-intensive approach is required for a hard segmentation mask. In addition, with varying organ structures and positions from patient to patient, the intensities of the pixels can vary largely, resulting in a poor and scattered segmentation outcome. Moreover, depending on the angle at which the needle is inserted into the body, the metal artifacts cause a huge shift in the intensity of the surrounding soft tissue. That can also cause an imperfect region of interest segmentation. As long as the model predicts a fuzzy mask with diminishing intensity towards the perimeter of the region, the needle tip can be localized with minimal error. This is not the case for hard segmentation. The shape of the predicted mask influences the center of the mask, in turn, the localization.

Along with the simple UNet, the TransUNet network used in this work for comparison consists of an encoder and a decoder. The downsampling is achieved only by a single patching convolution layer with large kernels. The latent features are passed through an MHA block before passing to the decoder segment. Figure 2 shows a block diagram of the TransUNet network architecture.

2.1   Data, annotation, and training setup

The work of this paper is carried out on CT volumes by scanning a phantom. A total of 22 iSequence CT volumes of 1mm slice thickness were captured using a SOMATOM X.cite CT (Siemens Medical Solutions, Erlangen, Germany). The volumes have pixel spacing of about 0.79 mm. Amongst them, 19 are used for training the model and hyper-parameter tuning, and the rest are used for testing. Each of the volumes is of shape 512×512 and has 36 slices. Two different types of needles, different angles, and depths of insertion were used before the scans were taken.

For training the networks, ground truth is generated in a semi-automatic way. To start with, programmatically two 2D projections are generated per volume by taking maximum intensity projection from the top (sagittal plane direction) and from one side (coronal plane direction) view. So each of these projections becomes a 2D image of shape 512×36. Afterward, both the projections are transformed using "HoughLinesP" implementation of OpenCV library [17], which adds postprocessing steps to the original Hough transform algorithm. The outcome of the augmented Hough transformation is the endpoints of all straight lines found in the volume. But depending on the insertion angle and the needle types the intensities throughout the needle in the CT scan vary over the volumes. Moreover, the Hough transform is a parametric and threshold-based transformation. Hence often, the outcome of the above-mentioned transformation is endpoint pair for more than one proposed straight line. Hence a manual and visual inspection needs to be done to select the correct endpoint that matches the actual needle tip. Combining the endpoints from both projections the true X, Y, Z coordinate of the needle tip is extracted. Then the ground truth fuzzy segmentation mask is generated for all of these 2D projections. Figure 3 shows an example of a sample 3D volume and its two maximum intensity 2D projections.

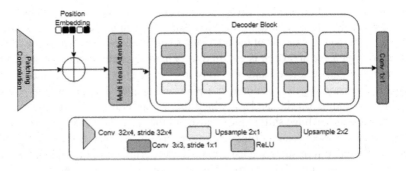

Fig. 2. Block diagram of the TransUNet network architecture.

Tab. 1. Quantitative evaluation results of the model, mean +- standard deviation.

Model	DSC (%)	Euclidean Distance (mm)
UNet	*0.9906* ±0.000013	2.96 ±4.95
TransUNet	0.9842 ±0.000116	*2.89* ±1.1

As there were only 19 volumes used for training, two projections per volume give rise to only 38 training images. To increase the number of training images, each volume is rotated between zero to 360 degrees with a step size of 0.5 degrees and for each rotated volume two 2D maximum intensity projections were captured. Hence 720 training images are generated from each of the training volumes. Also to generalize the learning process for the model, a couple of data augmentation techniques are used, namely random horizontal flip and small noise addition. A learning rate of 0.001 with an AdamW optimizer [18] having a weight decay of 0.0001 is used to train the models. Models are trained with NVIDIA GeForce RTX 2080 Ti GPU.

3   Results

The models are optimized using the Dice similarity coefficient (DSC) [19] based loss function. The predicted segmented mask undergoes an Argmax function which provides the coordinate of the center of the mask. So to test, we obtain two 2D projections of a test volume as described in section 2.1 and then a fuzzy segmentation mask is predicted by the model and furthermore, the coordinates are extracted by an Argmax function. The projection from the top provides the $\hat{Y}, \hat{Z}$ coordinates, and the projection from the side provides the $\hat{X}, \hat{Z}$ coordinates. As the $\hat{Z}$ coordinate is present in both predictions, hence we consider the average as the final prediction. Finally, for evaluation 3D euclidean distance is measured between the true X, Y, Z and predicted $\hat{X}, \hat{Y}, \hat{Z}$ coordinates. We also measure the DSC between the true fuzzy mask and the predicted mask. The DSC is calculated only for the segmentation mask, the background is ignored. Table 1 refers to the quantitative evaluation result for the applied models on the endpoint estimation task. Quantitative analysis shows that the TransUNet model, with no skip connection, achieves an average error of 2.89 mm between the predicted needle tip coordinates and the ground truth, whereas the average error for the UNet model is 2.96 mm. However, the standard deviation of the simple UNet is very high, 4.95 mm, compared to the TransUNet model. The higher standard deviation in simple UNet prediction is due to

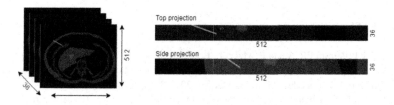

Fig. 3. A sample volume and its two maximum intensity projections.

Fig. 4. A, B. Predicted fuzzy segmentation mask overlaid on maximum intensity sagittal and coronal projections. C, D. Needle tip prediction overlaid on normalized test volumes (Images are cropped for visualization.).

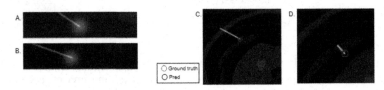

an outlier prediction. The outlier corresponds to a volume with a thin needle, which is susceptible to higher intensity variation compared to a thick needle. Figure 4 shows examples of the prediction of the needle tip by the TransUNet model and comparison with the ground truth.

4 Discussion

This work presents a novel method of converting a complex and hard task of 3D needle tip position regression to a relatively simpler 2D task. Also, it is shown that the hurdle of coordinate regression can be alleviated by means of a fuzzy segmentation of the region of interest containing the tip, and coordinates can be achieved cheaply from the segmentation prediction. A CNN model can achieve the fuzzy segmentation task efficiently. The simple UNet model predicts the needle tip coordinate with high accuracy, although, on our tested data, it is still inconclusive if the more complex transUnet model can perform better than the simple UNet. The reason for this could be the relatively less cluttered 3D CT scans from phantom. Hence as future work, this method needs to be applied to real patient CT scans which will increase the variance of the data significantly.

Disclaimer. This research study was conducted without any human subject data, hence no ethical approval was required. All authors declare that they have no conflicts of interest.

Acknowledgement. This work was funded by the Federal Ministry of Education and Research within the Forschungscampus STIMULATE (grant no. 13GW0473A)

References

1. Greffier J, Pereira FR, Viala P, Macri F, Beregi JP, Larbi A. Interventional spine procedures under CT guidance: how to reduce patient radiation dose without compromising the successful outcome of the procedure? Physica Medica. 2017;35:88–96.
2. Schreiter J, Semshchikov V, Hanses M, Elkmann N, Hansen C. Towards a real-time control of robotic ultrasound using haptic force feedback. Current Directions in Biomedical Engineering. 2022;8(1):81–4.

3. Yousef R, Gupta G, Yousef N, Khari M. A holistic overview of deep learning approach in medical imaging. Multimed Syst. 2022:1–34.
4. Mwikirize C, Nosher JL, Hacihaliloglu I. Convolution neural networks for real-time needle detection and localization in 2D ultrasound. Int J Comput Assist Radiol Surg. 2018;13(5):647–57.
5. Beigi P, Rohling R, Salcudean T, Lessoway VA, Ng GC. Needle trajectory and tip localization in real-time 3-D ultrasound using a moving stylus. Ultrasound in Med Biol. 2015;41(7):2057–70.
6. Mehrtash A, Ghafoorian M, Pernelle G, Ziaei A, Heslinga FG, Tuncali K et al. Automatic needle segmentation and localization in MRI with 3-D convolutional neural networks: application to MRI-targeted prostate biopsy. IEEE Trans Med Imaging. 2018;38(4):1026–36.
7. Ronneberger O, Fischer P, Brox T. U-net: convolutional networks for biomedical image segmentation. International Conference on Medical image computing and computer-assisted intervention. Springer. 2015:234–41.
8. Groves LA, VanBerlo B, Peters TM, Chen EC. Deep learning approach for automatic out-of-plane needle localisation for semi-automatic ultrasound probe calibration. Healthc Technol Lett. 2019;6(6):204–9.
9. Mukhopadhyay S, Mathur P, Bharadwaj A, Son Y, Park JS, Kudavelly SR et al. Deep learning based needle tracking in prostate fusion biopsy. Proc SPIE. Vol. 11598. 2021:605–13.
10. Chen S, Wang S. Deep learning based non-rigid device tracking in ultrasound image. Proceedings of the 2018 2nd International Conference on Computer Science and Artificial Intelligence. 2018:354–8.
11. Ernst P, Hille G, Hansen C, Tönnies K, Rak M. A CNN-based framework for statistical assessment of spinal shape and curvature in whole-body MRI images of large populations. Proc MICCAI. 2019:3–11.
12. Chen J, Lu Y, Yu Q, Luo X, Adeli E, Wang Y et al. Transunet: transformers make strong encoders for medical image segmentation. arXiv preprint arXiv:2102.04306. 2021.
13. Vaswani A, Shazeer N, Parmar N, Uszkoreit J, Jones L, Gomez AN et al. Attention is all you need. Adv Neural Inf Process Syst. 2017;30.
14. Liu R, Lehman J, Molino P, Petroski Such F, Frank E, Sergeev A et al. An intriguing failing of convolutional neural networks and the coordconv solution. Adv Neural Inf Process Syst. 2018;31.
15. Sun L, Chen M, Li G, Han L, Han J, Gu H et al. A positioning method of ablation needles in X-ray CT images. Proc IEEE CCISP. 2021:198–202.
16. Sarti M, Brehmer WP, Gay SB. Low-dose techniques in CT-guided interventions. Radiographics. 2012;32(4):1109–19.
17. Bradski G. The OpenCV Library. Dr. Dobb's Journal of Software Tools. 2000.
18. Loshchilov I, Hutter F. Decoupled weight decay regularization. arXiv:1711.05101. 2017.
19. Dice LR. Measures of the amount of ecologic association between species. Ecology. 1945;26(3):297–302.

Deep Learning-based Marker-less Pose Estimation of Interventional Tools using Surrogate Keypoints

Gino Gulamhussene, Jonathan Spiegel, Arnab Das, Marko Rak, Christian Hansen

Faculty of Computer Science, Otto von Guericke University, Magdeburg, Germany
hansen@isg.cs.uni-magdeburg.de

Abstract. Estimating the position of an intervention needle is an important ability in computer-assisted interventions. Currently, such pose estimations rely either on radiation-intensive CT imaging or need additional optical markers which add overhead to the clinical workflow. We propose a novel deep-learning-based technique for pose estimation of interventional tools which relies on detecting visible features on the tool itself without additional markers. We also propose a novel and fast pipeline for creating vast amounts of robustly labeled and markerless ground truth data for training such neural networks. Initial evaluations suggest that with needle base and needle tip localization errors of about 1 and 4 cm, Our approach can yield a search corridor that can be used to find the needle in a low-dose CT image, reducing radiation exposure.

1 Introduction

CT-guided interventions are a method for treating diseases like liver cancer through ablation or brachytherapy. The accurate placement of the needle or catheter is crucial for the outcome of such therapy. To assist the radiologist with navigation, several systems were proposed. They are usually based on either CT imaging or optical tracking. While CT images are accurate and allow a 3D view inside the patient, the high radiation dose applied to both patient and doctor during such interventions is undesirable. On the other hand, optical methods usually cannot account for needle bending. In addition, the markers which are used pose additional challenges, including more difficult handling of the instrument, the need for sterilization, and installation overhead in the workflow. While those existing optical tracking-based approaches usually make use of classical computer vision algorithms, most state-of-the-art approaches in computer vision utilize deep learning models. They have shown superior performance in a number of tasks, including image classification, segmentation, pose estimation, tracking, and more [1]. One important factor limiting such systems' applicability is the need for large labeled datasets. They are crucial for accurate predictions, but often difficult to acquire.

We propose a method for optical tracking of interventional needle-like instruments that combines deep learning with triangulation. Our segmentation-based deep learning approach detects visible key points on the needle axis in a multi-view registered camera system without additional markers. The 2D positions of these key points can be elevated to 3D using triangulation algorithms. As we detect points on the needle axis itself instead of detecting a marker on the handle, we can also determine if the instrument shaft is bent. While our accuracy cannot compete with marker-based tracking yet, our predictions can provide a search corridor as guidance for the more precise co-registered CT imaging to reduce the radiation doses applied during interventions. For the creation of ground truth data for our model, we have developed a pipeline for rapidly creating object pose and segmentation mask data without additional input like a 3D mesh of the tracked object. We make use of a calibrated multi-camera setup and optical markers for tracking, but we have also included a path in this procedure that allows us to create markerless data, thus avoiding any potential bias.

1.1 Related work

As listed in [2], there are several publicly available data sets that are commonly used as benchmarks for object pose estimation tasks. Many of those datasets were annotated in a manual or semi-manual fashion. [3] labeled their data by manually marking bounding boxes in a 3D point cloud and projecting them back into 2D images. In [4], the pose information was generated through the manual alignment of CAD models to the frames. As such fully manual approaches are very labor-intensive for larger datasets, it is common to use semi-automatic methods where only the first frame of a video is labeled manually through 3D model alignment ([5, 6]) or key point annotation ([7, 8]) followed by automatic propagation of the pose information through the rest of the scene. Some datasets feature fully automatic label annotation, which is usually achieved using optical markers ([9, 10]). While this requires minimal manual effort, the markers are visible in the ground truth images, introducing a potential bias. Even with these datasets and methods in existence, the amount of ground truth data available is lacking. This limitation can be overcome by using simulation techniques ([6, 11]). While this does mitigate the effects of too little training data, it can also open up a domain gap to real-world data, which can lead to poor generalization in deployment.

For a comprehensive overview of monocular deep learning-based pose estimation, we advise a look at a recently published review [2]. Directly regressing the poses without using a 3D model of the tracked object in the loss function is a difficult learning task. [12] proposed to circumvent this problem by reframing the regression into a fuzzy segmentation problem, which neural networks can solve reliably. Keypoints are extracted from the segmentations by finding the maxima of the mask.

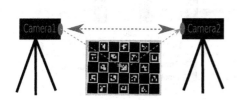 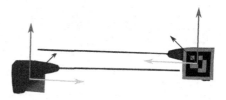

(a) Camera Setup with ChArUco board for extrinsic calibration.

(b) Left: Marker invisible, pose calculated. Right: marker visible, pose tracked.

Fig. 1. Calibration procedure and ground truth data.

2   Materials and Methods

2.1   Data labeling pipeline

We developed a novel fully-automated data labeling pipeline to create training data using optical markers. Our method has several advantages to the related work. Apart from being fully automated, it does not require a 3D object model. It is scalable and fast (we capture 30 fps per camera in a multi-camera setup), which allows large-scale datasets while being conceptually simple. Furthermore, it can generate non-synthetic data without visible markers, avoiding biases and domain gaps. We establish an extrinsic calibration between two or more cameras sharing a partial field-of-view (Fig. 1a). Next, a marker is placed on one side of the tracked object. For marker-less data, it has to be small enough to be completely covered by the object and thus can not be seen by the other camera. In our experiments, we used a small ChArUco [13] board for more stable and accurate tracking. The object pose is determined from the tracked marker in one camera and propagated into all other camera views that do not see the marker (Fig. 1b). In our experiments, the accuracy of the calculated poses is close to the original marker tracking and sufficient for approximate pose estimations. As we are not interested in the handle pose, but in the 3D position of the needle start and end points, we measure the 3D offset of the marker coordinate origin to the points of interest. This is done by placing the two points onto known coordinates of a calibration board. By measuring the poses of both the board and marker, the offset is calculated through a series of coordinate transformations. As small tracking errors can multiply through each of the transformation steps, a manual correction of the 3D offset might be required. This procedure only has to be performed once; the rest of the pipeline is fully automatic. Using our pipeline, we were able to capture more than 10,000 labeled video frames in less than 60 minutes. We integrated this method into a custom software tool, which can grab live stream data from all connected cameras, calibrate the cameras extrinsically, track the needle and save the data stream to a hard drive. We also implemented a live prediction mode to be used with our trained pose estimation model (Fig. 3).

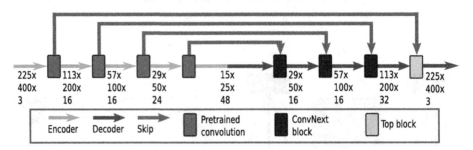

Fig. 2. Network architecture. The shapes are an example of using the Mobilenet backbone. Skips are branched off before the pretrained blocks and concatenated before the ConvNext blocks.

2.2   Needle pose estimation

2.2.1   Deep learning segmentation. For our deep-learning-based segmentation, we designed a network with a structure based on the famous U-Net [14] because of its strong performance on a wide variety of segmentation tasks. Figure 2 visualizes our model architecture; we omitted details to make the overview more concise. In the encoder part of the network, we decided to incorporate a backbone network pre-trained on imagenet classification to enable faster and better learning. This backbone can be of different sizes: To test configurations of different complexity, we used Tensorflow's MobileNetV3Small [15] implementation as a minimal example, EfficientNetV2B0 [16] as a middle-ground, and ConvNextTiny [17] as a large model. While even larger models might yield improvements in segmentation accuracy, we skipped further testing as our results were sufficient for a proof of concept. For the upscaling path of the network, we make use of the powerful ConvNext building block introduced in [17]. For details on how this block is constructed, we would like to refer the reader to the original paper. The final block is a single wide ConvNext block without repetitions to allow a large number of high-resolution feature maps before the output layer without using huge amounts of video memory. The output is a 3-channel segmentation mask of the original image for the axis, base, and tip of the needle. We trained our model using the Tensorflow implementation of the AdamW optimizer [18] with early stopping. As our needle mask is very thin and the points are just single pixels in the target masks, there is a strong bias for the model to predict completely black masks. To avoid that, we used the idea from [12] to apply a gaussian filter (sigma=5) to our targets and perform fuzzy segmentation.

2.2.2   Triangulation. To perform triangulation, we need the pixel coordinates of identical image points in multiple co-calibrated camera views. We used the maximum pixel intensities in the predicted segmentation masks of the same image in two different camera views for the start and end points of the needle as coordinates. For the triangulation of world coordinates, OpenCV's [19] TriangulatePoints method was used.

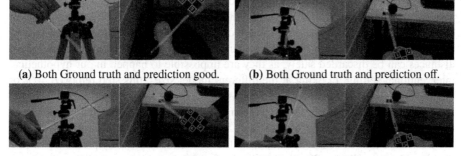

(**a**) Both Ground truth and prediction good.   (**b**) Both Ground truth and prediction off.

(**c**) Ground truth good, prediction off.   (**d**) Prediction good, ground truth off.

Fig. 3. Needle tip prediction, in a dual camera setup (left and right images). Images are cropped around the needle. Red mask shows the highest percentile needle masks. Green dots mark the needle base, blue dots the needle tip. Brighter color is prediction, darker is ground truth.

2.3   Experiments

For evaluation, we used about 60% of our 10.000 video frames for training and 20% each for validation and testing. Our data was captured by two different persons in front of ten different backgrounds. To ensure the model generalizes, we split the data so that the training data only contained needles on the right side of the images, while the validation and test data only contained needles that were entirely on the left side; any data overlapping both were discarded. We trained three different model sizes and evaluated them in terms of the Dice coefficient for each of the segmentation masks, the euclidean distance between triangulation and 3D ground truth, and the single sample inference time on our test machine using an NVidia GTX 1080Ti GPU. The triangulation results are based on a separate dataset of about 700 dual-image frames that do not follow the strict left-right split to preserve the correlation between two camera images of one frame. We evaluate using the median instead of the mean, as our results include lots of outliers.

3   Results

We present the results of our experiments in Table 1. Unsurprisingly, the larger models deliver better predictions at the cost of more parameters. While the median Dice score values for the needle axis and base are acceptable for the larger models, the standard deviation is often very high. This might be caused by samples for which part of the needle and a key point is covered or outside of the image, which is not yet represented in our ground truth. This hypothesis is supported by the fact that the needle tip, which is outside the image more often, scores much worse than the base. As we captured a sequence of frames, such an issue usually affects multiple frames at a time, leading to a high number of failed segmentations with mask values mostly close to zero (i.e. no point was found). To illustrate this problem: 43% of the predictions for the needle tip by the largest model on our test dataset had a Dice score of greater than .7, while for 32% the segmentation failed, leading to a score below .05. The issue is probably amplified by the fact that in contrast to the base point, the tip is harder to find as it does not have handle and hand as nearby visual clues.

   Our triangulation results show the same pattern. The base is much easier to detect than the tip. One issue is that a failed prediction quickly leads to a huge triangulation error, where the triangulated position is more than 100 meters away from the ground truth. We filtered outliers by removing distances above 50 cm for our evaluation. Larger distances can be discarded safely, as they are impossible to happen in our hypothetical interventional setting. Looking at the different model sizes, this step removed 40% of the tip and 13% of the base point predictions for our smallest model, 4% and 1% for the medium one, and 3% and 0% for the large one. Future versions of the method can utilize the temporal structure of the data to filter and smooth the 3D predictions. Even with those removals, our small model masks are too inaccurate for reliably predicting the 3D position of the needle tip. Please note that perfect 3D accuracy cannot be expected due to inaccuracies in tracking and low-resolution discrete pixel-based triangulation, which is why the errors of our medium and large model can be considered acceptable for the current proof-of-concept stage. With future applications in mind, we also evaluated the real-time capabilities of our system. Without further optimizations, we were able

Tab. 1. Evaluation of our three tested model architectures, given by median(std). We report the Dice score of the needle axis (A), tip (T) and base (B) segmentation masks, as well as the Triangulation errors (TE) in cm and the inference times in ms (Time).

Backbone	Parameters	Dice A	Dice T	Dice B	TE T	TE B	Time
MobileNet	1M	.68(.30)	.37(.38)	.78(.28)	29.30(15.91)	2.08(6.23)	71(5)
EfficientNet	7M	.71(.20)	.48(.40)	.88(.19)	3.84(8.23)	1.17(1.61)	105(5)
ConvNext	39M	.76(.18)	.48(.41)	.90(.16)	3.27(6.72)	0.88(0.96)	94(4)

to achieve about 5 frames per second on our machine using the smallest model. In Figure 3, we present screenshots from our live prediction tool with the needle mask and the maximum intensity key points overlayed for our dual-camera system. We visualize typical scenarios and sources of error. While both ground truth and prediction can be good, there are many cases in which either one of them or both can be off, limiting the accuracy of our approach. It should also be noted that the prediction quality on images without the marker (left images) was visually worse than on those with a visible marker. As we trained our models on more data with a marker included than without, this highlights the importance of avoiding biases in the training data.

4 Discussion

So far, we used simplified data. In future work, the training data could be diversified, by including different needle instruments, handled by radiologists in an interventional environment, bent and partially covered needles, and more data augmentation. We see further potential to improve our accuracy through more sophisticated model architectures, higher resolution, quality input images, and different methods for extracting key points from the segmentation masks (e.g. mean of strongest activations). It is also possible to improve the data quality by using Moiré Phase Tracking [20], and by eliminating calibration inaccuracies in the camera setup.

4.1 Conclusion

We have demonstrated a simple approach to estimate the 3D position of key points based on deep learning combined with triangulation. We introduced a pipeline for the rapid creation of labeled ground truth data without manual annotation and a 3D model.

Acknowledgement. This work was funded by the Federal Ministry of Education and Research within the Forschungscampus STIMULATE. (grant no. 13GW0473A)

References

1. Voulodimos A, Doulamis N, Doulamis A, Protopapadakis E. Deep learning for computer vision: a brief review. Comput Intell Neurosci. 2018;2018:7068349.

2. Fan Z, Zhu Y, He Y, Sun Q, Liu H, He J. Deep learning on monocular object pose detection and tracking: a comprehensive overview. ACM Comput. Surv. 2022;55(4).

3. A. Geiger, P. Lenz, R. Urtasun. Are we ready for autonomous driving? The KITTI vision benchmark suite. Proc IEEE CVPR. 2012:3354–61.

4. Hodan T, Haluza P, Obdrzalek S, Matas J, Lourakis M, Zabulis X. T-LESS: an RGB-D dataset for 6D pose estimation of texture-less objects. Proc IEEE WACV. IEEE, 2017.

5. Xiang Y, Schmidt T, Narayanan V, Fox D. Posecnn: a convolutional neural network for 6d object pose estimation in cluttered scenes. arXiv preprint arXiv:1711.00199. 2017.

6. Hodan T, Michel F, Brachmann E, Kehl W, GlentBuch A, Kraft D et al. Bop: benchmark for 6d object pose estimation. Proc ECCV. 2018:19–34.

7. Marion P, Florence PR, Manuelli L, Tedrake R. Label fusion: a pipeline for generating ground truth labels for real rgbd data of cluttered scenes. 2018 IEEE International Conference on Robotics and Automation (ICRA). IEEE. 2018:3235–42.

8. Liu X, Jonschkowski R, Angelova A, Konolige K. KeyPose: multi-view 3D labeling and keypoint estimation for transparent objects. Proc IEEE CVPR. IEEE, 2020.

9. Hinterstoisser S, Lepetit V, Ilic S, Holzer S, Bradski G, Konolige K et al. Model based training, detection and pose estimation of Texture-Less 3D objects in heavily cluttered scenes. Computer Vision – ACCV 2012. Ed. by Lee KM, Matsushita Y, Rehg JM, Hu Z. (SpringerLink Bücher). Berlin, Heidelberg: Springer, 2013:548–62.

10. Brachmann E, Krull A, Michel F, Gumhold S, Shotton J, Rother C. Learning 6D object pose estimation using 3D object coordinates. Proc ECCV. Cham, 2014:536–51.

11. Wang H, Sridhar S, Huang J, Valentin J, Song S, Guibas LJ. Normalized object coordinate space for category-level 6d object pose and size estimation. Proc IEEE CVPR. 2019:2642–51.

12. Ernst P, Hille G, Hansen C, Tönnies K, Rak M. A CNN-Based framework for statistical assessment of spinal shape and curvature in whole-Body MRI images of large populations. Springer, Cham, 2019:3–11.

13. Garrido-Jurado S, Muñoz-Salinas R, Madrid-Cuevas FJ, Marín-Jiménez MJ. Automatic generation and detection of highly reliable fiducial markers under occlusion. Pattern Recognit. 2014;47(6):2280–92.

14. Ronneberger O, Fischer P, Brox T. U-net: convolutional networks for biomedical image segmentation. Proc MICCAI. 2015:234–41.

15. Howard A, Sandler M, Chu G, Chen LC, Chen B, Tan M et al. Searching for mobilenetv3. Proc IEEE CVPR. 2019:1314–24.

16. Tan M, Le Q. Efficientnetv2: smaller models and faster training. International conference on machine learning. PMLR. 2021:10096–106.

17. Liu Z, Mao H, Wu CY, Feichtenhofer C, Darrell T, Xie S. A convnet for the 2020s. Proc IEEE CVPR. 2022:11976–86.

18. Loshchilov I, Hutter F. Decoupled weight decay regularization. arXiv:1711.05101. 2017.

19. Bradski G. The OpenCV Library. Dr. Dobb's Journal of Software Tools. 2000.

20. Gumus K, Keating B, White N, Andrews-Shigaki B, Armstrong B, Maclaren J et al. Comparison of optical and MR-based tracking. Magn Reson Med. 2015;74(3):894–902.

Abstract: Implementation of a Real-time 3D-thermometry Pipeline in Gadgetron for Easy Clinical Integration

Dominik Horstmann[1,2], Karen Meyer zu Hartlage[1,2], Daniel Reimert[1,2], Joaquin J. Löning Caballero[1,2], Othmar Belker[1,2], Frank Wacker[1,2], Bennet Hensen[1,2], Marcel Gutberlet[1,2]

[1]Hannover Medical School
[2]STIMULATE-Solution Centre for Image Guided Local Therapies
horstmann.dominik@mh-hannover.de

MR thermometry as measure for guiding thermal ablation of tumor tissue makes real-time imaging and arbitrary slice positioning possible while assuring precise knowledge of the size of the ablation zone. However, difficult clinical integration currently hamper the success of clinical thermometry. Purpose of this work was to implement a real-time 3D MR thermometry pipeline for easy clinical integration. The pipeline starts with fast data acquisition by a multigradient echo 3D stack-of-stars sequence. The acquired data is then sent to an external server where images temperature maps as well as necrosis maps are calculated from it via a modular Gadgetron pipeline running in a Docker container. Using Docker guarantees multi-platform portability and reproducibility of our pipeline whereas the ISMRMRD format makes it vendor independent. Parallel imaging, compressed sensing (PICS) as well as GPU accelerated reconstruction are implemented. Apart from that, the pipeline contains correction algorithms for noise, gradient delay, phase drift and phase errors. To test the pipeline, microwave ablations on nine static bioprotein phantoms were performed on a 1.5 T scanner. Fiber optical temperature sensors were used for gaining reference temperatures. Retrospectively, the calculated necrosis zones were compared to a ground truth. The pipeline yielded temperature accuracies of 1.15 °C ± 0.69 °C compared to the temperature sensors. The comparison of the ablation zone with the ground truth yielded dice scores of 84.02 % ± 2.36 %. For a 3D volume with 24 slices and 8 echoes the processing time was about 26 s. The experiments show that the thermometry pipeline is already close to real-time 3D thermometry. Further research will focus on optimizing it for moving phantoms as, in the future, it is planned to be used for clinical applications in moving organs such as the liver. The modular and opensource character of the pipeline makes future improvements and extensions easy to integrate [1].

References

1. Horstmann D. Implementation of a real-time 3D-thermometry pipeline in gadgetron for hepatic thermal ablation. 13th IMRI Symposium Leipzig, 2022.

© Der/die Autor(en), exklusiv lizenziert an
Springer Fachmedien Wiesbaden GmbH, ein Teil von Springer Nature 2023
T. M. Deserno et al. (Hrsg.), *Bildverarbeitung für die Medizin 2023*,
Informatik aktuell, https://doi.org/10.1007/978-3-658-41657-7_64

Matching Endoscopic 3D Image Data with 4D Echocardiographic Data for Extended Reality Support in Mitral Valve Repair Surgery

Juri Welz[1,3], Matthias Ivantsits[1,3], Isaac Wamala[2,3], Jörg Kempfert[2,3], Simon Sündermann[2,3], Volkmar Falk[2,3], Anja Hennemuth[1,3,4]

[1]Deutsches Herzzentrum der Charité, Institute of Computer-assisted Cardiovascular Medicine, Augustenburger Platz 1, Germany.
[2]Deutsches Herzzentrum der Charité, Department of Cardiothoracic and Vascular Surgery, Augustenburger Platz 1, Germany.
[3]Charité – Universitätsmedizin Berlin, corporate member of Freie Universität Berlin and Humboldt-Universität zu Berlin, Charitéplatz 1, 10117 Berlin, Germany.
[4]Fraunhofer Institute for Digital Medicine MEVIS
juriw@juriw.de

Abstract. Minimally invasive mitral valve repair is a common cardiac surgery procedure. Combining intraoperative stereo-endoscopic images with pre-operative 4D transesophageal echocardiography (TEE) can support surgeons in correlating surgical interventions with the functional implications in the beating heart. We propose a method for registering 3D point clouds reconstructed from endoscopic images with TEE by extracting and matching anatomical landmarks and refining the registration using the Iterative Closest Point Algorithm. The applicability of our method is assessed by the computation time and the registration accuracy.

1 Introduction

The mitral valve regulates the blood flow from the left atrium to the left ventricle. Mitral valve regurgitation (MR) is the insufficient closing of the mitral valve leading to abnormal blood flow to the atrium during systole. Significant MR affects about 2% of adults [1, 2] and, in the long run, leads to heart failure, arrhythmias, and pulmonary congestion. It is the second most common indication for valve surgery [3].

In minimally invasive mitral valve surgery, the mitral valve is accessed by small incisions through the thorax. The surgery is performed under cardiopulmonary bypass, so that heart and lungs do not move and the pressure caused by blood and air flow is eliminated. Commonly, mitral valve regurgitation is assessed by transesophageal echocardiography (TEE) and confirmed during surgery [4]. The expert mentally integrates TEE and the live endoscopic video output.

Extended reality (XR) approaches in this field (reviewed in [5]) mainly focus on pre-operative planning and outcome prediction. In particular, there is work on fitting annuloplasty rings into endoscopic and TEE images [6, 7].

While this work helps with an improved understanding of valve pathology, it is based on pre-operative images and does not yet take into account the actual physical valve analysis via endoscopy. Our XR approach aims to extend these solutions by fusing

© Der/die Autor(en), exklusiv lizenziert an
Springer Fachmedien Wiesbaden GmbH, ein Teil von Springer Nature 2023
T. M. Deserno et al. (Hrsg.), *Bildverarbeitung für die Medizin 2023*,
Informatik aktuell, https://doi.org/10.1007/978-3-658-41657-7_65

3D-reconstructed endoscopic scenes with the pre-operative TEE of the mitral valve to help the surgeons locate pathologies that can be seen in the TEE. It is based on landmark detection via segmentations of the endoscopic images of the mitral valve [8] and the corresponding presurgery TEE [9].

2 Materials and methods

In order to enable the registration of the endoscopic camera images with the 4D ultra-sound sequences, we reconstruct a 3D image from the endoscopic stereo image as a point cloud. This is registered to the 3D TEE image for each timestep of the 4D TEE sequence. The initial registration is done by identifying three corresponding landmarks on the annulus in the TEE and the endoscopic point cloud. The registration is further improved by using the Iterative Closest Point (ICP) algorithm (Fig. 1). The method requires segmentation masks and commissures landmarks in the endoscopic images, and annulus and aorta landmarks in the TEE, which all can come from interactive or automatic [8, 9] segmentation.

2.1 3D reconstruction

We first undistort the endoscopic images. Next, we rectify the images by using scale-invariant feature transform (SIFT) [10] and fast library for approximate nearest neighbors (FLANN) [11] to obtain a sparse matching between both parts of the stereo image. This is used to calculate the fundamental matrix, which relates the corresponding points of the stereo images. The depth map is obtained with a modified Hirschmüller algorithm [12] and used to create a point cloud representation of the 3D scene. Points outside a sensible coordinate range and points scattered loosely in space are removed with simple outlier removal methods. E.g., we remove points with less than 250 neighbors within a radius of 25 pixels. 2D masks for the valve and the annulus were created. The valve mask can be pulled directly from the segmentation masks. The annulus mask is created by improving the valve mask with morphologic closing and convolving it with the Laplace operator. Valve and annulus masks are mapped to the 3D point cloud using the correspondence of the pixels in the endoscopic 2D images to their counterparts in the 3D reconstruction. Thus we can extract a valve point cloud and an annulus point cloud.

2.2 Registration

As the initial registration step, three points are selected from the TEE annulus landmarks and the endoscopic annulus point cloud using the locations of the commissures. Annulus and commissures are projected onto a plane spanned by the annulus's mean m and the first two principal components. The three points p_1, p_2, and p_3 are selected so that the angles between the vectors $\vec{mp_1}$, $\vec{mp_2}$, and $\vec{mp_2}$ to the vector between the commissures, $\vec{c_1c_2}$ are closest to $0°$, $90°$, and $180°$.

The corresponding three points in the TEE are chosen based on the center of the annulus c and the aortic landmark a. We choose two opposite points p_j, p_k, on the annulus, for which the angle between the vector $\vec{ac}$ and the vector from c to the points is the closest to a right angle, minimizing $\left|\frac{\vec{cp_i}\vec{ac}}{|\vec{ac}|}\right|$. The third point is the annulus point p_i that maximizes this term.

We register the extracted triangles from TEE and endoscopy. The endoscopic triangle is isotropically scaled and then rigidly transformed with the Kabsch algorithm [13]. The ICP algorithm is used to refine the rigid transformation using either annulus or valve landmarks extracted from the endoscope point cloud and the corresponding TEE. All transformation steps are combined into a transformation matrix that enables the display of landmarks defined in the endoscopic scene in the TEE data and vice versa.

2.3   Implementation

All experiments were conducted on a 2013 Lenovo Thinkpad W530 with Windows 10 and an Intel Core i7-3840M processor at 2.8 GHz. Reconstruction is done with methods of OpenCV-Python 4.6.0.66 in Python 3.10.4. For the reconstruction, the endoscopic images were undistorted. Here, we achieved good results by picking the camera matrix of the zoom level 1.6, though the different zoom levels during surgery are not known. The

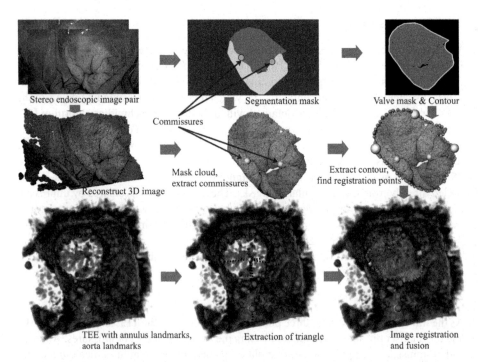

Fig. 1. Workflow of registration and transformation. From the stereo endoscopic image pair, a 3D point cloud is reconstructed, and masks for valve, annulus (dark green), and commissure points (light green) are extracted. With these, point clouds are extracted, and three registration points are calculated (yellow). Three registration points (red) are also calculated from TEE's aorta and annulus landmarks (pink). The modalities are rigidly registered with these points. The transformation is refined with ICP on the annulus pairs.

endoscopic images are converted to greyscale since color information could negatively impact reconstruction performance [14], and later added back to the point cloud. Outlier removal and export of the point clouds were done with Open3D 0.16.0. The registration, transformation, and fusion tools were developed in MeVisLab 3.5legacy[1].

2.4 Data acquisition and preprocessing

The stereo endoscope images used in the experiments were acquired with a B. Braun EinsteinVision 3.0 Aesculap system and captured with a DVI capturing card directly from the endoscope's output. The endoscope produces 1920×1080 interlaced RGB images, with each side having a size of 1920×540 and appearing stretched in the horizontal direction. The TEE images were acquired with a GE Vivid E95 ultrasound system.

2.5 Evaluation

A cardiologist annotated 4D TEE and the stereo endoscopic images from ten patients who underwent minimal invasive mitral valve surgery at the German Heart Center Berlin, DHZB (approval of local ethics committee: EA4/121/19).

The endoscopic annotation comprises the anterior leaflet, posterior leaflet, papillary muscles, and instrument classes as well as the commissure positions. The TEE annotation consists of a sparse set of landmarks, marking the positions of the mitral valve, annulus, and aorta.

The intrinsic camera parameters were collected for each zoom level by calibrating with a chessboard pattern. For 3D reconstruction, we downscaled the images from 1920×540 to 960×540, in order to achieve an isotropic pixel size and a correct display of the proportions of the image in the standard viewer.

We compared two approaches for landmark-based registration, one using the annulus points and one using the complete valve for the ICP algorithm. To quantitatively compare the performance of these scenarios, we applied the resulting transformation to the endoscopic valve landmarks and the endoscopic annulus landmarks and investigated how well they fit the TEE valve landmarks and annulus landmarks. We measured the mean of the distances of each point in the TEE point cloud to the closest point in the transformed endoscopic point cloud for each pair of landmark sets.

In addition, we compared computation times for registration with the original annulus vs. the computation time having the annulus downsampled by different degrees.

3 Results

Before applying ICP as an additional registration step, the mean distance between valve landmark sets was 7.26 ± 1.71 mm, and the distance between the annulus landmark sets was 5.69 ± 0.72 mm. When applying ICP on annulus landmarks, these distances were reduced to 6.41 ± 1.60 mm and 4.39 ± 0.35 mm. When using valve landmark sets as input for ICP, the distances were 3.39 ± 1.10 mm and 9.88 ± 1.65 mm (Fig. 2a).

---

[1]https://www.mevislab.de

We investigated the computation time of the processing steps of the image registration, varying the number of landmarks in the endoscope annulus point cloud. When
using the complete annulus point cloud of 2255 points, ICP takes the majority of
the computation time (649 ± 5 ms of 694 ± 7 ms total computation time). However,
downsampling the annulus to 70 points significantly reduced the ICP computation time
(22 ± 1 ms of 28 ± 2 ms total computation time) without affecting the registration result.
The calculation of the transformation matrix is possible in real-time (Fig. 2b).

4   Discussion

We presented a method to reconstruct a 3D point cloud from the endoscopic scene of
the mitral valve and register it with 3D TEE from the same valve. The registration of the
endoscopic point cloud and the TEE showed good results.

The registration using the annulus landmarks performed better than the one considering all the valvular points, which significantly worsened the annulus distances. This
could be explained by the differences in the valvular shape between the active and the
still heart.The overall effect of applying ICP as an additional registration step was lower
than anticipated, which accounted for a large part of the computational costs. Overall,
some differences will still occur with the best-possible linear method, as the images are
taken respectively before and during cardiopulmonary bypass.

The computation time measurements (including ICP) show that real-time (<33 ms)
calculation of registration is possible by downsampling while maintaining a good fit.
With this, interactively locating landmarks of the endoscopic scene in pre-operative TEE
is possible.

While the endoscopic point cloud is fitted nicely into the TEE annulus, some rotational deviations can occur. Matching the extracted commissures of the endoscopic
scene with the calculated ones in TEE can lead to this error. Finding the aorta in the
endoscopic scene for matching could be an alternative approach.

To extract the landmarks used in our fusion approach, the mitral valve has to be
covered completely in both imaging modalities with some margin to the image border.

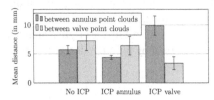

(a) Mean distances between point clouds.
For each of the TEE landmarkers, the distance to the closest point of the transformed
endoscopic point cloud was measured. The
mean of these distances was calculated.

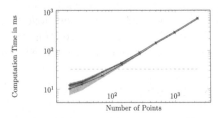

(b) Calculation times of Registration. Blue:
Complete registration. Red: ICP part of registration. The horizontal line is at 33ms. Ten
measurements per value.

Fig. 2. Evaluation Results. The evaluation includes distance and computation time measurements.

Usually, surgical instruments cover only small parts of the valve. When crucial parts are hidden, an incomplete annulus point cloud is produced, and the extraction of three points for registration is impossible.

The next step is integrating the automatic segmentation models to extract the landmarks for our extended reality approach. Further, scaling and rigid transformation should be replaced with a non-linear approach that considers the deformations of the anatomy caused by the cardiopulmonary bypass. At last, an extensive user study involving surgeons has to be conducted.

Acknowledgement. We thank Ann Laube and Chiara Manini for valuable assistance formulating and proofreading this manuscript.

References

1. Jones EC, Devereux RB, Roman MJ, et al. Prevalence and correlates of mitral regurgitation in a population-based sample (the Strong Heart Study). Am J Cardiol. 2001;87(3):298–304.
2. Dziadzko V, Dziadzko M, Medina-Inojosa JR, Benfari G, et al. Causes and mechanisms of isolated mitral regurgitation in the community: clinical context and outcome. Eur Heart J. 2019;40(27):2194–202.
3. Beckmann A, Meyer R, Lewandowski J, et al. German Heart Surgery Report 2021: the annual updated registry of the German Society for Thoracic and Cardiovascular Surgery. Thorac Cardiovasc Surg. 2022;70(05):362–76.
4. Jacobs S, Sündermann SH. Minimally invasive valve sparing mitral valve repair—the loop technique—how we do it. Ann Cardiothorac Surg. 2013;2(6):818–24.
5. Nanchahal S, Arjomandi Rad A, Naruka V, et al. Mitral valve surgery assisted by virtual and augmented reality: cardiac surgery at the front of innovation. Perfusion. 2022.
6. Engelhardt S, De Simone R, Zimmermann N, et al. Augmented reality-enhanced endoscopic images for annuloplasty ring sizing. Augment Environ Comput Assist Interv (2014). Cham: Springer International, 2014:128–37.
7. Ender J, Končar-Zeh J, Mukherjee C, et al. Value of augmented reality-enhanced transesophageal echocardiography (TEE) for determining optimal annuloplasty ring size during mitral valve repair. Ann Thorac Surg. 2008;86(5):1473–8.
8. Ivantsits M, Tautz L, Sündermann S, et al. DL-based segmentation of endoscopic scenes for mitral valve repair. CDBME. 2020;6(1).
9. Andreassen BS, Völgyes D, Samset E, et al. Mitral annulus segmentation and anatomical orientation detection in TEE images using periodic 3D CNN. IEEE Access. 2022;10:51472–86.
10. Lowe DG. Distinctive image features from scale-invariant keypoints. Int J Comput Vis. 2004;60(2):91–110.
11. Muja M, Lowe DG. Fast approximate nearest neighbors with automatic algorithm configuration. VISAPP 2009. SciTePress, 2009:331–40.
12. Hirschmuller H. Stereo processing by semiglobal matching and mutual information. IEEE Trans Pattern Anal Mach Intell. 2008;30(2):328–41.
13. Arun KS, Huang TS, Blostein SD. Least-squares fitting of two 3-D point sets. IEEE Trans Pattern Anal Mach Intell. 1987;PAMI-9(5):698–700.
14. Bleyer M, Chambon S. Does color really help in dense stereo matching? 3DPVT 2010. 2010:1–8.

Cross-modality Training Approach for CT Super-resolution Network

Wai Yan Ryana Fok[1,2], Andreas Fieselmann[1], Magdalena Herbst[1], Ludwig Ritschl[1], Marcel Beister[1], Steffen Kappler[1], Sylvia Saalfeld[2,3]

[1]X-ray Products, Siemens Healthcare GmbH, Forchheim, Germany
[2]Faculty of Computer Science, University of Magdeburg, Magdeburg, Germany
[3]Forschungscampus STIMULATE, Magdeburg, Germany
ryana.fok@siemens-healthineers.com

Abstract. In this work, we propose a U-Net-based super-resolution neural network, SRU-Net, to create emulated high spatial resolution (eHR) CT images from low spatial resolution (LR) CT images. As resolution could be defined by the modulation transfer function in CT reconstruction, we propose the novel approach based on CT reconstruction kernels to create realistic multi-detector CT (MDCT) synthetic LR images from high-resolution cone-beam CT (CBCT) scans. Keeping a constant sampling grid size of 0.20×0.20 mm^2, we reconstruct two types of MDCT-like LR images and one corresponding HR image from the same CBCT raw data and train two models respectively. We validated the performance of the trained models on unseen LR CBCT images. We then applied the trained network to MDCT images. Mean squared error, structural similarity index measures and peak signal-to-noise ratio of two models show significant improvements ($p < 0.001$) in the eHR images.

1 Introduction

X-ray as most widely available imaging modality carries high potential for artificial intelligence-based image analysis, however, often lacks annotated data. To overcome this limitation, annotated synthetic X-ray images (also called DRR, digitally reconstructed radiographs) can be generated from existing annotated computed tomography (CT) volumes [1]. However, the intrinsically lower resolution of clinical multi-detector CT (MDCT) limits the resolution of DRRs. Thus, we propose a novel way to increase the spatial resolution of MDCT scans for a further usage as high-resolution (HR) input to generate DRRs for deep learning applications. We propose to modify the modulation transfer function (MTF) by applying filter kernels during reconstruction to generate LR images from HR CBCT scans. Thus, the image resolution can be simulated more accurately than with the interpolation-based downsampling approaches in previous studies [2–4], as high frequency components remaining after interpolation could influence network training [5, 6]. The novelty of our approach, by using different CT reconstruction MTFs to simulate the actual MDCT resolution for SR network training, has three implications:

1. To remove high frequency components that do not exist in LRCT images.
2. Train on higher resolution dataset thus to enable a smaller in-plane sampling grid size, 0.20×0.20 mm^2, than existing SR models.

Tab. 1. Data distribution for training, validation and testing. Values indicate slices.

Networks	Training + Validation	Testing	
SRU-Net1	4237 (3296 + 941)	3520	
	LR_{K_1} and HR CBCT	LR_{K_1} and HR CBCT	1254 LR
SRU-Net2	4237 (3296 + 941)	3520	MDCT
	LR_{K_2} and HR CBCT	LR_{K_2} and HR CBCT	

3. To facilitate a cross-modality application on emulating HR MDCT images.

2 Materials and methods

Fig. 1 shows the overview of our approach which focus on improving CT in-plane resolution. It consists of: (1) training with CBCT images and (2) applying on MDCT images for synthetic X-ray generation.

2.1 Datasets and pre-processing

2.1.1 Frequency-based simulation of low-resolution data. Fig. 2 shows the three MTF kernels used in this study, which are common CT bone reconstruction kernels. LR CBCT images were reconstructed by 2 LR in-house kernel, namely K_1^{LR} and K_2^{LR}. They correspond to a resolution of 16.6 line pairs per centimeter (lp/cm) and 17.7 lp/cm respectively, to simulate MDCT resolution. Target HR images were reconstructed by K^{HR}, with a resolution of 30.7 lp/cm. All images are reconstructed with pixel size of $0.20 \times 0.20\,\text{mm}^2$ and 730×730.

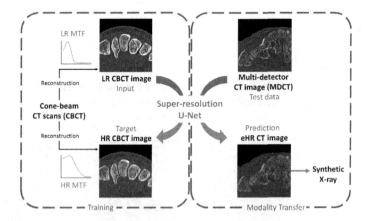

Fig. 1. Overview of our proposed method. LR: low-resolution, HR: high-resolution, eHR: emulated high-resolution.

2.1.2   Dataset. A subset of the CBCT and MDCT scans of formalin-fixed human wrists from body donors was used from this study [7]. The CBCT scans were acquired on a twin robotic X-ray system (Multitom Rax, Siemens Healthineers, Erlangen, Germany), the MDCT scans on a clinical MDCT scanner (Somatom Definition AS, Siemens Healthineers). 13 of the CBCT datasets acquired with the higher dose were selected for training (reconstruction described in next section). Four of the MDCT datasets, reconstructed with K_1^{LR}, pixel size of $0.23 \times 0.23\,\text{mm}^2$ and 512×512, are used for testing only. Table 1 shows the data distribution for training and testing.

2.2   Neural network and training

The SR U-Net [8] was implemented in PyTorch [9]. A region of interest of 512×512 pixels was calculated by the center-of-mass, to crop both the 2D LR input and HR target slice. Image intensity was normalized from Hounsfield unit range [-1500, 3500] to [0, 1]. SRU-Net was trained with a batch size 16, mean squared error (MSE) loss, Adam optimizer, maximum 300 epochs with early stopping patience of 30. SRU-Net1 was trained by LR_{K_1} reconstructed data, SRU-Net2 by LR_{K_2} reconstructed data.

2.3   Evaluation

We tested the SRU-Net1 and SRU-Net2 on five CBCT datasets unseen by the trained network. MSE, structural similarity index measure (SSIM) and peak signal-to-noise ratio (PSNR) metrics were evaluated on LR vs. target and eHR vs. target. A paired two-tailed Student t-test was evaluated on the LR and eHR images metrics. For cross-modality transfer, we applied both SRU-Net1 and SRU-Net2 on five MDCT datasets. We resized the MDCT images to the trained sampling grid size $0.20 \times 0.20\,\text{mm}^2$, and cropped to 512×512.

3   Results

3.1   Qualitative evaluation

3.1.1   Test on unseen CBCT data. Fig. 3 shows the intensity and difference images of a representative slice. The difference images were generated by subtracting the HR

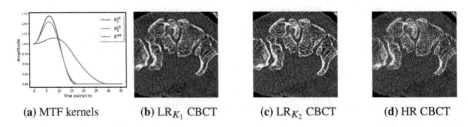

(a) MTF kernels   (b) LR_{K_1} CBCT   (c) LR_{K_2} CBCT   (d) HR CBCT

Fig. 2. (a) Resolution (line pairs/cm) of the modulation transfer function (MTF) in reconstruction kernels: K_1^{LR}, K_2^{LR} and K^{HR} and their corresponding reconstructed (b, c) LR and (d) HR images.

target with the respective LR or eHR intensity images. Both eHR CBCT images (Fig. 3b and d) showed improvements over their LR input (Fig. 3a and e). High resolution details in trabecular bone structures, and cortical bone edges could be better shown (Fig. 3, second row difference images). Both SRU-Nets could restore most of the high frequency components (Fig. 3b and d), which were removed by the kernels K_1^{LR} and K_2^{LR} (Fig. 3a and 3e).

3.1.2 Test on MDCT data. Representative slices of two MDCT test datasets are shown in Fig. 4 The left column shows the MDCT test input, the middle column shows the eHR predicted from model SRU-Net1, while the right column shows the eHR predicted from model SRU-Net2.

3.2 Quantitative analysis

Table 2 shows all evaluation metrics MSE, SSIM and PSNR. Lower MSE values, as well as higher SSIM and PSNR values are observed for the eHR than for the LR test images when compared to HR target images (Table 2). The p-value also showed statistically significance of such improvements.

4 Discussion

The intention is not to compare the performance between SRU-Net1 and SRU-Net2, but to show that it is important to consider the frequency behaviour of the MDCT input data, in this case, the reconstruction kernel, K_1^{LR}. K_1^{LR} and K_2^{LR} are the LR bone kernels and K^{HR} is the HR bone kernel. In Fig. 2a, we could see that all three MTF exhibit certain

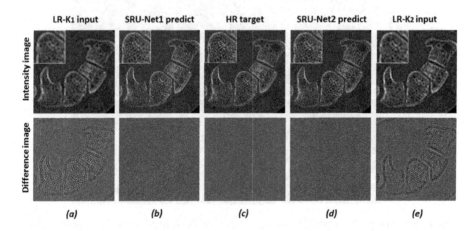

Fig. 3. The unseen CBCT test image and the eHR predictions by the two models. A more zoomed in image is shown at the top left. Same window level used for all intensity images: (600/1900 HU, center/width) and difference images: (0/600 HU, center/width).

Tab. 2. Quantitative analysis for the two SRU-Net models on respective unseen CBCT testing images (n = 3520). Values are shown as mean ± standard deviation. HU: Hounsfield Unit.

		LR vs. HR	eHR vs. HR	p-value
	MSE (HU)	10.21 ± 5.72	8.72 ± 4.84	
SRU-Net1	SSIM	43.53 ± 1.97	51.76 ± 1.01	$p < 0.001$
	PSNR	25.88 ± 2.90	26.48 ± 2.49	
	MSE (HU)	9.26 ± 5.62	7.57 ± 4.90	
SRU-Net2	SSIM	48.82 ± 1.37	56.09 ± 0.57	$p < 0.001$
	PSNR	26.90 ± 2.93	27.39 ± 2.88	

modulation characteristics across different frequency bands, which is also reflected by the difference images in Fig. 3a and 3c. When applied on MDCT data, SRU-Net1 shows higher sharpness in emulating the HR impressions than SRU-Net2.

Anatomical structures are affected by the partial volume effects in the thicker MDCT slices, as slice thickness of the MDCT is 0.60 mm, compared to CBCT with slice thickness 0.20 mm. In addition, the network might learn artifacts that exist in CBCT only, as the noise patterns of CBCT and MDCT are different. Moreover, our ultimate goal is to create DRRs from the generated eHR MDCT images, however, would be part of our future works.

The next step is to train a 3D SR network for improving both the in- and through-plane resolution, such as training on orthogonal slices [10]. One of the challenges include transferring the SR network training from LR isotropic CBCT volumes to MDCT volumes with anisotropic voxel size.

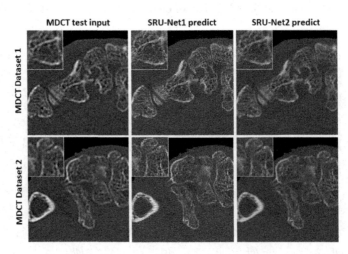

Fig. 4. The cross-modality MDCT test input and the eHR predictions by the respective models trained by the two types of LR CBCT images. A more zoomed in image is shown at the top left. Same window level used for all intensity images: (600/1900 HU, center/width).

5 Conclusion

We developed a SRU-Net for generating eHR CT images. The eHR images predicted from the two models, SRU-Net1 and SRU-Net2, show significant improvement in evaluation metrics and HR impression on unseen LR CBCT test data. Additionally early results for the cross-modality transfer to MDCT were shown. As a particular novel contribution, this study demonstrated the possibility of training a SR network for learning HR features on smaller sampling grid size than typically employed for SR networks.

Disclaimer. The presented methods in this paper are not commercially available and their future availability cannot be guaranteed.

References

1. Barbosa Jr EJM, Gefter WB, Ghesu FC, Liu S, Mailhe B, Mansoor A et al. Automated detection and quantification of COVID-19 airspace disease on chest radiographs: a novel approach achieving expert radiologist-level performance using a deep convolutional neural network trained on digital reconstructed radiographs from computed tomography-derived ground truth. Invest Radiol. 2021;56(8):471–9.
2. Umehara K, Ota J, Ishida T. Application of super-resolution convolutional neural network for enhancing image resolution in chest CT. J Digit Imaging. 2018;31(4):441–50.
3. Park J, Hwang D, Kim KY, Kang SK, Kim YK, Lee JS. Computed tomography super-resolution using deep convolutional neural network. Phys Med Biol. 2018;63(14):145011.
4. Yu H, Liu D, Shi H, Yu H, Wang Z, Wang X et al. Computed tomography super-resolution using convolutional neural networks. Conf Proc IEEE Int Conf Signal Image Process Appl. IEEE. 2017:3944–8.
5. Parker JA, Kenyon RV, Troxel DE. Comparison of interpolating methods for image resampling. IEEE Trans Med Imaging. 1983;2(1):31–9.
6. Hirahara D, Takaya E, Kadowaki M, Kobayashi Y, Ueda T. Effect of the pixel interpolation method for downsampling medical images on deep learning accuracy. J. comput. commun. 2021;9(11):150–6.
7. Grunz JP, Weng AM, Gietzen CH, Veyhl-Wichmann M, Pennig L, Kunz A et al. Evaluation of ultra-high-resolution cone-beam CT prototype of twin robotic radiography system for cadaveric wrist imaging. Acad Radiol. 2021;28(10):e314–e322.
8. Ronneberger O, Fischer P, Brox T. U-net: convolutional networks for biomedical image segmentation. Med Image Comput Comput Assist Interv. Springer. 2015:234–41.
9. Paszke A, Gross S, Massa F, Lerer A, Bradbury J, Chanan G et al. PyTorch: an imperative style, high-performance deep learning library. Advances in Neural Information Processing Systems 32. Ed. by Wallach H, Larochelle H, Beygelzimer A, d'Alché-Buc F, Fox E, Garnett R. Curran Associates, Inc., 2019:8024–35.
10. Peng C, Zhou SK, Chellappa R. DA-VSR: domain adaptable volumetric super-resolution for medical images. Med Image Comput Comput Assist Interv. Springer. 2021:75–85.

Abstract: MOOD 2020
A Public Benchmark for Out-of-distribution Detection and Localization on Medical Images

David Zimmerer[1], Peter Full[1], Fabian Isensee[1], Paul Jäger[1], Tim Adler[1],
Jens Petersen[1], Gregor Köhler[1], Tobias Ross[1], Annika Reinke[1], Antanas Kascenas[2],
Bjørn Sand Jensen[2], Alison Q. O'Neil[3], Jeremy Tan[4], Benjamin Hou[4], James Batten[4],
Huaqi Qiu[4], Bernhard Kainz[4], Nina Shvetsova, Irina Fedulova, Dmitry V. Dylov,
Baolun Yu[5], Jianyang Zhai[5], Jingtao Hu[5], Runxuan Si[5], Sihang Zhou[5], Siqi Wang[5],
Xinyang Li[5], Xuerun Chen[5], Yang Zhao[5], Sergio Naval Marimont[6], Giacomo Tarroni[4],
Victor Saase[7], Lena Maier-Hein[1,7], Klaus Maier-Hein[1,7]

[1]German Cancer Research Center, Heidelberg, Germany
[2]University of Glasgow, Glasgow, UK
[3]University of Edinburgh, Edinburgh, UK
[4]Imperial College London, London, UK
[5]National University of Defense Technology, Hunan, China
[6]CitAI Research Centre, University of London, London
[7]Heidelberg University, Heidelberg, Germany
d.zimmerer@dkfz.de

Detecting out-of-distribution (OoD) data is one of the greatest challenges in safe and robust deployment of machine learning algorithms in medicine. When the algorithms encounter cases that deviate from the distribution of the training data, they often produce incorrect and over-confident predictions. OoD detection algorithms aim to catch erroneous predictions in advance by analysing the data distribution and detecting potential instances of failure. Moreover, flagging OoD cases may support human readers in identifying incidental findings. Due to the increased interest in OoD algorithms, benchmarks for different domains have recently been established. In the medical imaging domain, for which reliable predictions are often essential, an open benchmark has been missing. We introduce the Medical-Out-Of-Distribution-Analysis-Challenge (MOOD) as an open, fair, and unbiased benchmark for OoD methods in the medical imaging domain. The analysis of the submitted algorithms shows that performance has a strong positive correlation with the perceived difficulty, and that all algorithms show a high variance for different anomalies, making it yet hard to recommend them for clinical practice. We also see a strong correlation between challenge ranking and performance on a simple toy test set, indicating that this might be a valuable addition as a proxy dataset during anomaly detection algorithm development [1].

References

1. Zimmerer D, Full PM, Isensee F, Jäger P, Adler T, Petersen J et al. MOOD 2020: a public benchmark for out-of-distribution detection and localization on medical images. IEEE Trans Med Imaging. 2022;41(10):2728–38.

Correction to: McLabel: A Local Thresholding Tool for Efficient Semi-automatic Labelling of Cells in Fluorescence Microscopy

Jonas Utz, Maja Schlereth, Jingna Qiu, Mareike Thies, Fabian Wagner, Oumaima Ben Brahim, Mingxuan Gu, Stefan Uderhardt and Katharina Breininger

---

Correction to:
Chapter 20 in: T. M. Deserno et al. (Hrsg.), *Bildverarbeitung für die Medizin 2023*, **Informatik aktuell,**
https://doi.org/10.1007/978-3-658-41657-7_20

The author's name Oumaima Ben Brahim has been corrected on page 82. An acknowledgement was added on page 87.

The updated version of this chapter can be found at
https://doi.org/10.1007/978-3-658-41657-7_20

Autorenverzeichnis

Printed in the United States
by Baker & Taylor Publisher Services